GROW IT
BACK

How Laser Phototherapy Stops
Hair Loss and Regrows Your Hair

By
Sayyid Tamim Hamid

ISBN (paperback): 979-8-218-09911-4
ISBN (eBook): 979-8-218-19171-9

Notable Endorsements

I've been in the hair growth profession for multiple decades now, and *Grow It Back* has, for the first time ever, definitively shaped the landscape of how we think about hair growth and loss. A must-read.

- John Ohanesian – Former CEO Bosley, 1990–2010

Grow It Back debuts the perfect accompaniment to the hair care treatment of your choice and sheds significant light on the subject of hair fitness.

- Mark Kress – Toppik Founder and former CEO

An authoritative and scientifically backed manual for hair care. Truly a game-changer.

- Chris Webb – Chief Editor Hair Authority Magazine

To have a NASA scientist compile the most innovative and comprehensive information on hair and scalp wellness in one complete resource is an invaluable tool for so many. *Grow It Back* is the book we've all been waiting for.

- Michael Napolitano – CEO Hair-U-Wear

Disclaimer Notice

Please note the information contained within this document is for educational and entertainment purposes only. All effort has been executed to present accurate, up-to-date, and reliable complete information. No warranties of any kind are declared or implied. Readers acknowledge that the author is not engaging in the rendering of legal, financial, medical, or professional advice. The content within this book has been derived from various sources. Please consult a licensed professional before attempting any techniques outlined in this book. By reading this document, the reader agrees that under no circumstances, is the author responsible for any losses, direct or indirect, which are incurred as a result of the use of information contained within this document including but not limited to errors, omissions, or inaccuracies.

Legal Notice

This book is copyright protected. This book is only for personal use. You cannot amend, distribute, sell, use, quote, or paraphrase any part of the content within this book without the consent of the author or publisher.

Table of Contents

To my wife, Shamack, who is a true angel and has supported me over the past three decades. You are my love and best friend, you are and always will be my perfect wife and mother to our children.

To my three children, Sheen-Sheen, Samo, and Deeno, you are all the light that fills my brightest days. I am extremely proud of each one of you and how you have all become amazing, accomplished human beings.

PREFACE

What would make a former NASA biomedical engineer working at Kennedy Space Center invent a device that regrows hair? Maybe you've guessed the answer. I was losing my hair! About two decades ago, I realized my hair was thinning. While it wasn't that bad, or so I told myself, it was enough to make me look for a product that could restore what I'd lost and prevent it from getting worse.

The options I came across were discouraging. All were costly or inconvenient; they couldn't regrow the lost hair; and some, I discovered, even sped up hair loss! I definitely wanted to keep what I had. Wasn't that the point?

After an exhausting (and useless) search for something that worked, I decided to create a safe, affordable, and effective solution *myself.* It dawned on me that the millions of other people experiencing hair loss must have gone down the same dead-end path. So, what started out as a quest for a viable solution to my own hair loss soon became an endeavor to help others.

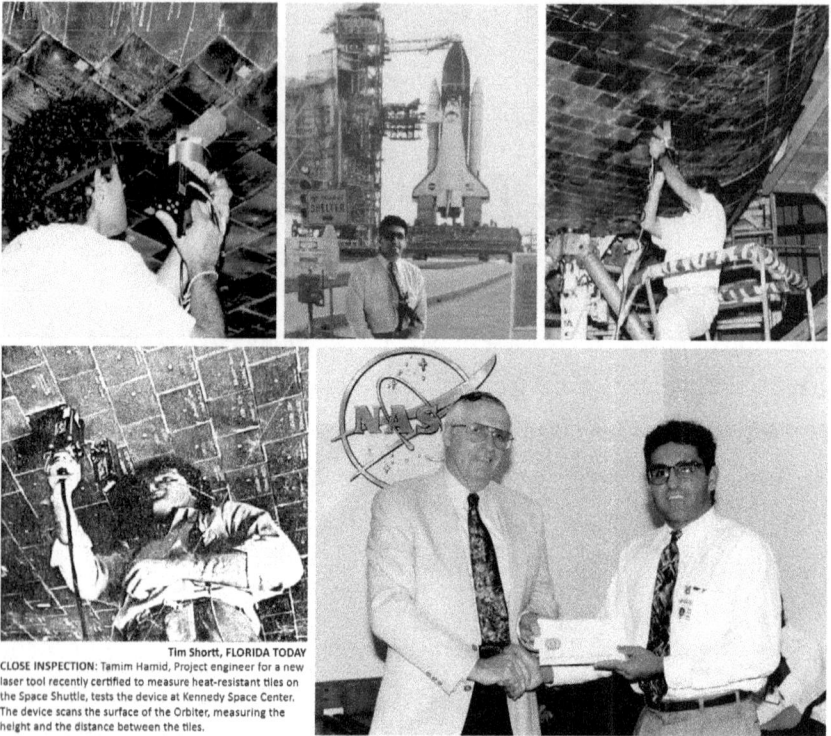

CLOSE INSPECTION: Tamim Hamid, Project engineer for a new
laser tool recently certified to measure heat-resistant tiles on
the Space Shuttle, tests the device at Kennedy Space Center.
The device scans the surface of the Orbiter, measuring the
height and the distance between the tiles.

Tim Shortt, FLORIDA TODAY

Figure 0.1 Photos of the Author (from upper left to right): The author
under the space shuttle; in front of the space shuttle; developing
a laser measurement device for space shuttle thermal system tiles;
featured in *Florida Today* article; receiving the engineer of the year
award.

That's when my biomedical engineering background and experience with NASA came to my rescue (and now yours). I knew enough about medicine, engineering, and photonics (the science of light) to research how light can treat human health conditions—particularly hair loss. In fact, I had twenty-five years of laser-design experience. This expertise led me to grow our own proprietary lasers (yes lasers are grown, just like crystals, and Silicon Valley is the world's headquarters for growing semiconductors). Our goal was to develop the perfect laser device that not only effectively reduces hair loss but also regrows it!

I quickly realized that I was onto something, and the next step was to gather a group of skilled engineers, technology specialists, and hair loss experts from Silicon Valley, California. Working as a team and using my proprietary lasers, we developed a cutting-edge laser device. With my initial construction and technology, I researched a prototype. My team tweaked and tested it to make improvements before its launch in 2013. Our unique device, a wearable hair regrowth helmet called the Theradome, was cleared by the Food and Drug Administration (FDA) as the first, over-the-counter (OTC), wearable, clinical-grade medical device of its kind.

My father and grandfather were physicians, and I grew up watching them save lives. Some of those people were cancer patients who had experienced severe hair loss. I saw firsthand the gratitude they expressed when they were restored to health—pies, cakes, and other gifts filled our home. It made a powerful impression on me, and my goal in studying laser phototherapy (LPT) was to inspire the same type of gratitude in others while at the same time making a global impact on medicine. I have not been disappointed. Since we began offering our LPT device, I have witnessed happiness and increased self-esteem from numerous people who've experienced hair regrowth thanks to my research in laser therapy. This has brought me untold joy.

Note: I avoid the word "baldness" in this book because it has negative connotations. Instead, I prefer "thinning" or "hair loss." After all, women don't really go bald; their hair thins over time. And most men find the word "bald" offensive.

INTRODUCTION

Can Lasers Really Restore Hair?

Since ancient times, a full head of hair has been associated with youth and vitality. When we notice lots of hairs on our pillow or in the drain or if our hair looks thin when reflected in the mirror, we ask, "Why am I losing my hair?" and "Can I get it back?" We frantically start searching for solutions without understanding the cause of our hair loss or the science behind treating it.

The truth is there are things to do and *not* to do, and that's something many of those in the business of hair-restoration products won't tell you.

When people meet me, they ask similar questions about laser phototherapy (LPT) and our LPT helmet. Does this device really help grow hair? How does it compare to other hair-restoration alternatives? Is it safe? How does it work? Does it hurt? Lasers do hurt, don't they? What is laser-therapy hair restoration? I've never heard of it. How long will it take to show results? Even though it works for others, will it work for me? Will I have to use this for the rest of my life? What if I'm not experiencing hair loss yet and simply want to maintain my hair? How does it compare to other products—the ones I know—like Minoxidil and hair transplants?

These are all excellent questions. I had many of the same concerns. That's why I've written this book about using light (lasers) to treat hair loss. And all the answers are here.

As an expert in the field and as someone who used to worry about my thinning hair, I give precise answers to questions about safety, side effects, results, effectiveness, and overall knowledge about hair and lasers. This book will enlighten you on the science of laser therapy without sounding like a physics textbook. It's written with an emphasis on complete and clear explanations so anyone can understand how laser phototherapy treatment works. You'll get an overview of light, its uses for treatment, where lasers come in, hair growth, and much more. I discuss how hair regrowth and reduced hair loss occur and how to use this therapy. This book also explores the different types of laser lights (cold and hot).

This book is unique because it talks about what works for hair growth— instead of merely sharing a bunch of home remedies that *might* help. And the science (or lack of science) behind all of them.

I am committed to eliminating the social media and internet noise about miracle hair loss cures and hair growth technologies. As a result of all that racket, many people experiencing hair loss are confused and overwhelmed by the range or the efficacy of the remedies offered. Unfortunately, many of these approaches and gadgets are fake. They thrive on deception and swindle ordinary people whose fear about their hair loss has gotten the best of them.

We're all concerned about hair appearance. And social media counts on that and uses it to manipulate us.

My mission and goal are to provide the most complete resource on laser phototherapy ever created. I aim to resolve everyone's concerns—and I genuinely mean everyone's—about hair loss and hair growth.

Yet unlike a tent preacher's call, my message is based on scientific evidence, and it can be easily understood by anybody of any age.

One Woman's Hair Loss Story: A Case Study

Melba, age sixty-eight, was suffering from severe hair thinning—so much so that the condition was bringing her embarrassment and stress. After years of struggling, Melba was finally ready to take action and treat her hair loss. When she presented to a hair-restoration specialist about our LPT laser helmet, Melba had already tried all the usual treatments, from home remedies to special shampoos and beyond. The specialist, who had come highly recommended, was able to successfully diagnose Melba with advanced androgenetic alopecia, a condition that in all likelihood was genetic.

The specialist, a hair-restoration practitioner known as a trichologist, assessed her situation and was able to offer her hope in the form of a treatment newly-cleared by the FDA: a laser phototherapy helmet. After answering Melba's questions and reassuring her that the process would be painless, relatively convenient, and safe, Melba agreed to try the helmet on for size, promising she would take photos to document her journey.

Six months later, Melba returned to the same office less than satisfied—she told the specialist that, despite consistent and appropriate use of the helmet for half a year, she hadn't noticed any results.

The specialist, who had come across reactions like Melba's before, understood, explaining how it often takes time to notice any difference in hair thickness given that the changes are incremental and occur slowly over time. Luckily, the specialist was prepared, having taken photos of Melba before her treatment and saved them for just this scenario.

After taking a photo of Melba's hair six months later for comparison, the specialist brought out the original photos, taken before Melba had begun wearing the helmet, and held them up, side-by-side with the latest images for Melba to see.

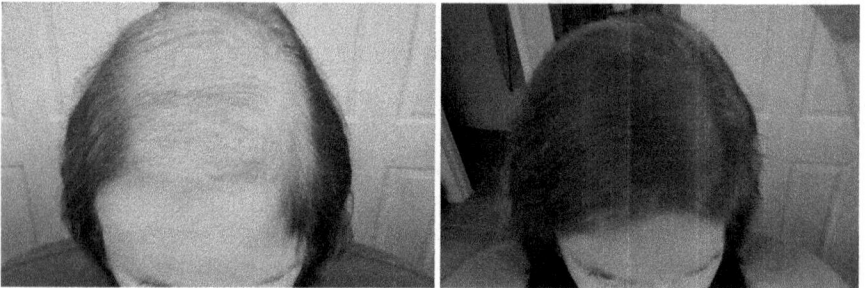

Figure 0.2. Melba: Before and After Using Our LPT Helmet: The picture on the left (before) shows mostly white hairs on Melba, and the image on the right (after) shows her natural hair color. The gray hairs are still there, just not as prominent.

Melba's response was immediate: "That can't be what my hair looked like six months ago! It's so thin!" she said, reacting to the before and after photos alongside each other. The before photos clearly showed a scalp covered in thinning, almost all-white hairs. This was the condition of Melba's hair before she began treatment, when she walked into the trichologist's office six months previously. The after photos, however, were night and day by comparison. Hairs that were once white and sparse had been replaced with a consistent layer of new, darker (red) hair—her natural hair color!

After confirming that the specialist hadn't tampered with the photos—that they really showed that much hair growth over half a year—Melba was relieved. The specialist explained how our brains and eyes are trained to automatically integrate new information over time, which makes it difficult for us to notice gradual changes over time. Melba admitted that she *had* noticed *some* improvements, but because they were pretty subtle, she had started to doubt the efficacy of her hair growth regimen. Melba's husband, then spoke up for the first time and said: I told you, Melba, that thing has been working these past few months and you didn't believe me!

Melba's confidence in the helmet was renewed, and they both left the office with future plans to continue the LPT therapy and take plenty of pictures along the way.

CHAPTER 1

Light Is the Foundation of Growing It Back

"Everything is the Light" — Nikola Tesla, Inventor, 1899

Light Through the Ages

In the beginning, there was light. Light is energy. Humans have always been obsessed with light. Our ancestors worshipped it because they knew it was life-sustaining. Their reverence led them to build enormous temples arranged by meticulous calculations to capture light at the perfect moment and magnify it into a cascade of brilliance. This reverence for light is seen across continents, throughout religions, and in various cultures, including in Hindu temples, Jewish synagogues, Muslim mosques, and Christian cathedrals. Light is associated with goodness, creation, and knowledge.

Where there is light, there is life.

Besides lighting our path and illuminating spaces, light warms us, tans our skin, and relaxes us. Animals seek out the sun's rays to rest and sleep. And so many of us flock to the beach for our annual vacations. Summer is the season of fertility, abundance, and joy. We break up the summertime with cultural and religious festivities. So, it's almost impossible to be melancholy on a warm, sunny day when the light is at its most brilliant.

We use light to decorate our homes, and keep winter's darkness at bay. Light comforts us and makes us feel safe. In the depths of winter or the dark of night, we find comfort in knowing the sun will rise again. We feel protected and restored in the light of day. We even use special therapy lights to drive away the winter blues. No wonder humans adore light!

It should come as little surprise that we've found ways to heal our bodies with light and solve many of our health problems. I'm confident you'll be amazed when I teach you what light can do for your body.

Let me ask you a question: What is light? Can you describe it? We love it, bathe in it, and crave it when it's absent, but what do we really understand about it?

Light is the substance that makes up all of existence. Light is photons. Photons compose subatomic particles, and subatomic particles compose particles, and particles compose matter, and matter composes you and me and everything we see and touch and smell and taste and even eat. So light really is everything. And everything is light.

The car you drive is made of light; your last meal was all light; even this book is light. The cellulose extracted from trees that became paper pulp to produce this book is made of light. So too is the linseed or soybean oil that became ink for this book—light, all of it light. If you're reading this book on an e-reader device or app, the backlight that allows you to read these words are photons, and those photons illuminate these pages, which allows you to read. For those with an audiobook version of *Grow It Back*, you need a power source to listen on your electronic device. Plus, if your power grid relies on or is supplemented by solar energy, then, in a way, the audiobook too is light.

Light is the building block of the entire known universe. It's energy that also comprises matter. Light is a wave and a particle simultaneously that moves however it wants. Visible light makes up the range that human eyes can see. However, light also exists in other forms invisible to the human eye. Light goes beyond the limited range of humankind's senses.

We can achieve (almost) anything we want with light. All that's necessary is to learn how to harness light to accomplish each unique goal.

Healing with Light: Light as a Treatment for Many Ailments

Early humans harnessed fire for warmth and protection. Staying warm with firelight is the earliest known use of light for health purposes. Ever since, humans have used light to heal.

Records show the ancient Egyptians built temples dedicated to healing with sunlight and colored light beginning in about 500 BC. Likewise, ancient Chinese and Indian texts refer to the healing power of different colored lights. In fact, light therapy has been practiced in every major civilization in human history. The Assyrians, Babylonians, and Egyptians recognized that sunbathing had therapeutic effects. Interestingly, the ancient Egyptian city of Heliopolis, a name that translates to *City of the Sun*, was fortified with light rooms and healing temples. The temple windows were covered with cloth dyed in various colors to bring about different healing effects. It was the center of worship of the sun god, Ra.

As civilizations advanced, light therapy became more standardized. Civil War General Augustus Pleasonton used blue light to stimulate secretory glands and the nervous system. He documented this system's effectiveness in treating diseases, especially those that presented with pain. Later, Dr. Niels Finsen, a physician and scientist from the Faroe Islands, proved ultraviolet (UV) light treats tuberculosis scarring. Moreover, he used red light to treat smallpox scars. This achievement earned him the Nobel Prize in Medicine in 1903.

It's no surprise that sun worshipping is a thing!

Florence Nightingale, English reformer and founder of modern nursing theory and training, regarded light as therapy. She first began advocating for plenty of sunlight to treat the sick and wounded during the Crimean War (1853 to 1856) and continued to do so throughout her long nursing career.

Later, Dr. Kate Baldwin, chief surgeon at Philadelphia Women's Hospital (1903 to 1926), declared that color therapy worked faster and better than any other treatment. She also attested that phototherapy produced the least strain on patients.

There's enormous data on the curative powers of the light of the sun. In fact, in 1918 during the influenza pandemic in Boston, they conducted successful experiments by taking patients who were in the hospital outside to sit in the sun. They called this "open-air therapy" and showed that the mortality rate decreased from 40% to about 13%.

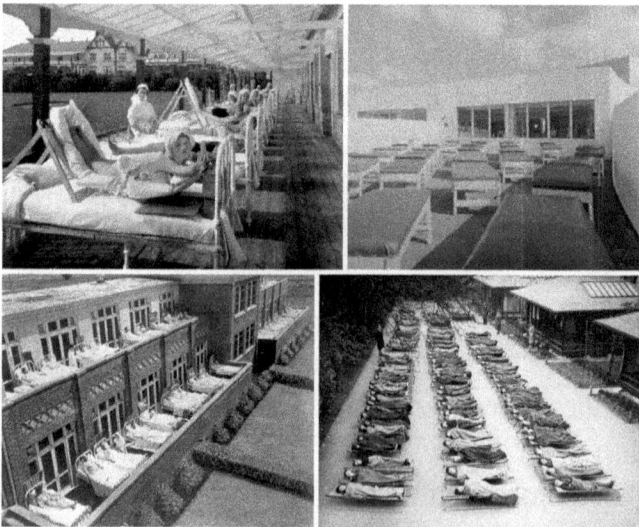

Figure 1.1. Nurses Bringing Patients into the Sunlight to Heal: The concept of using the sun to help heal medical conditions was very popular in the early 1900s.

By the 1950s, phototherapy gained ground, and ultraviolet light was being used to manage dermatological conditions. The use of light therapy continues today in many wondrous ways—too many to be discussed in this book, the focus of which is hair loss and hair growth, which we will explore together.

Light is Life

We feed on sunlight, and we see echoes of photosynthesis in humanity. Humans absorb sunlight in much the same way plants do. We need sunlight for nutrients such as vitamin D3, which regulates almost every part of our minds and bodies. People with seasonal affective disorder (SAD) take synthetic vitamin D3 to simulate sunlight and get them through winter.

A trial conducted to see how light affected SAD patients took place above the Arctic Circle where they wouldn't be exposed to outside light. Light was shined behind the knees of half the patients so they could not see if it was being beamed onto their bodies. Half of the patients received no light at all. No one knew what they received. At the end of the study, 100% of the patients who received light had normal levels of serotonin (a key hormone that when raised can boost mood and help other brain functions). People need sunlight so badly that even artificial light is better than nothing at all.

In some ways, we rely on plants to fuel us. They absorb even more sunlight than we do through proper photosynthesis, and we gain their stored light by eating them. You can say we rely on plants to maximize our light absorption. The light they absorb allows them to draw in trace minerals from the ground, in turn providing us with nutrients we otherwise wouldn't have access to. Part of healing from disease and injury is giving the body nutrients it may be lacking and providing adequate doses of essential vitamins and minerals. Proper nutrition also helps boost and build a healthy immune system. The more light our food gets, the healthier we become. Light enriches our food while powering and healing our bodies and mentality. Is it a coincidence that citrus fruits rich in vitamin C deliver these valuable goods at the exact same time as the flu and cold season when we need these the most?

Interestingly, recent studies show that humans and other mammals can convert sunlight into chemical energy through a process similar to photosynthesis. All mammals have unique light-absorbing pigments called chromophores, which are similar to chlorophyll, the green pigment in plants. A chromophore in mammals you might be familiar with is called melanin. Melanin is the pigment in skin responsible for tanning and the different pigments in every shade of skin.

Mammalian and plant pigments work by triggering reactions in the cell and converting sunlight to energy. Once absorbed by chlorophyll in plants or chromophores in mammals, light energy is sent to the mitochondria. The mitochondria are where the energy that cells need to function is produced.

Light exists in a range of intensities and energy called a spectrum, which is composed of differing wavelengths. All of these forms of energy such as X-rays, visible light from the sun, microwaves, radio waves, and TV waves, are made of light with a broad spectrum of wavelengths. The difference between these wavelengths is how long or short they are. Shorter wavelengths are more powerful and longer wavelengths are less powerful. Some we can see; others we can't see, but light is always there.

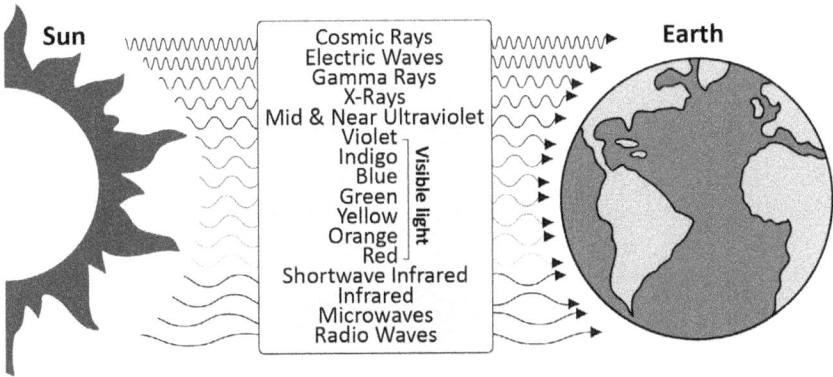

Figure 1.2. The Sun and All Its Wavelengths Emitting EMF onto the Earth: These are the ones we know of at this time, but there might be additional emissions that have not been discovered.

The photon is where the magic happens. The photon is the starting point, the most elemental building block for all the wondrous things that light does. Many believe the definition of a photon is just a packet of energy, but that's way too broad and not entirely accurate. Without delving deeply into physics—and the fact that no one has technically seen a single atom with their naked eyes let alone a photon (which also moves way too fast to "see")—trying to picture the size of photons can be challenging. Imagine it this way: If an atom were as large as a skyscraper, a photon would be approximately the size of a small garden shed. This comparison helps illustrate the incredibly tiny scale of photons in relation to even the most basic elements of matter.

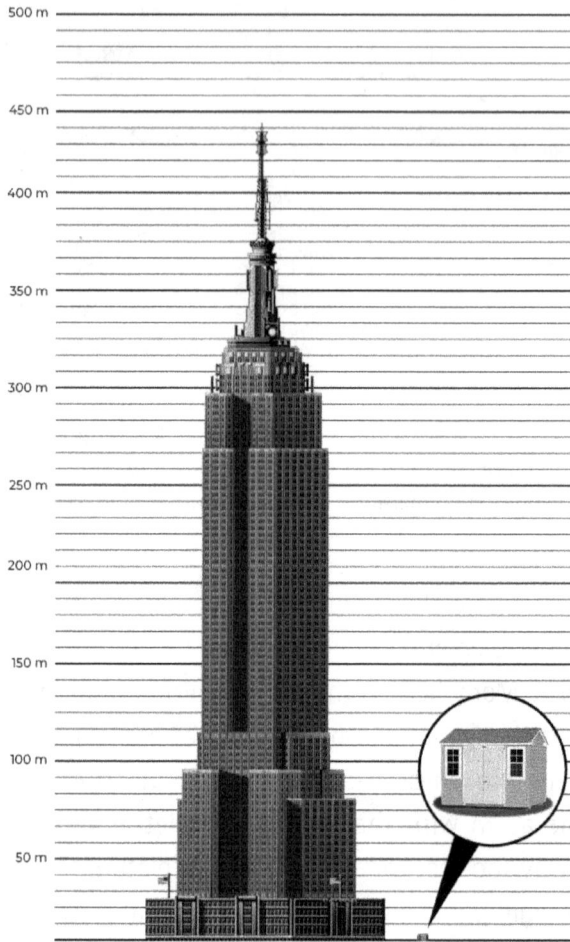

Figure 1.3. Comparing the size of an atom to a photon is equivalent to comparing a skyscraper to a small garden shed.

It is important to know that photons comprise not only light but also exist across the electromagnetic spectrum. Gamma rays, X-rays, radio waves, and so on are all made up of photons.

We've figured out how to adjust the light in a laser and tune it to the correct wavelength and power to accomplish a specific goal. All light can impact an organism, but we know lasers powerfully affect biological matter. And there are many different types of lasers.

If a red laser or near-infrared light is aimed at the right spot on your body and held there long enough, it can reduce swelling, help cells repair themselves faster, improve circulation, and decrease pain. In effect, our cells are taking the extra energy the laser provides and using it to heal themselves.

Lasers, of course, do not occur in nature. They are strictly, 100% man-made. And their sole function is to penetrate matter—any type of matter. This is why a laser is more effective in healing the body than any other light source. *And* it can be controlled.

The sun's intensity varies by season. Its intensity, for example, can't be easily adjusted. Fickle weather-related and seasonal changes forfeit healing in our modern medical practice. That makes natural sunlight limited in its use.

Fortunately, the advent of artificial light sources has allowed phototherapy to be offered year-round.

We can now use light to treat many diseases, injuries, and other conditions. Breast cancer, colorectal cancer, cardiovascular disease, metabolic syndrome, Alzheimer's, autism, type 1 diabetes, multiple sclerosis, seasonal affective disorder (SAD), neonatal jaundice, and myopia are a handful of the conditions treatable with the application of light, and some we haven't yet discovered.

Humankind has always worshipped light *and* craved the ability to harness its power. We've come a long way, and our ancestors would be utterly astounded by the lasers we use today. In fact, we've improved upon light since the invention of lasers. And we are finding new ways of using laser light to substantially improve our lives all the time. Hair regrowth is just one.

Lasers: Science Fiction to Science Fact

LASER is an acronym for *Light Amplification by Stimulated Emission of Radiation.* Don't let that word radiation scare you. In physics, it simply means "the emission of energy as electromagnetic waves or is moving subatomic particles, especially high energy particles which cause ionization" (Oxford Languages Dictionary).

American engineer and physicist Theodore Maiman invented the first working laser at the Hughes Research Laboratory in 1960. It didn't take long for people to recognize that this new form of light could solve many problems. For example, in 1963, American dermatologist Leon Goldman pioneered laser treatment to destroy unwanted black hairs. He also described the potential for lasers in removing tattoos and treating melanomas, vascular malformations, and skin damage. Goldman's work formed the background for later medical applications of laser phototherapy.

Understanding Medical Lasers

Different lasers are tuned for different uses. There are those lasers that burn such as surgical lasers which necessarily must cut. This takes great precision. Calculating the precise wavelength and power necessary to destroy tumors or seal an incision, for example, is crucial. There are also cool lasers such as those used in LPT. Using lasers on human tissue is always a delicate balancing act. Enough energy must be applied to stimulate the targeted tissue for healing without adding so much heat that tissue is damaged. It is a delicate balance dependent on many factors.

Lasers can be tuned to stimulate biological tissue via a method called photobiostimulation, which doesn't burn or even get warm. Instead, it suffuses the tissue with light, like sunbathing. Imagine doing all your summer sunbathing at once while it causes your cells to regenerate and strengthen in the process. It's one of the many effects lasers can accomplish.

Are Lasers Safe?

Many question the safety of lasers. People picture science fiction films like *Resident Evil* and *Star Wars*, in which people are sliced to pieces by lasers or zap each other to death. Hollywood has made it easy to imagine something going wrong with a laser device and accidentally causing chaos or burning your skin. Some lasers can be dangerous at specific wavelengths, power outputs, and particular divergences. However, a new type of laser known as a *cold laser* (classified as Class 3R by the FDA) is safe to use on humans. As you can guess from the name, cold lasers produce no heat and put out less than five milliwatts (mW) of optical power. To give you an idea of just how low-level the power in these lasers is, a typical incandescent light bulb of 100 Watts is about 20,000 times more lumens (light energy) than a 5 mW cold laser—so yes, these are safe.

Consequently, the usual four risk factors (burns, scarring, pain, and infection) contributing to the damage other lasers cause become a non-issue. Cold lasers are incredibly safe and don't cause any damage because they *cannot* cause harm. For instance, a regular flashlight cannot damage your eyes. Even though it might be uncomfortable or annoying to have a flashlight shine in them, there's no permanent damage done. It's the same with cold lasers.

An example of a cold laser is the typical red laser pointer used during presentations. Laser pointers have been around for decades, and you might have one in your home right now. We sometimes hear people say, "Be careful, or you'll blind someone with that!"

In 1998, the European press worked itself into a panic after learning that some young boys had been aiming laser pointers at people's eyes while they were driving. Train engineers were also targeted. There were claims of a vision reduction of as much as 20% because of these pranks, but laser pointers are far too weak to damage your vision, especially over the distances involved in these incidences.

Eyes have a built-in defense mechanism from mischievous kids armed with laser pointers: the blink reflex. Blinking, which limits the eye's exposure to about one-tenth of a second, protects the eyes from bright light.

Even when college kids pointed red lasers at each other's eyes to see who could go the longest without blinking, the only negative effect was dry eyes, which was caused not by the laser pointers but by not blinking. Fun fact: The world record for not blinking is twenty-two minutes.

Airplane pilots, too, were sometimes targeted by kids armed with green laser pointers (green lasers are stronger than red lasers and can travel longer distances). This is dangerous not because it will blind the pilots, but because it distracts the pilots, which is why authorities are right to ban the practice.

In the more than fifty years laser pointers have been available to consumers and with millions sold worldwide, no one has ever suffered severe injury from a red laser pointer or any other consumer-grade, red, cold-laser product. That's a fact, not just my opinion.

Laser Phototherapy

Using a laser or another light-emitting device in therapy is a form of photobiomodulation (PMB). This is a fancy word that refers to the stimulation of biological tissue with light. The sun does this every morning when its rays reach the plants in your garden. Plants and trees convert and absorb that light which triggers a photochemical response turning energy (light) into chemical energy (glucose). We call that process photosynthesis—another type of photobiomodulation necessary to all green plants.

Humans have a chemical pathway of their own (digesting food into nutrients). And humans still rely on the sun for vitamin D as well as mood and circadian rhythm regulation.

There are structures in the body that require a specific light source. Certain wavelengths of light trigger specific responses in cells. For example, gamma rays destroy messenger Ribonucleic Acid (mRNA), microwaves stimulate water molecules, and certain UV wavelengths destroy bacteria.

For hair rejuvenation, a laser must be properly tuned to a specific wavelength (680 nanometers) to stimulate all parts of the hair follicle, which include melanin and non-melanin components. The laser must also be controlled enough to prevent harm and powerful enough to be absorbed by the follicle to regrow hair.

Sound complicated? It is!

A rare skillset combining expertise in medicine, physics, and electronics is a prerequisite for building a cold laser that is successful for hair growth. That's probably why no one has created a light-therapy device—designed to regrow hair—in their garages until I did it in mine! I gathered a group of the best techs in Silicon Valley around me—engineers and scientists. We would troubleshoot and brainstorm at the dining room table over Afghani food my wife, Shama, cooked for us.

I tested four or five generations of lasers on my own head to discover the optimal design that would stimulate hair follicles by mimicking the effects of the right type of light.

Our new patented LPT helmet invention had to be fitted with eighty laser diodes of the optimized wavelength. Even with all those diodes, the designers demanded that it be lightweight. Each laser must have optimal scalp penetration to reach the base of hair follicles for powerful, effective energy absorption. The helmet had to have maximum scalp coverage with cool airflow and still be one-size-fits-all with safety and comfort designed in.

Our expertise allowed us to build treatment tracking into a cordless and mobile model. It has a user interface with voice reminders announcing product status such as session timing (with automatic off), and battery charging, in multiple languages. It's even easily updated with the latest software via internet access.

The result was a safe, award-winning, FDA-cleared laser hair regrowth technology that stops hair loss in the comfort of your home designed by experts in their field. And it's still made right here in Silicon Valley.

The Father of Laser Phototherapy

Some scientific discoveries are the result of deliberate research and experimentation, whereas others occur by accident. In the case of lasers and their effects on hair growth, it was the latter. The story begins with Endre Mester, who was born in Hungary in 1903. A violin enthusiast, he studied medicine at the University of Budapest and laser phototherapy at Semmelweis in 1965. Lasers had already been employed in surgery, but Professor Mester wanted to use them to destroy malignant tumors. He implanted tumor cells under the skins of lab rats and exposed them to a customized laser.

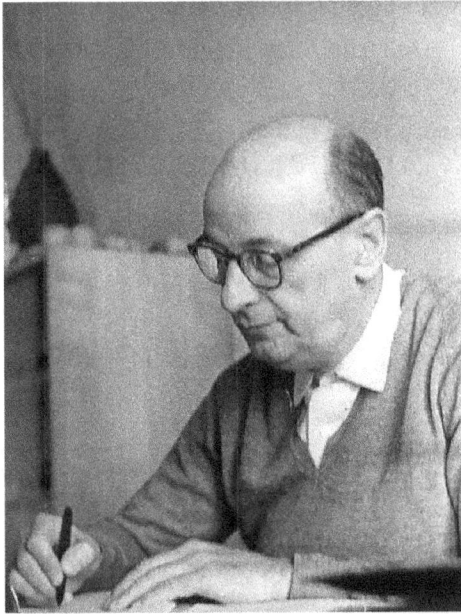

Figure 1.4. Dr. Endre Mester, regarded as the father of laser phototherapy, first accidentally discovered that hair follicles could be stimulated with cold lasers and published his findings in 1965, which was forgotten until recently.

The lab technician in charge of this new laser unknowingly set the laser at its lowest level instead of emitting a higher power unbeknownst to Mester. He noticed that the rats' incisions healed faster than those of rats not exposed to lasers. Further lab experiments explored red light's effects on the healing of surgical incisions. Mester confirmed that treatment with red light resulted in higher healing rates. Consequently, he expanded his experimental focus to include the effect of laser light on skin defects, burns, diabetic ulcers, venous insufficiency, and infected wounds. These conditions all healed faster with laser phototherapy.

Our understanding of lasers has increased significantly over the past six decades. During this time, laser hair stimulation, now called laser phototherapy (LPT), has been studied extensively. What was accidentally accomplished by a violin-loving scientist in 1965 can now be reproduced with remarkable consistency. Today, laser phototherapy is so safe that you can do it while relaxing in the comfort of your own home.

Cold Lasers: An Unexpected Invention

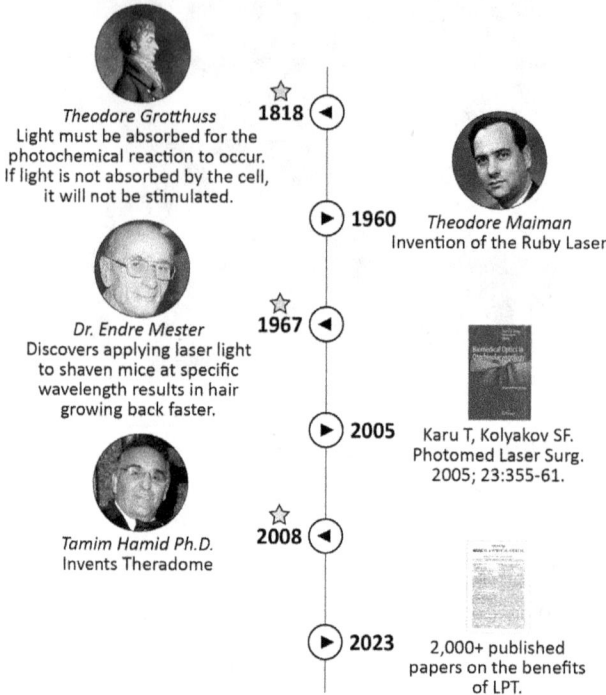

Figure 1.5. LPT Timeline from 1818 to 2023. Many scientists contributed to bringing LPT to the forefront of science. Dr. Mester is regarded as the Father of LPT.

The discovery of cold lasers dates back to the 1980s, a time when physicians used hot lasers for hair removal. More and more patients started complaining of sudden unwanted hair growth outside the targeted area. Although unwelcome hair was successfully removed by laser treatment, hair started growing on the skin nearby. For instance, if a top lip was targeted, hair growth on the cheeks or chin unexpectedly increased. This was a real problem, so research was done to find the root cause.

The results were surprising and would later prove to be groundbreaking. Reflection from the powerful, heatless lasers acted as a pseudo-application of red light, stimulating hair growth in adjacent areas. Despite this discovery, it took another thirty years until the first laser hair growth product was launched. The initial research paper from Dr. Mester was the main reason I pursued this very exciting discovery, and why I was so surprised that no one else had taken advantage of Dr. Mester's finding about fifty years later!

LPT, LLLT, LED: The Important Differences

Laser Phototherapy – LPT

LPT is a new term emphasizing the fact that only lasers are used to treat specific medical conditions like hair loss/growth. So, we will be using LPT throughout the book and we use LPT when discussing hair regrowth, halting hair loss, and maintaining volume. Another word that is also being promoted is photobiostimulation, but unfortunately this word does not specify if the light source is a laser or another source of light, so we rarely use this term when describing the process.

Low-Level Light Therapy – LLLT

You'll find many clinical papers and materials that market hair growth products speaking of LLLT, which refers to the use of low-level light energy as a treatment. This can be misleading since the word "light" could refer to LED or any other source of photons, including your car's headlights! That's why you won't find that term used here.

I also disagree with the phrase "low level." That's because it refers to the use of energy. If light is used to direct energy into human tissue over an extended period, it accumulates and becomes a large volume of energy. Therefore, even though publications and other references use the term

LLLT, which can mean photomedicine, broadband polarized light therapy, and other non-laser-based light therapies, it is more precise to refer to laser phototherapy as LPT. In this book the word photobiomodulation is also not frequently used since this too does not clarify which type of light source it uses.

Light Emitting Diode – LED

An LED is a semiconductor device that emits light when an electric current passes through it. It is used in digital devices, traffic signals, camera flashes, toys, etc. Although some companies advertising their LED-powered products would like you to think they have similar capabilities to laser-powered lights, lasers and LEDs each come with distinct properties and are not interchangeable. Thus, it is important to understand the difference between lasers and LEDs when selecting the best light-powered product for your purposes. Devices that use LEDs are not considered LPT devices.

The difference between Theradome's laser light and typical LED light comes down to three key attributes: coherence, wavelength, and energy density. To illustrate these three differences, we'll use the analogy of comparing a medical syringe (laser) to a topical ointment (LED).

Coherence

The concept of coherence simply refers to the ability to align light in a concise column or beam of light, like the needle of a syringe that, once injected, can reach deep below the skin's surface. Only laser light has the coherence necessary to focus its energy in this way. LEDs have absolutely no coherence in that the light emanating from LEDs is more like a typical light bulb that when illuminated spreads light around a room. If we apply the same analogy to LEDs, LEDs are like a topical ointment that is spread across the skin's surface in a diffuse and unfocused manner.

Wavelength

Taking the syringe analogy further, the wavelength is the medicine inside the syringe and if the wrong medicine is used, then it will not have the desired effect. In this example, the ideal, most effective wavelength for hair growth is 680 nm, which falls in the red color of the light spectrum and is the wavelength of our VL680 lasers in our helmet. This specific wavelength of light is delivered via the needle deep below the surface of the skin, up to 5 mm under, where it's needed most (the depth at which hair follicles reside). LEDs, however, use the wrong medicine so to speak, with a wavelength that is fewer than 630 nm. LED light, therefore, barely penetrates the skin's surface, much like a topical ointment, rendering it completely ineffective.

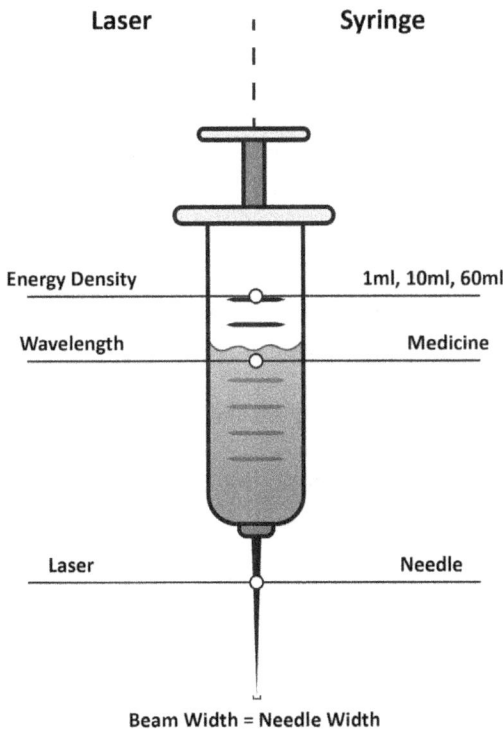

Laser | **Syringe**

Energy Density — 1ml, 10ml, 60ml

Wavelength — Medicine

Laser — Needle

Beam Width = Needle Width

Figure 1.6. Lasers and Syringes. Laser light and syringes are a great example of how both can penetrate deep and deliver the right dosage. LEDs, in comparison, are a little more like topical ointments.

Energy Density

Finally, the energy density or dosage of the laser light "medicine" is similar to the size of the syringe. The larger the syringe, the more powerful the dosage. For example, a 1 ml syringe is small and commonly used by diabetics, while a 60 ml syringe delivers a higher dose. In this analogy, we made sure that our lasers have the largest syringe size, and therefore the most powerful dosage of any LED, or for that matter, any laser on the market. And, since LEDs have no comparable syringe or targeted (coherent) light delivery, their dosage or energy density can never come close to that of a laser.

These three attributes directly reflect how laser phototherapy is used for applications such as hair growth. A hair laser phototherapy device must have at least these three attributes optimized and combined to be effective at stopping and regrowing hair.

Lasers Are Here to Stay

It takes at least ten years for any technology to move from the lab into the hands of consumers. We are now in a time where safe, reliable laser hair growth technology is accessible, easy to use, and really works. Even if other treatments have failed you previously, today's lasers will help you increase and maintain hair growth and substantially reduce your hair loss.

What we have discovered is that a specific type and color of laser light is specially designed just to stimulate our hair, so it slows the hair loss and starts regrowing. You can take advantage of this newfound fact and finally see the results you've always wanted. Just read ahead to see what's in store.

How Does LPT Work?

Red light or near-infrared light, like that found in lasers, has been known for decades to have curative powers. Held on a spot long enough, lasers can reduce swelling, help cells self-repair faster, improve circulation, and decrease pain.

You may be asking yourself, "Why lasers and not sunshine?" The explanation is simple: Lasers can be controlled, whereas sunlight's healing uses are limited. The sun's intensity varies by season. Natural light has qualities that can't be easily adjusted—its intensity, for example. Our modern medical practice cannot afford to be subject to seasonal and weather-related changes or we forfeit healing. Fortunately, the invention of artificial light sources has allowed phototherapy to be offered year-round.

Now, we can use light to treat many diseases, injuries, and other conditions. Breast cancer, colorectal cancer, cardiovascular disease, metabolic syndrome, Alzheimer's, autism, type I diabetes, multiple sclerosis, SAD, neonatal jaundice, and myopia are a handful of the conditions treatable with the application of light. And some we haven't even discovered yet.

People picture science fiction films like *Star Trek* and *Star Wars* in which lasers are used to zap each other to death. And we're used to hearing about lasers in surgery, which we associate with cutting. So how are they used in the first over-the-counter (OTC), clinical grade, wearable hair loss device, without causing pain? The *cold laser* (classified as Class 3R by the FDA). As you can guess, cold lasers produce no heat and they put out less than 5 milliwatts (mW) of optical power, making them safe to use on humans. So, the usual four risk factors contributing to the damage other lasers cause—burns, scarring, pain, and infection—are not an issue. Cold lasers are incredibly safe and don't cause any damage because they *cannot* cause harm.

The cold laser then has to be properly tuned to a specific wavelength, 680 nanometers (nm), in order to stimulate all parts of the hair follicle, including melanin and non-melanin components, to be controlled enough to prevent harm, and powerful enough to be absorbed by the follicle and regrow hair. Then, the designer with the right skill set combining expertise in medicine, physics, and electronics must consider the therapeutic window which measures the minimum dosage a person needs to get an effect versus the maximum dosage they can tolerate before harm occurs.

LPTs or devices sold as LPTs that contain lasers without the proper wavelength can cause damage with too much heat buildup beneath the helmet or hat. Or if they contain lights (in the case of LED lights which can be made to simulate lasers), they can have no effect at all. On the other hand, our LPT device has been thoroughly tested and FDA-cleared to meet the proper requirements for wavelength depth, and cooling. When you use this LPT with laser lights specifically designed just for hair, you will increase and maintain hair growth and substantially reduce your hair loss. Best of all, you can do it while relaxing in the comfort of your own home.

Actual Customer Success Stories

Let There Be Light

Diane grappled with the discomforts of menopause, many of which she hoped were temporary. She disliked drugs and chemical treatments and decided she would have to accept her hair loss as part of the aging process. However, when she read about laser hair treatment, she was inspired. Her imagination lit up at the thought of using something as natural as light to nourish her scalp. As a keen gardener, she truly appreciated the power of photosynthesis and light in general. She purchased a wearable LPT device, which she sometimes uses while she cleans the house or tends her rooftop garden. She was most pleased when she visited her hair stylist, who told her that new hairs were coming in not previously seen.

CHAPTER 2
Human Hair 101

"When you have exhausted all possibilities, remember this: you haven't." — Thomas Edison, Inventor, 1899

Psychology of Hair

Hair can be one of the most attention-grabbing parts of our body. It can make an outstanding first impression. Is it neat and tidy? People will see you as neat and tidy. Is it messed up as though you just got out of bed? That's how people will see *you*. Is your hair dull and lifeless? That, again, is how people will see you. People are more likely to remember what your hair looks like than what you wear.

Unfortunately, as far as the body is concerned, hair isn't a high priority because it's not a necessity for survival. Hair condition is frequently one of the first things to decline when the body experiences illness or distress. Society's preoccupation with hair, sadly, can have negative results.

Having personally communicated with tens of thousands of worried people, it is fascinating to hear all of the issues surrounding their insecurities and stigmas with hair loss. We worked a lot with aspiring actors who gave us great insight into their feelings regarding hair loss. This group tended to be active on social media and relied heavily on their perceived looks or attractiveness for their careers. The most common emotional aspects associated with hair loss are self-consciousness, embarrassment, frustration, and jealousy. The psychological stress is felt more acutely in women than men. Any sign of hair loss can be traumatic for a woman's self-esteem and identity, especially when affected at a younger age. Hair loss also is perceived to be a sign of early aging for women, which adds extra anxiety.

What is interesting is that about 100% of women who might see signs of thinning will attempt to do something about it, whereas only 5% of men will try to do something about their hair loss issue. Men have the advantage of being able to shave it all off, and some men look great with shaven heads. Women for the most part are discouraged from taking this step, and solutions for women are a lot more limited than what are available for men. Therefore, hair loss for women is very traumatic and many men also are extremely concerned about their hair loss. My conclusion is that that hair loss has such a traumatic effect on certain human beings that some people truly lose their minds as they lose their hairs.

What's Your Hair Worth?

The concern over hair loss isn't a new phenomenon, and solutions of various kinds have abounded for years. The classic symbolic story occurs in the Old Testament when Samson loses his strength after Delilah cuts his hair off. Today, many people lose their confidence and self-esteem because of hair loss, and they are willing to pay a fortune to save their hair.

Hair loss affects men and women alike, and there are plenty of scammers taking advantage of people's vulnerability promising hair growth miracles. There are only three FDA-cleared solutions for hair growth: two drugs and laser phototherapy (LPT). Almost everything else is suspect—and not FDA-cleared.

Did you know that the American Association of Dermatologists (AAD) says that the average person—that's you—loses between fifty and one hundred hairs *every day!* That amounts to almost 3,000 hairs per month. *Three thousand!*

Now, what does that mean if we look at the cash value to *replace* that hair? In other words, what is your hair worth? Assuming you're in North America or Europe, the average cost today for a transplant is about $5 to $7 per hair.

Average transplant cost...

$5-7 per hair

100 hairs lost a day x 30 days = **3,000 hairs**

$15,000-$21,000 a month in value lost

100,000 hairs on your head

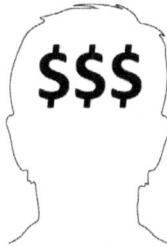

$$$

A full head of hair has a potential value of $500,000 to $700,000

Figure 2.1. Average Value of Hair: The cost of replacing lost hair can amount to thousands of dollars—the value of hair.

So, those 3,000 hairs you lost were worth about $18,000 (between $15,000 and $21,000). If your hair loss is greater than average, your cost is higher. And where you live changes the cost as well. With 100,000 hairs on your scalp, a full head of hair has a potential value of $500,000 to $700,000.

More than half a million dollars for hair? That sounds insane! But some people would be willing to pay that if it meant a lifetime with a full head of hair. A research study showed that 63% of men reported that their hair loss, or visibly thinning hair, had negatively affected their careers. Some people compare the trauma of hair loss to be similarly devastating to that of a death in the family or loss of a job and some have even contemplated suicide. In a German survey, men would even give up sex to keep their hair! It puts the cost of hair loss into perspective.

Hair Loss vs. Hair Growth—Know How to Tell the Difference

This topic has not been discussed in any other publications or anywhere since hair loss and hair growth are vastly different from each other. Before you start thinking of growing back your hair, you must stop or slow down hair loss.

It's obvious that hair *loss* starts first. Over time, most people start seeing the effects of hair loss when about 30–40% of their hair has already been lost. Once you start noticing that something isn't quite right with your hair, panic usually sets in. The immediate thought is: How do I stop my hair loss? This sentiment is very different from "I want to grow new hair!"

Most people want to keep what they have and just want the hair loss to stop. They have negotiated this in their minds and are looking for easy-to-solve solutions to stop or slow down their hair loss. They turn to vitamins, shampoos and thickeners, and leave-in scalp solutions to help. Hair regrowth is something people don't even think of when seeking quick fixes.

Customers who are concerned about hair *growth* are the more advanced hair loss patients. They want to fill in patches or certain areas of thinning.

It is important to understand that hair growth and hair loss occur simultaneously and to understand the difference between the two. Because laser phototherapy (LPT) will stop hair loss while renewing hair growth, a healthy balance between the two processes maintains the overall hair density. When hair loss outpaces hair growth, it leads to thinning hair, while a robust hair growth phase can make hair appear fuller and healthier.

Stopping hair loss is actually mathematically the most advantageous, especially if started early and you're still losing hair. As we calculated earlier, about 3,000 hairs are lost per month with regular hair loss. Since hair loss tends to occur in different stages, it can be as low as fifty to as high as 150 hairs per day during certain times of the year. That is about 36,000 hairs per year that are being saved when you *stop* hair loss!

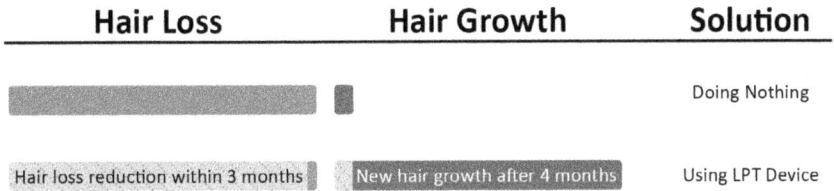

Hair Loss	Hair Growth	Solution
		Doing Nothing
Hair loss reduction within 3 months	New hair growth after 4 months	Using LPT Device

Figure 2.2. Hair Loss vs. Hair Growth. Hair loss and hair growth are vastly different from each other and one must focus on stopping hair loss first. Hair growth takes four months per hair follicle.

Hair growth is a much more time-consuming process to achieve than stopping hair loss. It means areas of the scalp that have had no activity for many months or years need to be "re-awakened." We get frequent calls from desperate customers who call us on a Monday (for example) and ask us to ship our LPT product via next-day air shipment since they claim they have a very important date or event and they need to make sure they have hair by the weekend. In this world of instant gratification, options like LPT should be carefully considered. Hair growth takes some time—but LPT will work. Take a look at the before and after pictures in Appendix A.

If a person wants to do hair transplant surgery, they need to prioritize stopping their hair loss. When they suddenly get more hair, they must do everything they can to keep it. The transplant surgery doesn't protect against the risk of future hair loss from their newly transplanted hairs or their non-transplanted hairs. LPT does.

The Luxury of Hair

We are born with all the hair follicles we'll ever have. An average scalp has about 100,000 hair follicles. These follicles are buried in the skin, each beginning as a root that grows to form the external hair strand. Blood circulates to the follicle and supplies oxygen and nutrients to the hair root to facilitate growth. As hair develops, it pushes through the skin and is lubricated by oil glands that make it shiny and soft. All hair exposed on the scalp is dead but remains anchored in the follicle as it grows. That's why we should trim our hair regularly. Otherwise, the ends of our hair can get unruly with split ends.

People often blame a lack of blood flow to hair follicles when they experience hair growth issues. This is a myth. It is true that our body treats our hair poorly. It pushes hairs out when they're too old, shoves them aside when illness strikes, and gives them the dregs of nutrients left at the bottom of the pot once the rest of the body has had its fill. That's because, as far as the body is concerned, hair is expendable. It's simply *not* a priority.

A good analogy can be made with mountain climbers trying to conquer Mount Everest or other exceptionally high peaks. After climbing past 12,000 feet, oxygen levels drop substantially. Since Mount Everest is about 29,000 feet, the human body starts focusing on preserving the core body parts, including the heart, lungs, liver, and kidneys. As the climber ascends higher, the body's heat pulls away from non-essential parts like the toes, fingers, nose, and ears to keep the most important parts of the body—lungs, heart, brain—as warm as possible while the limbs get frostbite. The body no longer supports them because they're not essential to survival. It's the same in daily life. As we age or develop underlying health conditions, hair is the first thing the body stops sustaining (along with your nails). The fact is that hair is the last thing our bodies need so we have to know how to stop our bodies from getting rid of our hairs every time we are stressed or have to fight underlying medical conditions.

Hair Types from Head to Toe

There are different types of hair on your head and body. "Terminal" hairs are the larger hairs on the scalp, and these have a distinctive color. The tiny, fine hairs on every other part of the body—except on the palms of the hands and soles of the feet—are called "vellus" hairs.

During puberty, vellus facial hair in men thickens into beards and becomes terminal hair. This is one of the amazing transformation processes demonstrating how hormones can change hair types.

Even though women have amazing hair in their third trimester of pregnancy, this does not carry on after a few months of giving birth. The hormonal changes women face during menopause when their child-bearing years end also affect hair. These changes are both due to the hormone estrogen which increases during pregnancy and decreases with menopause.

Although transformation can cause beneficial results for hair, the downside is that scalp hairs can shrink in size and density to become vellus hairs. This results in noticeable hair loss. In most cases, it's not that the hair is gone; it has merely been transformed.

Structure of the Human Hair

Each hair follicle has its own bulge, which contains all the stem cells for that hair. Stem cells have the all-important job of producing new hair follicles. These, in turn, produce hair shafts (this happens when hair is in its growth phase—more on this below). The (dermal) papilla in the hair structure is made up of cells that play a key role in regulating hair growth. While the papilla decides how long your hair will grow (a few inches or a couple feet), the bulge determines how long your hair will stay on your scalp—an average of two to eight years.

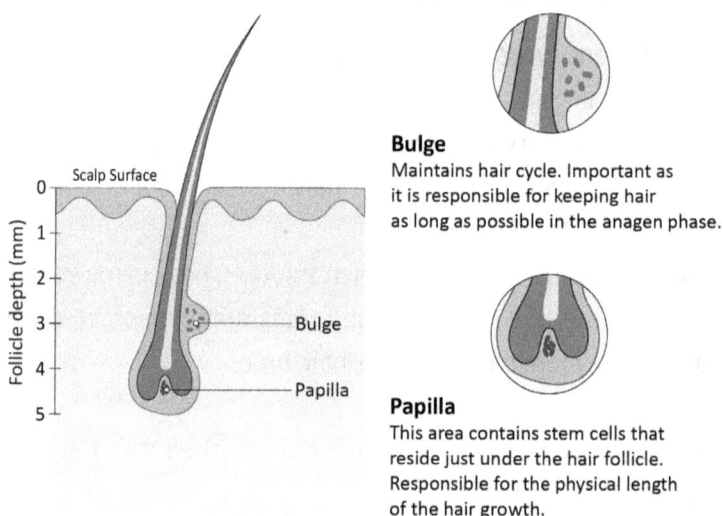

Bulge
Maintains hair cycle. Important as it is responsible for keeping hair as long as possible in the anagen phase.

Papilla
This area contains stem cells that reside just under the hair follicle. Responsible for the physical length of the hair growth.

Figure 2.3. The Bulge and Papilla: The two most important and active structures of the human hair follicle. Stimulating these two will result in hair staying on the head longer with greater thickness and length.

Mitochondria: The Powerhouse of Hair Growth

The mitochondria are the powerhouse of the cell because they produce the energy for the cell's functioning and survival. In the human body, there are an estimated 37.2 trillion cells. Inside each of these cells, there are many mitochondria, depending on the specific organ or type of tissue.

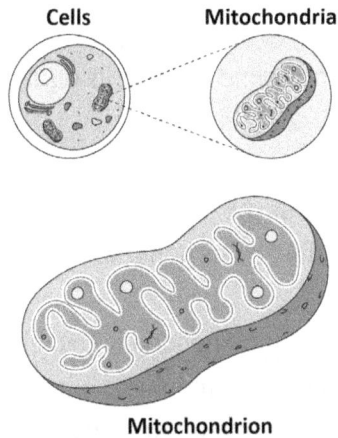

Figure 2.4. All human cells contain mitochondria, which makes energy called ATP, and hair follicles use ATP to grow.

Perhaps you're wondering just how many mitochondria are required to power the hair follicle cell. Researching the precise number of mitochondria in each cell was an undertaking, since this information was not readily available. But we finally found a couple of key papers that estimated the number of mitochondria in the bulge and dermal papilla. As you can see, the two key areas of the hair follicles have an incredible number of mitochondria compared to any other organ in the body. Other organs, except for the heart, have far fewer mitochondria. The brain has the highest number of mitochondria per cell of any organ. The always-working heart cells have the fourth-highest concentration of mitochondria per cell, tied with the skin.

The number of mitochondria in hair varies because some structures need more energy to do their job. The key structures in the hair follicles are the dermal papilla and the bulge. Scientists are still studying the exact number of mitochondria in hair cells. The only published information on these to date has been from Polymerase Chain Reaction (PCR) tests. PCR tests are a way to find and study small pieces of DNA since mitochondria have their own DNA.

Even though PCR tests can give us an idea of how many mitochondria are in hair follicles, it's not a perfect way to count them. PCR tests were the main methods used around the world during the COVID pandemic to detect the SARS-CoV-2 virus.

Hair cells that are outside of the scalp are dead cells and no longer active and do not have any active mitochondria.

An astonishing fact about mitochondria is that they make up about 10% of a human's body weight. This amount of mitochondria power produces an immense amount of energy for trillions of cells in our bodies. It's equivalent to the amount of energy, gram for gram, coming from the sun.

Cell Type		Mitochondria
Brain		2,000,000 Mitochondria per Cell
Kidney		1-2 million Mitochondria per Cell
Human Egg		100,000 - 600,000 Mitochondria per Cell
Bones		30,000 - 50,000 Mitochondria per Cell
Skin		5,000 Mitochondria per Cell
Heart		5,000 Mitochondria per Cell
Liver		1,000 - 2,000 Mitochondria per Cell
Hair Follicles	Hair Shaft (above scalp)	0 Mitochondria per Cell
	Papilla	1,000 Mitochondria per Cell
	Bulge	500 Mitochondria per Cell
Small Intestine		21 - 42 Mitochondria per Cell
Stomach		3 - 5 Mitochondria per Cell

Figure 2.5. Mitochondria per Cell. This chart shows the number of mitochondria per cell and hair follicles contain the most in the papilla where hair length occurs.

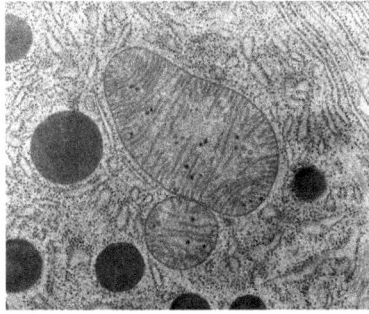

Figure 2.6. The following image depicts a healthy mitochondrion in a hair follicle cell, photographed via a scanned transmission electron microscope.

The Three Phases of Hair Growth

Human hair is one of the body's fastest-growing tissues. If a hair is plucked from its follicle, another hair immediately begins growing in its place and forms in around four months. Scalp hair grows at about 0.4 mm or 0.0157 inches per day and 15 cm or 6 inches annually. This means if you have 100,000 hairs on your scalp and each hair grows at 0.4mm or 0.0157 inches per day, the combined growth would be approximately 4,000 cm or 131 feet a day!

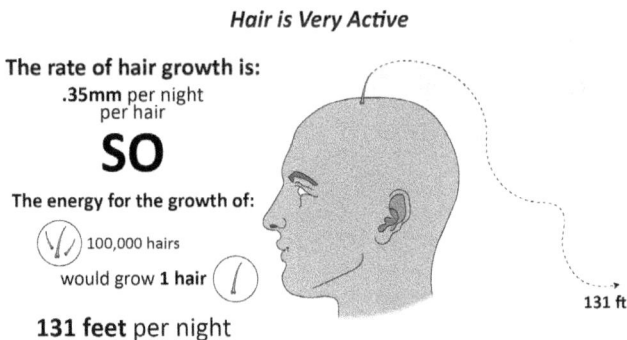

Figure 2.7. Hair Growth Per Night: Hair grows extremely fast—if all the growth from all of the hairs on the body went into one hair, that one hair would grow 131 feet every night!

Hair has active (anagen) and dormant (catagen) phases. During the active phase, cells in the hair root divide rapidly, resulting in faster growth. New hairs are formed that push old, inactive strands out of the hair follicles. A human scalp stays in this phase for two to eight years when hair grows at a rate of 0.35 mm or 0.0138 inches daily. Some people's growth phase is on the shorter side of that spectrum, and they have difficulty growing head hair. It's interesting to note that one square inch (6.45 square cm) of the scalp contains anywhere from 800 to 1,300 hairs, but not all will result in hair growth.

Some people have more active hairs on their scalp, while others have very few active hairs. Those with few active hairs usually suffer from thinning scalp, or alopecia.

Conversely, the dormant (catagen) phase is a transitional period in the hair growth cycle. All growth stops, and the outer root sheath of the hair shrinks and attaches to the root. At any given time, roughly 3% of scalp hairs are in this dormant phase, which lasts for about three weeks.

There's also the resting, or telogen, phase. Lasting about one hundred days, 10% to 15% of head hairs are in the resting phase at any time. In this stage, the hair separates from the papilla (cells contained in the follicle—see Figure 2.5) and is pushed until it falls out completely. Hair cells then start multiplying again to replace the shed hair, and the hair growth cycle begins again.

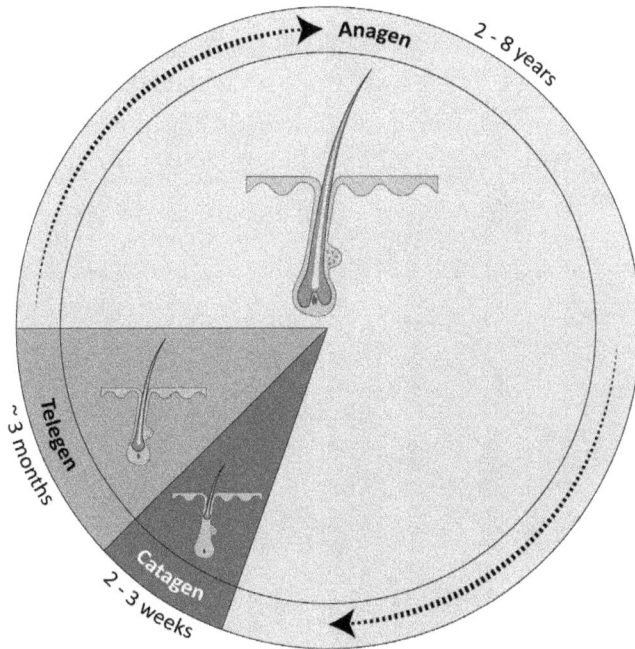

Figure 2.8. Phases of Hair Growth. There are three major phases for a hair follicle and the most important one is the anagen phase which lasts from two to eight years.

Older adults can enter a period when hair is no longer being lost and replaced. When you stop losing hair, your scalp has reached a final resting phase. Your grandpa, with his slick, shiny scalp, is no longer losing hair. Active hair loss indicates an active scalp. Nor is he growing any back. To regrow hair, you must lose hair. That train has left the station.

When hair loss no longer occurs, the hair cycle is nearing its end. This is the final resting phase, during which all hair growth may cease. This usually happens after you reach sixty years of age.

If you're currently losing your hair, that's good news. You just need to halt the loss and then improve the regrowth. That's doable. Once you understand hair growth, all you have to do is learn how to manage it.

It takes time to overcome what's been happening in your body. Just as a baby takes about nine months to fully develop, a single hair needs about four months to grow. This period can't be shortened. However, I've got a method that can help you to regrow your hair like never before. The goal isn't perfect hair tomorrow; it's great hair for *the rest of your life.*

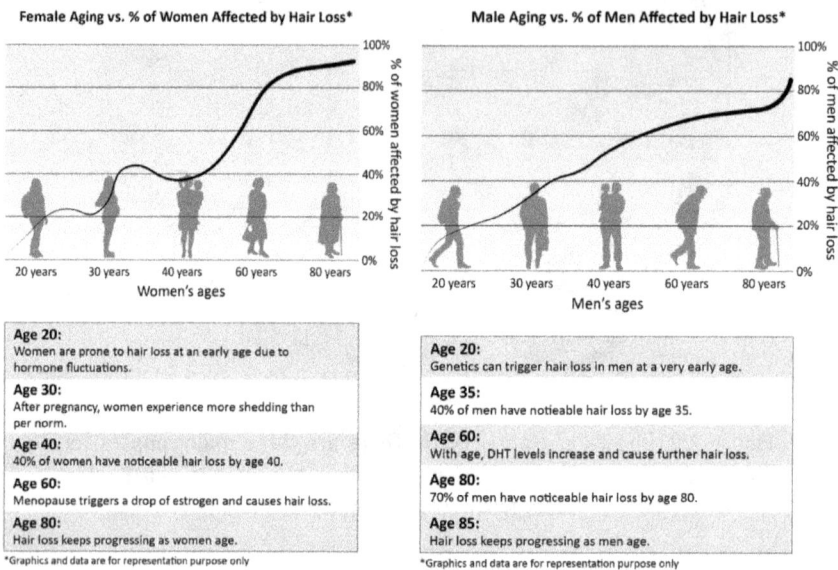

Female Aging vs. % of Women Affected by Hair Loss*

Age 20:
Women are prone to hair loss at an early age due to hormone fluctuations.

Age 30:
After pregnancy, women experience more shedding than per norm.

Age 40:
40% of women have noticeable hair loss by age 40.

Age 60:
Menopause triggers a drop of estrogen and causes hair loss.

Age 80:
Hair loss keeps progressing as women age.

*Graphics and data are for representation purpose only

Male Aging vs. % of Men Affected by Hair Loss*

Age 20:
Genetics can trigger hair loss in men at a very early age.

Age 35:
40% of men have notieable hair loss by age 35.

Age 60:
With age, DHT levels increase and cause further hair loss.

Age 80:
70% of men have noticeable hair loss by age 80.

Age 85:
Hair loss keeps progressing as men age.

*Graphics and data are for representation purpose only

Figure 2.9. Hair Loss in Males and Females over Time. This chart clearly shows that hair loss gets worse as one ages regardless of gender.

Introducing the Bullseye Growth Effect (BGE)

As we know, tracking hair loss is difficult, so it should come as no surprise that tracking the progress of hair regrowth is also a difficult task. The fact is, until now, we've never really needed to measure hair growth because nothing worked well enough to make it worthwhile. There have been hundreds of books written on hair loss and not one discusses how hair growth really works! As part of researching previous books on hair loss, I discovered that the majority of the authors who wrote books on hair loss had either completely lost their hair or had advanced hair loss themselves. In my personal situation, I have provided my before and after images (see Appendix A) showing how my LPT stopped my hair loss and re-grew the thinned-out areas. Just to be clear, I personally use my LPT device every day and have fully incorporated this routine as part of my regular lifestyle.

LPT works so well that we're breaking new ground in measuring hair growth. What is remarkable is that there is no previous method for measuring hair growth. That speaks volumes about archaic hair growth products and claims.

In the introduction of this book, *Grow It Back*, I told the story of Melba, a sixty-eight-year-old hair loss patient who used the Theradome as instructed for six months, but who struggled to see any noticeable results. It took showing Melba the before and after pictures of her former sparse, thin hair next to current photos for her to appreciate just how much her hair had grown. Because the change came on slowly, Melba didn't even notice that her hair looked much thicker now, as the before and after comparison revealed.

The human eye automatically adjusts to daily growth over time, so we don't have a good reference point by which to measure new growth. Monitoring progress is akin to using a child's height growth chart, where gradual advancements need to be documented over time, allowing for clear visualization of development and the identification of trends or patterns.

Similarly, we have to create references for hair as well. One of the easiest ways is with global photography as previously mentioned. The key is to take consistent pictures to provide a careful record of growth.

Or reduction of loss.

Reducing hair loss versus growing new hair—there is a difference. When hair loss is reduced substantially, hair looks thicker. For the first three months, this is just an illusion since hair takes four months to grow.

When we look at before and after pictures of a hair loss patient, our eye automatically focuses on the most pronounced area of hair loss, which we refer to as the bullseye effect. This area also tends to be the longest-affected area making it the last area to fill in. The first area to fill with regrown hair is the most recent area of hair loss, often, hair loss that has occurred within the last three to five years.

The image below shows hair regrowth from the outside inward for both the male and female models. In this case, the inside is the oldest area of hair loss, so this is the area that takes the longest to fill in. This new pattern of growth is significant for laser phototherapy (LPT) patients. My personal observation is that hair density is related to the length of time a patient has experienced active hair loss. For women, hair loss or thinning generally starts at the part line, mainly at the center of the scalp. Over time, it tends to gradually spread from there. Therefore, the part line is the oldest area and usually has a much lower hair count per square centimeter than areas farther out. Regrowth is a slow, frustrating process.

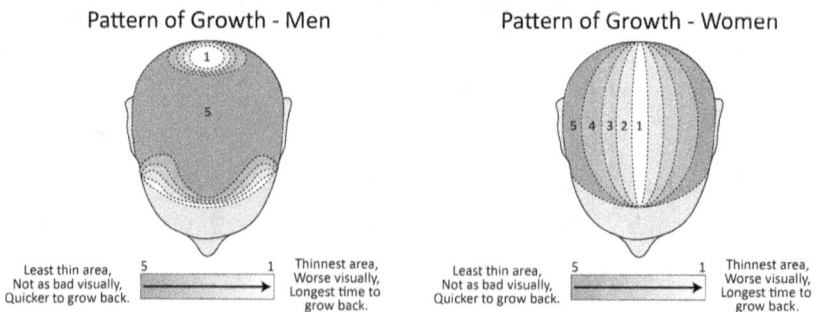

Pattern of Growth - Men

Pattern of Growth - Women

Least thin area, Not as bad visually, Quicker to grow back. 5 → 1 Thinnest area, Worse visually, Longest time to grow back.

Least thin area, Not as bad visually, Quicker to grow back. 5 → 1 Thinnest area, Worse visually, Longest time to grow back.

Figure 2.10. Pattern of Hair Growth Illustrated for Men. The lower numbers (e.g., 1) represent the oldest area suffering from hair loss and higher numbers (e.g., 5) represent the most recent hair loss area. Higher numbers will start filling in first before the lower numbers.

Male and female hair loss typically occurs in concentric circles with the circle's center becoming the barest. As hair loss expands outward, the areas that have thinned the least make up the outermost circles. They are the farthest from the part line.

The hair count up and down the part line varies from an average of ten to fifty hairs per square centimeter. In comparison, areas farther away from the part line can have as many as 400 hairs per square centimeter (depending on the person's age and health). While this loss pattern varies from patient to patient, the number and density of hairs in the growth phase are much lower on the part line.

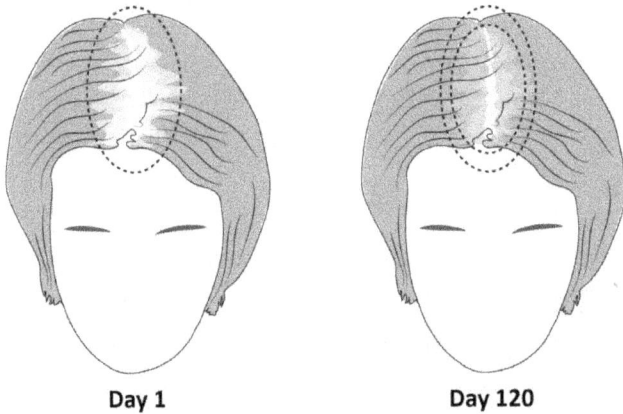

Day 1   **Day 120**

Figure 2.11. Female Hair Loss and Regrowth Occurring in Oval Areas, with the Part Line at the Center. The outer part of the oval fills in first, and then about three to seven months later, the part line will start filling in.

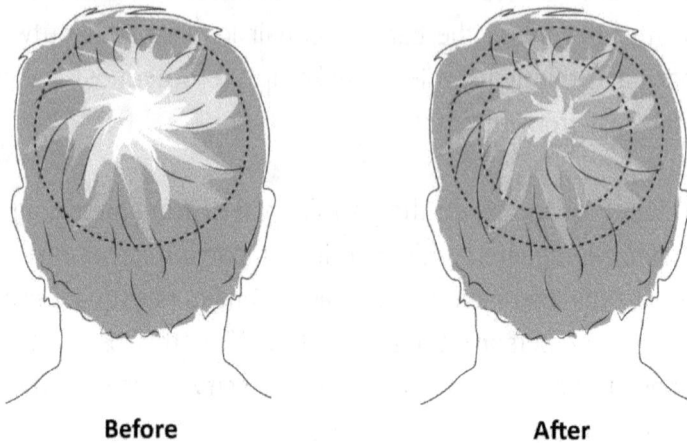

Figure 2.12. Male Hair Loss and Regrowth Occurring in Circles, with the Crown at the Center. The outermost part of the circles will start filling in (within three to six months) and the center (bullseye) will take anywhere from six months to one year (depending on the severity of their hair loss to fill in).

The photos below show an LPT patient on day one and after 120 days. This woman's part line was spreading, especially toward the front. After 120 days of LPT (she used the LPT device at least twice per week), the outer edges of her part line started to fill in. Notice in the right-hand photo how the concentric circle has decreased. This circle will continue to shrink until the part line fills in, which usually takes about six to nine months.

That doesn't mean LPT should be discontinued. LPT is a lifetime commitment. Remember that hair loss gets worse as one ages—this applies to every human being. The body constantly produces excessive levels of 5-alpha reductase which creates excess DHT. Once hair regrowth reaches a maximum, patients should continue treatments three to five times a week to slow or prevent any further hair loss. Without ongoing treatment, the hair loss process will start again.

Generally, in men experiencing hair loss, spreading begins at the crown, not along the part line.

Both examples show that reducing the speed and spread of hair loss is the fastest, most reliable way to reverse and regrow hair as well as to prevent further hair loss. The progress can be seen in concentric circles of gradual improvement. The outermost circles fill in first because LPT affects the outer areas first.

Understanding human hair, factors contributing to hair loss, and how to maintain a healthy head of hair, are vital for understanding the myths and misconceptions about hair regrowth. We know that measuring the amount of daily hair loss and hair growth is difficult, but we know that the use of LPT produces long-term results. Now, it's time to dig a little deeper and discuss how LPT actually works.

Actual Customer Success Stories

Your Hair Deserves a Break

When Janine noticed her ponytail had suddenly got much thinner, the thought of it kept her awake at night for weeks. She was used to her pretty hair attracting attention when she walked down the street. She was not ready to give this up. At the salon, she asked her stylist not to use thinning shears as she had been for years. She yearned for a fuller crown, not the expanding parting line that had become all too visible. She read about laser therapy and was thrilled to learn that there was still a way she could reverse this nightmare. Now, she wears her laser device while she drives her kids to school daily. If she gets out at the school gate, she turns heads! Her hairdresser compliments her on her hair and tells her there are more striking styles open to her to try than ever before.

CHAPTER 3

Hair Loss: Causes and Consequences

"The more you understand the reasons for things, the less you fear them." — Marie Curie, Scientist, 1923

All the Reasons for Hair Loss

Let's untangle the mystery of hair loss. Finding solid scientific studies is nearly as difficult as building a rocket. It seems that most funding for hair studies is more interested in charting hair growth than tracking hair loss.

According to the calculations in this book and the American Academy of Dermatologists' website, we shed around fifty to one hundred strands of hair every single day. Who conducted this study? And how? Not all of us shed the same amount of hair. It's a mystery no one has a firm answer to.

Picture this: You're engrossed in one of those thrilling crime scene investigation shows, and what do the detectives find? Hairs everywhere! Usually, they pick them up with tweezers. To measure hair loss accurately, we'd have to wear a cone around our neck each day coated in adhesive to catch all the dropping strands to find out the true number of hairs that have fallen from our heads.

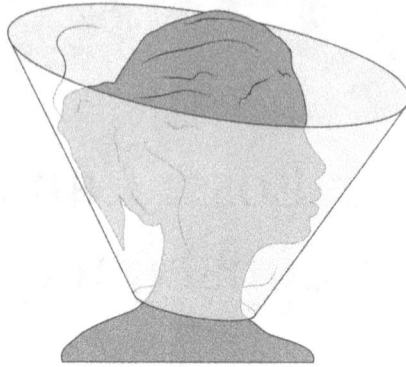

Figure 3.1. The only effective way to measure hair loss would be to wear a cone with adhesive attached every day!

The truth is, nobody's willing to shell out the expenses for a study on hair loss. Most products out there promise significant growth, not saving us from a strand Exodus. A study like that would cost a fortune and be more complicated than it's worth. It would require a big budget and lots of patience, something those of us with hair loss just don't have.

We can make the following simple calculation to come to an educated guess of fifty to one hundred strands per day. Keeping in mind that this is an average, some people will lose more, some people will lose less. We'll base this on the total number of hairs on the human head and the percentage in the telogen phase. This phase is like a hair vacation, where the follicles take a break from growing.

About 10,000 to 15,000 hairs of the 100,000 hairs or so on the human head are in the telogen phase at any given time. When this phase is completed, the hairs begin a whole new growth cycle. This may take around two to four months (sixty to 120 days).

This telogen phase and the number of hairs in it vary from person to person. We normally lose around 7,000 hairs in three months. If we crunch the numbers, that's about 77.8 hairs per day (dividing 7,000 by ninety days). Pretty close to seventy-five, which is right in the middle of fifty and one hundred. So, it seems that the estimated range of fifty to one hundred hairs lost daily reflects the average amount of hair strands being lost during the telogen phase.

This calculation hasn't been published anywhere. We hope you find it useful.

Types and Causes of Hair Loss

While it's true that the rate of hair growth declines as people get older, anyone can lose hair at any time. Hair loss isn't restricted to a particular age group, gender, or race. Hair color and type have no effect on hair loss either. Anyone is at risk of hair loss for various reasons, including hormonal changes, genetics, and medical conditions.

The fact is that hair loss typically becomes noticeable when approximately 50% of the hair density has diminished, making the thinning areas more apparent to the naked eye. That's bad news for all of us!

Let's take a deep dive into the reasons for hair loss.

Gray Hair vs. Hair Loss

What about gray hair? Much research has gone into understanding why we go gray, and the process is now fairly clear. Pigment-producing cells in the scalp give hair its distinctive color. These cells, however, have a limited lifespan. As they wear out or are damaged, they stop producing melanin, the pigment that gives hair (and skin) its color. New hair has no coloring, making it appear white, silver, or gray.

It's generally agreed that graying hair results from aging. Hair loss, however, can have many underlying causes primarily unrelated to aging, including genetics, hormones, and certain diseases. Despite appearing to go hand in hand, graying and thinning hair are two distinct processes. What is very interesting is that in Melba's case, the only hair that would grow from the top of her hair prior to starting LPT was gray/white hair. But once Melba started to use LPT, her natural hair came back instead of more white hairs. This phenomenon suggests that within each square centimeter of her scalp are both white/gray hairs as well as her dark red hairs. We see this phenomenon all of the time; that people with white/gray hair state that after wearing the LPT device, their white hairs have nearly disappeared. The fact is, the same number of white hairs are there, but now more naturally colored hairs are present, giving the illusion that their white/gray hairs have been reduced.

Pattern Hair Loss (Genetics)

Hair follicles are the structures from which new hair strands grow. When hair follicles shrink, the hair growth cycle begins to weaken. This process is called "miniaturizing." The weakened hair follicles produce shorter and more delicate strands of hair. At the end of the growth cycle, these hairs are shed, and no new hairs replace them. This process takes years to accomplish and hair that normally lasts two to eight years on the scalp stays on the head for a much shorter time.

The illustration in Figure 3.2 shows that terminal hairs (on the very far left side) start diminishing after each hair cycle. Eventually, over the course of several years, the hair follicle gets covered up by a new skin called Epidermal Growth Factor (EGF). The hair follicle is not dead, but it will not be able to break through the new skin. We will be discussing this concept throughout the book, as it plays a major role in whether someone can reverse their hair thinning or not based on how advanced this miniaturization process has progressed.

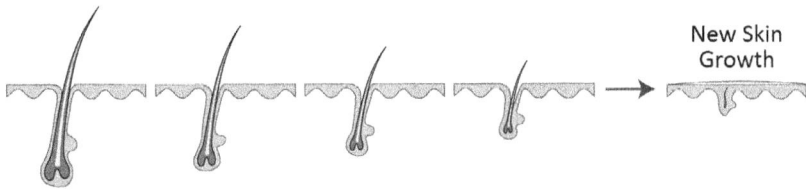

Figure 3.2. Shrinking Hair Follicles or Miniaturization in the Hair Growth Cycle. This process starts with a thick hair (far left), which miniaturizes over the years and eventually gets covered up by new skin growth.

In order to determine if someone has a genetic versus a non-genetic hair loss condition, there are many methods of analyzing the level of hair loss, such as a pull test, tug test, and microscopic analysis can only determine the hair's strength, color, and texture. To confirm female pattern hair loss (FPHL)—or male pattern hair loss (MPHL), more in-depth tests, such as bloodwork and scalp biopsies, must be conducted (in the medical community, genetic pattern hair loss is referred to as androgenetic alopecia).

Weak hair hints at a higher risk of hair loss but we can't specify whether the hair loss is actually due to the weakening of hair follicles. Consequently, hair analysis doesn't provide any information about determining the outcome of hair loss from pattern hair loss.

Men tend to lose hair at the crown and front of the scalp, extending to the areas near the ears. Women usually lose hair along their part line, and the thinning is restricted to the top of the scalp. In terms of surface area, women on average lose much less hair than men.

Androgenetic alopecia is the most common form of hair loss and represents about 93% of all hair loss diseases. It affects up to 50% of both men and women. By age seventy, up to 80% of men are afflicted with this condition. For women, the incidence of androgenetic alopecia increases after menopause. This condition, as you may remember, is what caused Melba's thinning hair. The terms "male pattern hair loss" (MPHL) and "female pattern hair loss" (FPHL) are derived from the gender-dependent patterns hair loss creates.

Hair problems for both men and women are worse in some families than others. Androgenetic alopecia is caused by a combination of maternal and paternal genetic factors. One source claims that men whose fathers suffered hair loss are up to six times more likely to develop the condition. The mitochondria, however, are inherited exclusively from the mother because they are present in the egg, which contributes to the fetus's development, while the sperm contributes only its genetic material. Therefore, today, androgenetic alopecia is not classified as a mitochondrial disease (coming from the mother's side), as there is only some evidence pointing towards a possible connection between mitochondrial dysfunction and hair loss. If this link is proven, it could imply that inheritance from the mother may play a key role in a child getting androgenetic alopecia. However, further study needs to be done.

Stress

Did you know stress is a leading cause of hair loss? Yet, being stressed out is practically the national pastime in America. Everybody experiences stress. Stress is such a constant that it might be easier to think of a time when you weren't stressed!

Think about all the stress we must cope with today. The COVID-19 pandemic was a source of extreme stress. Firstly, there were the fears of the virus itself and the imposed isolation. Aside from coping with sickness and, in many cases, grief, people lost their jobs, businesses, homes, and in some cases, close relationships. Financial difficulties like inflation, legal problems, and other strife associated with quarantine were compounded by political arguments with family, friends, and even strangers on the internet. In addition, a rough economy caused entire industries to disappear. This led many to worry about losing their jobs to automation. All the while, political trouble, murders, threats of war, demonstrations, protests, and riots—already present before COVID-19—made our anxiety even worse. No wonder we were strained to our limits.

Social media can also trigger a good deal of stress. People can quickly become influenced by what they see. They soon feel pressured to buy more expensive things, live a luxurious lifestyle, be seen with products with famous brand names, and develop an unhealthy self-image. This adds to financial difficulties and greater stress factors. Even though most of us will never own, or even desire, private jets, supercars, or tropical vacation homes, we make unconscious comparisons. We may subconsciously feel like we're supposed to pursue a celebrity lifestyle.

Human beings aren't made to handle so much stress. The way we live today dramatically affects our health and, consequently, hair loss. Our ancestors didn't have to cope with the same stress levels. Nor did they die from stress. Their needs were straightforward: find shelter, food, and a mate. Although we have the same basic needs, they are much more difficult to meet today. The economy, financial demands, more complex social structures, and other modern complications mean life is much more difficult.

If you're thinking, "Surely prehistoric humans were seriously stressed out by things like adverse weather and wild animals," you're right. But that was acute stress, whereas today, we live with chronic stress. Chronic stress means we're constantly under pressure without a gap in which to hang a hammock and relax. We spend all our time trying to figure out how to pay the rent, mortgage, or car loan, cover food and gas costs, find a better job, keep our mates happy, or any number of other challenges. On the other hand, prehistoric humans could relax and have regular downtime, which helped them lower their stress levels.

People who have the gene for androgenetic alopecia are more affected by stress-triggered hair loss. If they are struggling with today's cut-throat, competitive, chaotic society, hair loss can occur at a younger age than normal.

In all, stress accounts for a good deal of the hair loss in our modern world.

Hormones

Hormones are potent chemicals secreted by special cells in the body. While hormones have many functions, several studies have proven they contribute to hair loss no matter your gender, age, or race. Various hormones regulate the hair cycle and determine hair structure. Since these hormones are responsible for hair growth, hormone imbalances will result in hair loss. Here are the hormones directly implicated in hair growth.

Androgens and Anti-Androgens

Androgens are a particular type of hormone known as steroids. Androgens are the hormones responsible for the development of secondary sex characteristics. They are produced in several places in the body, including the adrenal glands, gonads, brain, and placenta. Androgens, especially dihydrotestosterone (DHT), are involved in hair growth and in producing hairs on the face, underarms, and pubic area during puberty. But they've also been shown to hinder the growth of scalp hair. In general, men tend to have higher androgen levels than women.

You may have heard of anti-androgen drugs, which, as their name suggests, block the effects of androgens. Women should avoid them since there are severe side effects including low estrogen levels, menstrual irregularities, osteoporosis, and fetal abnormalities. Even for men, the probability of side effects must be weighed carefully against the potential benefits. These can include acne, male pattern hair loss (MPHL), and prostate cancer.

And an overactive sex drive can be treated with anti-androgens. The side effects, however, include increased breast size, shrinking of the prostate gland, and low sex drive. Women can use anti-androgens to treat hair issues, female pattern hair loss (FPHL), skin conditions (such as acne), and excess facial and body hair. The side effects, however, particularly for women of childbearing age, are severe. These include low estrogen levels, menstrual irregularities, osteoporosis, and fetal abnormalities.

Sex Hormones

Hair loss is more prevalent in men because certain sex hormones present in women can protect them from it. These hormones include estrogen, progesterone, and prolactin, which are known to inhibit the effects of an enzyme called 5-alpha reductase. Let's call it 5-alpha for short. It helps with turning testosterone into DHT. Higher levels of DHT aren't good if you want to grow a fuller head of hair.

For transgender individuals who are undergoing hormone therapy, male pattern baldness can be an unwelcome side effect that can impede their transition goals. Laser phototherapy can be a non-invasive and effective option for combating male pattern baldness, as it can stimulate hair growth and improve the thickness and quality of existing hair. This can help trans individuals achieve a more traditionally feminine appearance, if that is their desired outcome, reduce feelings of dysphoria and lessen some of the mental health and well-being feelings associated with hair loss. Laser phototherapy can also be a non-invasive and affordable option for those who may not be able to undergo more extensive procedures or hormone therapy. Similarly, individuals assigned female at birth looking to make the transition to a masculine gender identity may be worried about newfound hair loss associated with going on testosterone, as increased levels of this hormone can in turn increase DHT levels, leading to hair loss. For transgender men or non-binary individuals looking to undergo hormone replacement therapy (HRT), LPT can be used to treat hair loss from heightened testosterone and DHT levels resulting from such treatment.

Thyroid Gland Hormones

Referred to as T3 and T4, triiodothyronine and thyroxine, respectively, are the thyroid hormones that increase the concentration of hair cells (keratinocytes) and make the growth phase (anagen) last longer.

Melatonin

Melatonin can inhibit hair growth but it can also promote it. For example, it can interfere with the effects of certain hormones, such as prolactin and estrogen, which may then decrease hair growth.

DHT

This is a particular type of testosterone. Both men and women have it, although men usually have more. When the scalp becomes irritated, DHT attacks and kills hair—that's its only purpose. Think of it as a hair follicle assassin. Currently, there's nothing that stops or even lowers DHT levels without side effects. Hormones are powerful and they're practically unstoppable. Think of women with Premenstrual syndrome (PMS), of the driving power of hunger, of the insanity of sleep deprivation. No shampoo, lotion, cream, or pill helps stop DHT any more than there's a pill to prevent any of those.

Scientists have found that 5-alpha reductase, the enzyme that speeds up the rate at which testosterone is turned into DHT, is more active in thinning scalps. DHT is a hormone that shows no mercy and prevents nutrients from reaching hair cells. Without nutrients, hair cells can't provide energy to hair follicles. DHT also controls the hair follicle through each passing hair cycle, shrinking the follicle still more. This results in hair loss. It should come as no surprise that scalps suffering from hair loss show higher levels of DHT.

What is it that causes an increase in DHT levels? One key factor is sickness or certain medical conditions that trigger the body to focus on healing itself. Remember, disease and hair loss are closely linked. When we get ill, our bodies put all their energy into ensuring survival. Since hair is expendable, the body responds by releasing DHT into the scalp to prevent hair cells from using up nutrients. Therefore, many people lose hair while suffering from an illness. Their hair isn't merely falling out; it's being purged to help the body preserve what it needs to stay alive and fight off disease. Since hair is the fastest-growing part of the body, the body gets rid of it first.

High DHT levels can also be genetic. You can be perfectly healthy and still suffer from hereditary hair loss. If your relatives have struggled with thinning hair, it may mean the same fate awaits you, so it's a good idea to take preventative measures as early as possible.

Men have higher DHT levels which drop steadily every decade after age thirty. Hair loss for men also tends to be much more severe than for women. Nonetheless, despite having less DHT, women can also experience hair assassination. Even small amounts of DHT can cause hair loss. While women rarely experience advanced hair loss, DHT is still a factor.

What can we do? Many claim that reducing DHT levels can stop hair loss. Current research doesn't support this idea. Remember that DHT's purpose is to assassinate hair. But hair loss doesn't always align with the body's DHT levels. People with normal levels of DHT can still experience hair loss, just as people without a family history of hair loss might lose their hair. No one understands specifically how hormones affect the hair cycle or why, other than that in the case of poor health the body sends DHT to kill hairs. All that's known is that if the health of a hair follicle is improved, DHT has a much tougher time trying to get rid of the hair. We'll address this issue in later chapters of *Grow It Back*.

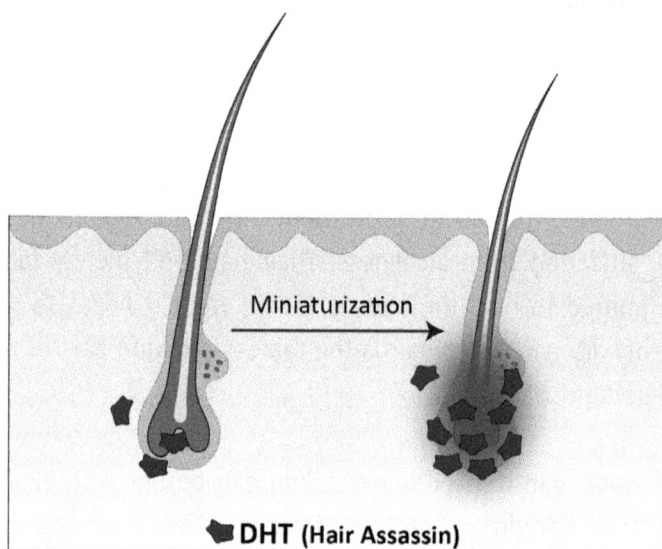

Figure 3.3. Hair Follicle Being Attacked by DHT Hormone and Programmed to Miniaturize Over Each Hair Cycle.

Brushing, Pulling, Wigs, and Weaves

The arrector pili is a tiny muscle that supports each hair growing out of the skin. It's not meant to hold more than a hair's weight, so it's not very strong. It's only capable of making the hair stand up during a stressful moment or easing it back down when calm returns. Recent findings have connected this muscle with maintaining hair follicle strength. In people with normal hair or people experiencing reversible hair loss, the arrector pili stay connected to the follicles. Simple pressure can break the connection between this muscle and hair follicles.

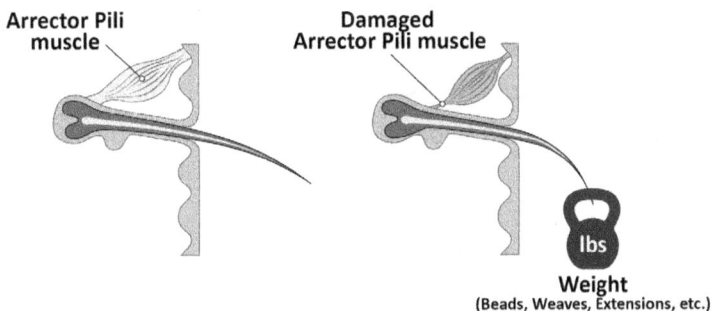

Figure 3.4. The arrector pili muscle is responsible for contracting in response to cold or fear, and adding excessive weight to the hair can damage these muscles leading to hair loss.

How often do you brush or run your fingers through your hair? You probably never think about it. Tugging, rubbing, and friction can pull hairs from their follicles. Putting pressure on an area of the scalp can cause hair loss. This is called pressure-induced alopecia. Symptoms of hair loss caused by pressure include broken hairs, redness, and sores.

Hair extensions and weaves can damage hair if they are not used cautiously. Braiding, adding, or attaching extensions involves tugging on the hair. This tugging can cause hair breakage and loss. It can also damage the follicles, resulting in permanent hair loss. This type of hair loss is known as traction alopecia. It's common in people of African descent who wear beads, weaves, and extensions.

Think Twice before You Heat

High temperatures, such as those used in hair styling (think of hair dryers, flat irons, and curling irons), can damage hair. Dandruff is not the only cause of hair loss. High temperatures can dry out hair and harm the cuticle—the protective outer layer. High heat makes hair more brittle and makes it break. Hair can also be damaged and split at the ends as well as have a rough or stringy texture, making it hard to style or straighten.

We all learned in our high school science class that we can change the state of a molecule or compound—say, from a solid to a liquid—by heating it. Hair follicles are also affected by heat: the growth phase of the hair cycle gets much shorter, and your hair falls out more quickly.

How Important Is Vitamin D to Great Hair

I can't overstate the importance of vitamin D. We need vitamin D to absorb calcium and phosphorus—minerals that are necessary for normal bone and heart health. According to scientists, there are twenty-seven diseases associated with a lack of vitamin D. Without adequate exposure to the sun, mobility becomes limited and aging speeds up. Consider older folks living in nursing homes—less time spent in the sun quickens the aging process. Vitamin D deficiency impacts mood, hormone levels, and energy. Another critical role of vitamin D is to build and maintain hair health since it is involved in nurturing hair follicles. Deficiencies in vitamin D may cause hair loss, particularly a form called "spot hair loss" (alopecia areata).

Contrary to popular belief, the sun doesn't actually *produce* vitamin D. Instead, sunlight is needed to bring about certain chemical reactions to enable the body to make vitamin D.

Although there's a limit to how much vitamin D your body can make each day, you can't overdose on vitamin D no matter how much time you spend in the sun. People who are in the sun all day, such as construction workers, never get vitamin D poisoning. The sun, however, does present other dangers. After all, no one wants to develop skin cancer or look older than they really are. Can you get vitamin D from the sun without risking cancer and wrinkles? I believe you can.

It is important to note that many people associate sun exposure with skin cancer, but research has found that *insufficient* exposure to UV radiation, the kind of light you get from the sun, may also be linked to other types of cancer, so there is a balance here that must be better understood.

Vitamin D plays a significant role in hair follicle growth and hair loss prevention. Hair loss, or alopecia, is directly linked to reduced levels of vitamin D. Studies have confirmed that men with higher rates of hair loss usually have lower vitamin D levels. There are some indications that vitamin D supplements can reduce hair loss. Unfortunately, research into the relationship between hair loss and vitamin D levels in women has so far shown inconsistent results.

Although no one has been able to prove that vitamin D *stops hair loss* in everyone, activated vitamin D contributes to *hair growth* for everyone. Exposure to sunlight, vitamin D supplements, and artificial ultraviolet light all help activate vitamin D. In fact, human hair actually contains vitamin D receptors (VDRs), that increase during the hair growth phase (anagen phase), when VDRs are the most active.

Ultraviolet A (UVA), ultraviolet B (UVB), and ultraviolet C (UVC) are the three types of ultraviolet light. All are invisible to the human eye. UVA has the longest wavelength. Ninety-five percent of the ultraviolet light that reaches the earth's surface is UVA. It is present during daylight hours year-round and is the wavelength that causes the skin to age. It can also worsen skin cancer caused by its cousin, UVB. UVA penetrates more deeply into the skin and causes more damage to material in the cell nucleus than UVB. It's also harder to protect yourself from UVA light.

Whereas UVB is blocked by a good sunscreen or glass (such as the glass in your windows at home), we only get UVC exposure from artificial sources. It's the shortest wavelength of the three UV lights, blocked by the ozone layer—unlike UVA, which can pass right through windows and some clothing.

UVB is the middle wavelength of the UV spectrum. While it's thought to be the main cause of skin cancer, it's also the wavelength that produces vitamin D. The atmosphere blocks most UVB coming from the sun, so only a little gets to the Earth. UVB penetrates only through the outer layer of the skin. Since it can't penetrate glass like UVA, you can't get any UVB light indoors even on the brightest day. People with dark skin are less able to make vitamin D because the melanin in their skin blocks UVB just like sunblock. During winter, as well as in the morning and evening during summer, the angle of the Earth to the sun prevents UVB from reaching the ground. Generally, the farther you live from the equator, the less UVB reaches you in the winter.

How Much Vitamin D Do You Need?

Vitamin D provides many health benefits, including improved cardiovascular and immune functions. Ways to get more vitamin D include increasing sun exposure, taking vitamin D supplements, and using artificial UV light sources.

According to doctors, bloodwork should show about 20 to 50 micrograms per liter of vitamin D to ensure continued hair growth and prevent hair loss. However, a Yale Medicine report suggests that taking a vitamin D supplement isn't the same as getting out in the sun. This is because the body doesn't absorb vitamin D supplements in the same way as it does when sunlight hits your bare skin. According to the study, both are absorbed quickly, but the supplement vitamin D is quickly cleared from your body, while the sunlight-absorbed vitamin D stays in your body, continuing to release its goodness for up to seven days. That's powerful.

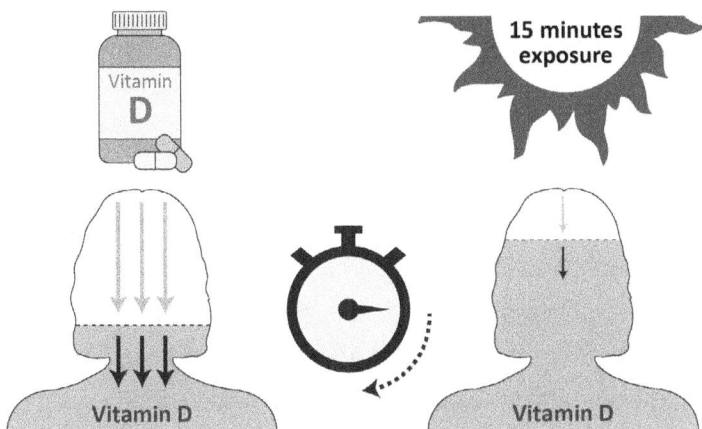

Figure 3.5. The Effects of Vitamin D Supplements vs. Sunlight. Getting fifteen minutes of sunlight daily has been shown to be more effective than consuming vitamin supplements.

Conversely, vitamin D supplements can be lethal if overdosed, but vitamin D overdose is simply not possible with the sun.

On the downside, you run the risk of getting sunburn or even skin cancer, especially if you're prone to sores on your skin, lesions, masses, tumors, cancerous growths, or don't have hair on your head—remember the photoprotective effect of hair?

On average, we need about fifteen minutes a day of exposure to sunlight. It's important to have the sun shining on areas of your skin for that time. Studies suggest the best time to get your daily dose of natural sunlight during the summer months is before 9 am or after 2 pm. This is when your body will do the best job of absorbing sunlight and the sun is least likely to cause sunburn.

Be sure not to wear any sunglasses and avoid taking in sun through a glass window or windshield when getting your daily dose, as the majority of sunlight is absorbed by the retina. As such, sunglasses and other see-through barriers will only confuse the brain, which will no longer be able to accurately gauge how much light energy the body is really taking in. The fact is the body loses its natural ability to sense the amount of light in the environment when wearing sunglasses or looking through a tinted glass structure. This is a little counterintuitive—when we wear sunglasses, we're tricking out brains, which then cannot protect the skin and body by signaling the point at which enough sunlight has been taken in. Without our brain's ability to let us know when we've had enough sun, we risk causing more damage, including increasing the likelihood of developing skin cancer, sunburns, wrinkles, and so on.

If you live in an area where there's not much sunlight, sitting under artificial UV lights can help you get enough vitamin D levels for a healthy body and to fight depression if you suffer from Seasonal Affective Disorder.

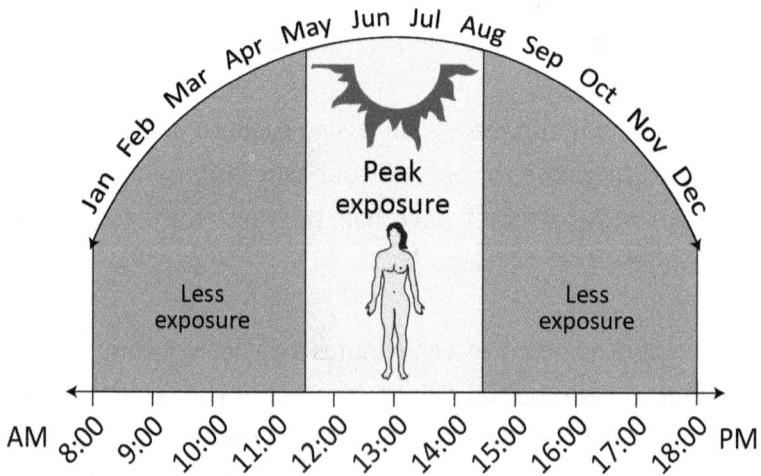

Figure 3.6. Sunlight Exposure Times: The best time to get the most sunlight is during mid-day and during the summer months.

Thankfully, we've got several options for getting this lifesaving nutrient. Another study proved that the artificial lights used in tanning salons can also give the body what it needs to produce vitamin D. Researchers saw an increase in vitamin D levels in patients who were regularly exposed to the rays of a sunbed over eight weeks. However, be wary of overexposure. A burn does not equal a "good base tan."

One interesting fact is that above natural vitamin D levels, cancer is extremely rare . . . if not altogether non-existent. On the other hand, a total deficiency of sunlight causes, among other things, toxins. Toxins allow a great environment for cancer to thrive. Therefore, the relationship between hair health and vitamin D levels is something hair experts closely monitor.

Chemotherapy

Cancer cells reproduce extremely rapidly and steadily. Unlike normal cells, they don't have limits on how long they live. This means they continue forming immature cells, which grow into abnormal masses, lesions, neoplasms, and tumors. Doctors often prescribe chemotherapy drugs to kill these rapidly reproducing, tumor-forming cells. Chemotherapy drugs are powerful medications and have many side effects. The most common and visible side effect is hair loss from the scalp and the rest of the body.

The problem is that cancer cells aren't the only quickly growing cells in the body. Other rapidly growing cells, such as hair cells, which are similar in structure to cancer cells, and chemotherapy drugs get confused and instead, kill hair follicles. Worse, these drugs don't just target hair cells; they attack the entire structure of the hair follicle. When hair cells are destroyed, the hair strands fall out—but no new hairs take their place. As more and more hairs are lost and not replaced, the patients end up with partial or total hair loss.

The good news is that once chemotherapy treatments have finished, within four to six months, hair follicles do grow back. However, not all patients are so lucky, and sometimes their scalp hairs do not come back the same quality, thickness, texture, or density.

There are many ways to prevent hair loss caused by chemotherapy. One of the most effective is LPT. Research was conducted on women who received chemotherapy to treat breast cancer. LPT devices and placebo devices were given to participants. The entire study group had to use the device for twenty-five minutes daily for twenty-four weeks. At the end of twenty-four weeks, the LPT group showed more hair growth than the placebo group, which didn't receive any treatment.

How does it work? Well, LPT rays are directed at the areas of the scalp that show hair loss. These cool rays are taken in by the scalp and hair follicles, and energy is produced during the process. The cells use the energy to repair themselves and grow back. As the cells regain their functions, they start to divide again, producing new hair cells and strands. That's how LPT helps prevent hair loss from chemotherapy, increase hair density, and promote new hair growth. It's also how it works on anyone else who experiences hair loss and wants new hair growth.

Seasonal and Other Shedding Events

Hair loss is a natural process that doesn't play favorites. Awareness of normal shedding prevents panic or that dreaded stress that comes from finding hair on your shoulders or in your hairbrush, particularly for people already struggling with hair loss. Hair goes through phases, as I've mentioned. But constant shedding without regrowth is a real problem. A quick look at pictures of yourself taken some years ago may reveal changes to your hairline.

Shedding increases during certain times of the year. Humans shed according to the season, like dogs. The body instinctively casts off unneeded hair. Unlike dogs, we shed our hair to save nutrients that might be siphoned off during the winter months, when a food shortage would most likely occur, especially in centuries past.

In the northern hemisphere, the worst time for shedding is between November and December; while in the southern hemisphere, it's between May and June. That's when dogs are hoarding their hair to keep warm. Between March and April or between September and October, we shed again. This one is lighter, and helps to rid us of the excess hair that kept us warm during winter. That's also when dogs are shedding their winter warmth hair. So, houses with dogs are a real mess.

The fluctuation of hair growth according to the season is also likely due to human hibernation practices in prehistoric times when humans survived the harsh cold by sleeping through the winter months. Bet you didn't know we once hibernated, did you? Archaeologists have found fossil remnants displaying seasonal bone-growth disruptions, which supports this theory. There was also an old Russian practice, akin to hibernation, of sleeping through the winter when food and resources were scarce.

Apart from seasonal shedding, there are many other reasons humans might shed their hair. We shed in the resting (telogen) phase of the hair cycle. Most of the time, the hair you shed is just an end to a chapter in your hair growth story. If all is well, your hair will grow back with the same intensity and speed at which it fell out. It becomes an issue, though, if something disrupts the cycle of regrowth.

Several medical issues can cause shedding as well, including fevers, thyroid problems, inflammatory bowel disease, cancer medication, and treatments such as chemotherapy. Weight-loss surgery is another reason for hair loss. Patients experience excessive hair shedding after these high-risk procedures.

More recently, there is a new rash of hair loss cases from the new class of weight loss drugs such as semagultide (a.k.a. Ozempic®) and tirzepatide (a.k.a. Wegovy®)—both have reported three times to six times more reports of alopecia compared to 1% of those who got a placebo in testing.

Humans Shed 2x a Year

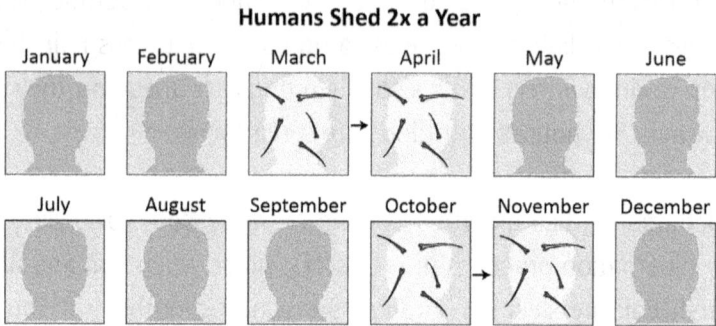

Figure 3.7. Seasonal Shedding. Humans naturally shed twice a year, with fall being the worse shedding period and spring the lighter shedding period.

In addition, the ketogenic (keto) diet can inadvertently contribute to hair loss by causing nutrient deficiencies and the stress of rapid weight loss on the body. Yet another group risking accelerated hair loss as a side effect are athletes that are using anabolic steroids, particularly if they are genetically predisposed to male or female pattern hair loss.

Humans shed hair all the time. It's a normal response to unusual circumstances. The trick is to stimulate the natural regrowth cycle and keep the hairs in the growth phase as long as possible. This way you regain your full head of hair. A balanced diet, regular exercise, and minding your mental health are all beneficial to healthy hair.

Telogen Effluvium

It can't be emphasized enough: Heat is an enemy of hair follicles. Applying too much heat to the hair follicles and the reaction of the hair follicles to that heat are examples of telogen effluvium (TE). TE can sometimes cause temporary hair loss due to increased shedding. Resting hairs, also called telogen hairs, can get pushed out by growing (anagen) hairs. Childbirth, illness, injury, surgery, psychological stress, endocrine disorders, and medication changes may cause old hairs to be shed for new ones.

TE can affect up to 50% of scalp hair—*half*—at once. Hair loss is usually noticeable two to four months after a stressful event. The primary causes of TE are usually a hormone imbalance or, as mentioned above, a scalp exposed to too much heat.

Recipients of hair transplants may also experience TE. Unfortunately, once these hairs are shed, the chances the hairs will grow back are low since the scalp technically has no hair follicles in that area. The good news is that for normal, healthy scalps, hair loss because of TE usually grows back in six to nine months. In some cases, though, the hair may not entirely return.

Dandruff and Malassezia Furfur (MF) and Their Role in Hair Loss

Everyone hates dandruff, but few people know what it really is or what causes it. This is an important point because dandruff is the main reason that we lose our hair. Most researchers think androgenetic alopecia (AA)—hair loss—is a genetic disease. But what if it's not as simple as that?

The fungus Malassezia furfur (MF) makes up over 80% of the fungi that live on human skin. It's a yeast. And it causes many common skin diseases such as psoriasis and dermatitis. One such condition is seborrheic dermatitis—the cause of dandruff. The fungus feeds on sebum, an oily substance secreted by the scalp. Dandruff results when Malassezia grows too rapidly, and the fungus's waste products interfere with the way scalp cells are normally recycled. The scalp develops sticky patches and becomes itchy and flaky.

Dandruff affects up to 50% of males and females of all races. It usually appears during our teenage years, so it may be connected to hormone levels. Certain weather conditions can worsen symptoms, especially in winter. In addition to causing itching, dandruff can make your hair and scalp look unattractive. Its impact on both self-esteem and scalp health can be severe.

In serious cases, flakes of dandruff get enmeshed in the hair. There are two types of dandruff flakes: wet and dry. The wet ones are more visible and less attractive. These trapped flakes can lead to triple the normal daily amount of hair loss! Finding solutions has been a challenge. Various studies have shown patients with dandruff can develop AA.

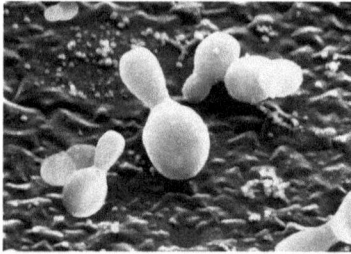

Figure 3.8. Malassezia Furfur (MF) Scanning Microscope: MF is thought to reside between the dermal/epidermal junction on the scalp and causes dandruff and eventually hair loss.

I'd like to share two independent studies that demonstrate that hair loss, MF fungus, and dandruff are closely connected. One was done in South Korea, the other in Iran, both measuring the amount of fungus on the scalps of patients. Some were suffering from hair loss; others were not. Both studies found that 100% of the hair loss patients had large amounts of MF on their scalp, whereas non-hair loss patients had very little. Given this evidence, I think we can agree that controlling MF is critical in preventing hair loss.

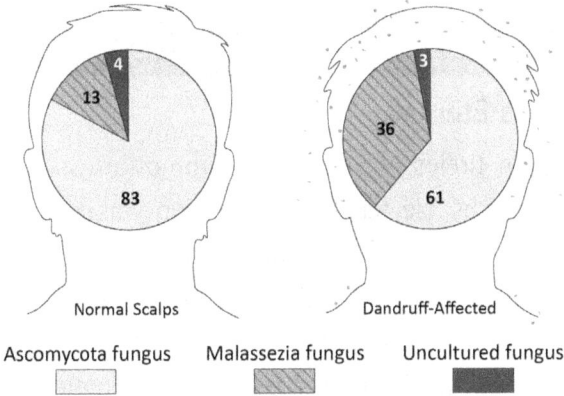

Figure 3.9. Normal Scalps vs. Dandruff-Affected Scalps. This study from Iran showed that scalps with dandruff all suffered from Androgenetic Alopecia (aka hair loss), where scalps with normal MF loads had normal hair loss and were not diagnosed with Androgenetic Alopecia.

About 50% of the world's population is allergic to MF. The same 50% has AA. No wonder Head & Shoulders'® anti-dandruff shampoo has been the best-selling shampoo worldwide since 1955! Here is clear evidence that dandruff is common in people who are losing their hair and that these same people have MF on their scalps.

I believe that MF is the root cause of AA and that an allergy to MF is a genetic trait handed down from one generation to the next. Patients who are allergic to MF suffer from hair loss, while patients who aren't allergic to MF don't. If I'm right and an allergy to dandruff (MF) causes AA, which is the leading cause of hair loss, then dandruff is the leading cause of hair loss. Unfortunately, antifungal (dandruff) shampoos such as Head & Shoulders®, only treat the symptom—not the cause. In addition, these shampoos such as Head & Shoulders® contain caustic ingredients which we will discuss in Chapter 7, that further exacerbate the thinning scalp. So, the antifungal ingredients help in minimizing scalp inflammation but the ingredients such as surfactants and preservatives cause even more damage.

Actual Customer Success Stories

Youth Springs Eternal

Brian had been tirelessly pursuing a promotion, sacrificing social outings for months. He felt that something was just not right—he knew he had been overdoing it. Though he was still in his twenties, he began to feel old. He looked in the mirror and saw his hairline receding like his father. Concerned, he consulted a physician who diagnosed him with elevated stress and a vitamin D deficiency. Recognizing the need for change, Brian committed to spending more time outdoors and reducing his stress. After reading some glowing reviews of laser therapy devices, he impulsively ordered a helmet. He soon had new hair growth along his receding hairline. Brian was so delighted that he joined a great health club, proudly showing off his full hair.

CHAPTER 4

Fungus and the Five Whys

"Fungi have a quiet and unassuming presence, yet their impact on the world is profound." — Peter McCoy, Mycologist, 2016

The Answer You've Been Searching For: Why You've Lost Your Hair

If you still have doubts, let's try looking at hair loss another way. I used to be head of research for a Japanese medical device company, Pentax (in the video gastrointestinal endoscopy division). When I was sent to Japan to study their research techniques, one of the things I learned was a method of problem-solving called "The Five Whys." A simple way to find the answer as to why something works is to answer the question "why?" at every level, five times. Most of the time, a question cannot be answered beyond the second or third why. For example, no one can answer why fire works, or why gravity happens, or anything about the universe, or how humans came to this world and so on beyond the second or third why. If someone can answer all five whys, then the ultimate answer of the secrets of our existence, and everything surrounding us, can be answered.

The Five Whys

Here, for the first time, are the answers to your burning question: "Why do people lose their hair?"

The First Why – "Why do people lose hair?" Androgenetic alopecia.

The Second Why – "Why do people get AA?" It is a genetic condition referred to as male pattern hair loss or female pattern hair loss.

The Third Why – "Why is this a genetic condition?" Unfortunately, no one has ever answered this question. I've asked dozens of physicians and hair experts, and not one of them could get past the second why.

I decided to do intensive research on the subject which led me to the conclusion above that people with excessive amounts of Malassezia furfur suffer from AA. Yet that still doesn't explain why 50% of the world's population has a genetic allergy to MF, though it does lead to solutions for AA. Studies from Iran and Korea have shown that high concentrations of MF and hair loss are highly correlated.

The Fourth Why – "Why does fungus grow on the scalp?" MF lives on all parts of the body, but it thrives in areas that have high heat and moisture. Think of someone wearing tight shoes during physical activities, such as running or playing basketball. Their feet get hot and sweaty. This often results in athlete's foot, and, non-breathing underwear can cause jock itch in men and fungal (yeast) infections in women. Women with larger breasts may suffer from fungus infections (MF) under their breasts due to the high heat and moisture from sweating. It's no surprise these fungal conditions have the same symptoms as dandruff—itchy, flaky skin—just not on the scalp.

Head hair, like tight shoes, retains heat and moisture. The head, in fact, has the highest temperature of the body; that's why we check the forehead when a child has a fever. A high temperature plus excessive moisture creates a perfect environment for MF.

Wearing a hat can raise your scalp temperature by 10° to 15° F. The higher temperature can cause fungus to grow out of control, while the heat can damage the hair. You should avoid wearing a hat all the time if you want to keep hair loss to a minimum. Hats or head coverings increase scalp temperature and can cause heat to build up. This, in turn, promotes the growth of MF fungus. Again, if you are allergic to MF, then the likelihood hair loss will occur increases.

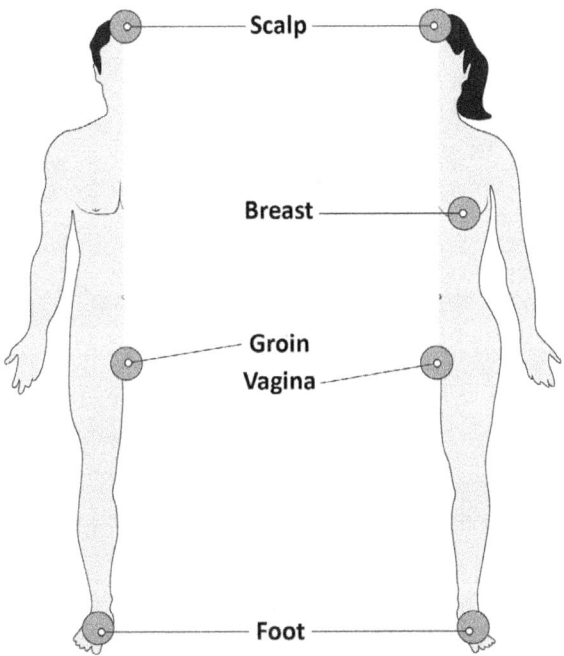

Figure 4.1. Areas on the Body That Are More Likely to Be Moist: All of these areas have the same characteristics—high heat and moisture areas. It is advisable to not wear tight shoes or tight undergarments or headgear that might encourage higher than MF loads.

During our research investigating the effects of heat and hair loss, we used a very sensitive thermal-imaging device to photograph the scalps of numerous patients. The pictures showed that patients with early to advanced cases of AA all had scalps with slightly higher temperatures.

Not all patients with higher temperature scalps had hair loss. But *all* the people genetically allergic to MF had hair loss.

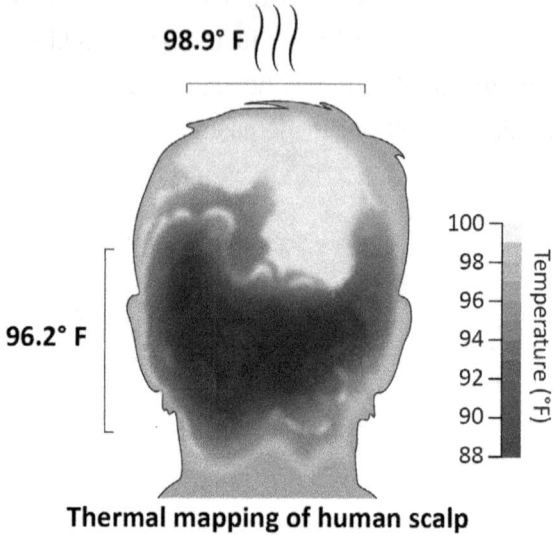

Thermal mapping of human scalp

Figure 4.2. Thermal Mapping of the Human Scalp: The human head behaves like a chimney—the majority of the heat escapes from the top of the head.

The Fifth Why – "Why does MF cause hair loss?" MF feeds on sebum, which is oil secreted by glands under the scalp. The waste created by this fungus causes inflammation between the epidermis (the outer layer of skin) and dermis (the middle layer of skin) resulting in dandruff. There are hair follicles and sebaceous glands, which secrete sebum, in the dermis. The body sends DHT, a steroid responsible for creating male characteristics in the first place, to hair follicles that have been weakened by dandruff. And then it assassinates them.

It's often asked why men have plenty of hair on the sides and in the back but not on top. MF attacks those areas highest in heat and moisture. DHT is then sent only to those areas (not to the sides or back of the head). Men's hair loss can get to the point where all the hairs on top are gone, but the sides and back still have hair. Women have less testosterone, and so have less DHT, but the effects are the same: Women lose hair from the top of the head (along the part line where part lines are dead center the top of one's head), although, unlike men, they don't lose all the hair on top. What is also interesting is that almost everyone will suffer from hair loss as they age; this is because the immune system weakens over time and fighting off fungus infections such as MF becomes more difficult to manage.

Not surprisingly, if the scalp is shaved clean, dandruff disappears because the heat and moisture MF needs to grow are no longer trapped beneath the hair in the ideal growing conditions. A good experiment would be to test a set of young (around sixteen years old or so) male identical twins with confirmed AA and have one keep their hair short, as well as use anti-dandrufff topicals and perform period hair counts. Both twins would be receiving a 1 square square centimeter-sized permanent tattoo in the same location and both twins would be measured for comparing hair counts over time. The other twin would of course, have no restrictions about hair length or type of topicals

This concept is very new, but could open up fresh research possibilities on the relationship between MF, heat, and moisture. One simple clinical trial would be to have two groups of patients: one with confirmed Andro-genetic Alopecia (at different hair loss levels, age ranges, and genders) versus another group with no hair loss. Researchers would perform allergy tests for the MF for each group. Validating that MF and hair loss are correlated would be straightforward. If the group with confirmed Androgenetic Alopecia all were allergic to MF, and the second group was found not to be allergic to MF with no hair loss, then this would be a great starting point.

If this concept holds true, then we can test people early on and if they test positive after an MF allergy test. Then, we can give them a warning and advise them to start using antifungals very aggressively. If the MF allergy test could determine the severity of the MF allergy of an individual, then it would be very useful for designing the proper clinical strategy for higher-than-normal MF allergies.

Such an approach would completely shift the way we address Androgenetic Alopecia, increasing the role of antifungals in an individual's hair loss protocol. In fact, there is a certain breed of dog (e.g., West End Terriers) that have chronic hair loss. In order to treat it, veterinarians prescribe the dogs ketoconazole baths to minimize the amount of MF (yes, the same fungus!) on their skin so they can regain their hair and have a comfortable life.

The reason why I have included a full section on topicals and vitamins is because of how important it is to control MF in one's body. To provide some guidance, I'll discuss how to reduce hair loss by using the right product to control dandruff.

After all, we want a long-term solution, and shaving one's hair is not the solution to a clean scalp. Not all of us want to walk around with a shaved head. Don't worry. We don't have to go to that extreme to have healthy hair.

Actual Customer Success Stories

Radiant Revival

Amelia was frustrated with her hair—dull, dandruff-ridden, a source of constant discomfort, and worse of all, steadily disappearing. She contemplated shaving it all off. But her dermatologist recommended a prescription strength anti-fungal shampoo, looked at her symptoms for hair loss, and suggested laser hair phototherapy. As the months passed, the transformation was astonishing. Not only did her hair fill in the bare spots, but it was glossy and beautiful as it had been when she was a child. Her scalp was clear, and the itchiness a distant memory and she could go back to wearing black clothing.

CHAPTER 5

How Much Hair Have I Lost?

"Before anything else, preparation is the key to success."
— Alexander Graham Bell, Inventor, 1898

Measuring the Level of Hair Loss

The sun is very harsh on delicate scalp skin, and sunburn can be excruciating. Hair protects one of our most sensitive areas, the head, from the damage sunlight can inflict on it. This is called the photoprotective effect. While light—sunlight included—helps us heal and thrive, hair filters how much sunlight we get so that we receive just the right amount.

All things considered, it's fair to say that hair has a value equal to the photoprotection it provides and the self-identity it allows us to express. You are not your hair, but your hair reflects who you are.

Many things damage, weaken, and destroy your hair. Washing, pulling, styling, and brushing cost us up to one hundred hairs daily. Heat exposure, radiation, and certain chemicals can also accelerate hair damage, as do ultraviolet radiation and aging. Additionally, 10% to 15% of scalp hairs aren't growing at any given time. The world's a nightmare for our hair. To stop hair loss, we've got to take responsibility for how we treat it.

There are two ways of measuring hair loss that have been developed for both men and women.

Hamilton-Norwood Scale

Mainstream medicine has had a way of assessing the amount of hair loss for decades. In the 1950s, Dr. James Hamilton developed the Hamilton-Norwood Scale to assess MPHL. It uses images of different stages of alopecia to help medical professionals gauge patients' hair loss. The Hamilton-Norwood Scale includes seven stages of MPHL.

- Stage One: Minor hairline recession, often goes unnoticed. It needs no treatment unless there's a family history of hair loss.
- Stage Two: Characterized by a triangular pattern of hair recession along the front of the head and the temple. Hair loss gradually becomes apparent at this stage.
- Stage Three: The lowest level of hair loss to qualify as "thinning." The temples are covered only with sparse hair.
- Stage Four: The hair loss pattern from stage three continues. The front of the head forms a more prominent crown.
- Stage Five: The band of hair extending toward the crown thins. There is more significant and more noticeable hair loss.
- Stage Six: The bridge of the hair across the crown is lost entirely.
- Stage Seven: Advanced hair loss. The characteristic horseshoe-shaped hair pattern develops on the scalp. In some cases, patches of hair may form a semicircle over the ears.

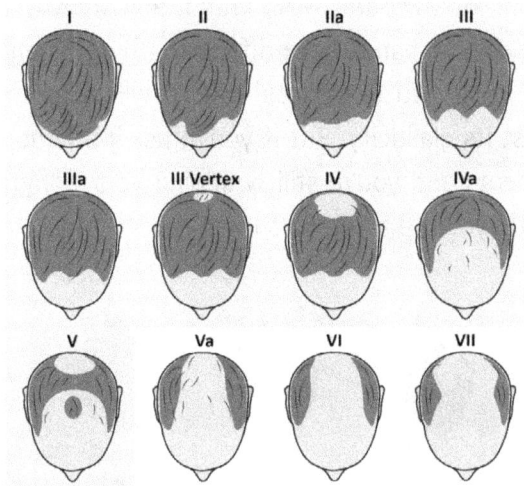

Figure 5.1. The Hamilton-Norwood Scale. Men's hair loss is reversible up to level V, but beyond this, they will require a hair transplant.

Over time, the scalp forms a new skin called the epidermal growth factor (EGF). This layer of skin contains many oil and sebaceous glands with few or no hair follicles. When too much oil and sebum are secreted, the scalp appears shiny. This happens most frequently with men, which is why you see men whose heads look slick and shiny.

The Ludwig-Savin Scale

The Ludwig-Savin Scale, or Savin Scale for short, measures hair loss in women. The Savin Scale can also assess hair thinning in addition to hair loss. This method uses stages similar to the Norwood version.

A quick way for women to estimate hair loss is by tying a ponytail. The number of rubber-band ties indicates how thick or thin the hair has become. A hair shaft is actually oval-shaped and not perfectly round. That makes the thickness of the ponytail a great way to tell whether hair density has increased or decreased. Are you wrapping the elastic more times than the last time you did this on clean, dry hair? Be sure to use an elastic of the same size, brand, and thickness and that it's new each time. Elastic bands have different strengths and they tend to stretch over time. If you use an old one, it will wrap more times just because it's lost its elasticity. But if you're using a band that meets all these requirements and you're still wrapping your ponytail more times than last month, you're having hair loss.

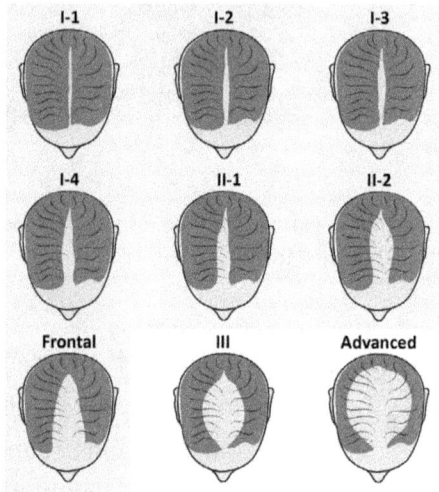

Figure 5.2. The Ludwig-Savin Scale. The pattern for women's hair loss starts at the part line and expands as shown in the images. Phase III and Advanced hair loss are the most difficult to reverse.

Clinical Methods of Measuring Hair Loss

Measuring increases in hair count, density, and thickness is vital to treating hair loss. Unfortunately, hair regrowth is difficult to measure since it's affected by many factors. Although dermatologists have different ways of diagnosing hair loss, many are based on opinion. Because measuring only starts after a person has been losing hair for long enough to notice a problem, we can't get a true starting point for the hair count, density, and thickness. That's why there's never been a comprehensive hair loss study that resulted in someone shouting, "Aha! This is the specific cause!"

Nevertheless, identifying the cause of hair loss the best we can is the key to finding the right treatment. This means taking an in-depth medical history or interviewing the patient about their life, especially as it relates to hair loss. Pull tests, tug tests, laboratory tests, and scalp biopsies are also helpful, all described briefly below. Bloodwork may also show a connection to hair loss.

There are additional ways to determine the strength of hair and diagnose hair loss. These methods include:

Pull Test	The pull test is simple and just involves gently pulling hair strands and noting the number of strands that fall out. Pulling out six or more strands out of forty indicates active hair loss.
Tug Test	This is done to determine the brittleness or fragility of hair strands. The doctor grasps a section of hair from both ends and tugs them to see whether any strands break.
Daily hair count	This requires the patient to collect shed hair for seven consecutive days. These hairs are then counted to establish daily hair loss.
60-S hair count	Hair is combed onto a sheet for sixty seconds and the shed hair is counted.
Target-area hair counts	These counts measure hair density. Hair is clipped in a circular patch one inch in diameter from one targeted area and hair is cut again from the same area in the next visit. The two samples are counted, and the numbers are compared to whether hair loss is ongoing.

Scalp Biopsy	A small section of scalp tissue is taken for analysis during a scalp biopsy. The analysis looks for damage to hair follicles, infection, or scalp inflammation, which could have harmful effects on hair growth.
Hair Weight	Hair is removed from one square centimeter of scalp. After six weeks, the hair that has grown back is clipped, washed, dried, and weighed. This test determines hair growth rate (length), diameter, and hair count.
Float Test 2-4 min (sink or float)	Hair health is tested by simply placing a hair strand in a clear glass of water. If the hair strand floats on top of the water, the hair does not hold moisture; if the hair sinks, the hair will dry quickly and is prone to breakage, frizziness, split ends, and hair loss.
Card test	This test is used to determine hair health and evaluate the number of hair strands in the growth phase. The doctor holds a small, rectangular card covered in felt against a section of the scalp, and newly growing hair is counted and examined.
Wash test 5 Days	In this test, the patient doesn't shampoo their hair for five days. Then when they wash their hair, all the hairs that fall are collected and analyzed. The severity of hair loss and the percentage of hair not in the growth phase can be determined.
Phototrichogram Density	This is the best non-invasive method to determine hair density and growth rate. It's performed on a specific area of the scalp. Hair follicles are studied thoroughly at regular intervals. A phototrichogram helps record the differences in hair growth on different scalp sites.
Global photographs	Global photography of the full head of hair is a subjective means of detecting changes in hair count, diameter, or growth rate.

Figure 5.3. Various Hair Health Tests. There is an art in measuring hair loss and many methods can be used by a hair loss professional. This is still an evolving field of study.

These testing methods help determine average hair loss. However, hair analysis can't determine whether hair loss is a result of male pattern hair loss (MPHL) or female pattern hair loss (FPHL). Only scalp analysis bloodwork provides this essential information.

Other clinical techniques for measuring hair loss include questionnaires and dermoscopy (also called a trichogram), in which a scalp camera greatly magnifies hair follicles. This can be useful to show inflammation, sebum status (the oiliness of the hair), stage of growth of hair follicles, hair shaft diameter, body hair versus head hair ratios, empty hair follicles, and conditions such as telogen effluvium (diffuse non-scarring alopecia). More invasive scalp biopsies can be used as well, but these are for cases of more serious hair loss conditions.

Although it's easy to perform hair analysis, the results are not standardized, so findings differ from one researcher or clinician to another. Measuring daily hair counts can be helpful in guessing whether hair loss is normal or due to deeper issues. Still, counting hair loss is so complex that no proper study has yet been done. Also, there is no standard method of measuring hair loss.

This is not the case with scalp analysis and thorough bloodwork, which are both consistent, validated, standardized, and objective. While scalp analysis is painful and invasive, it can accurately diagnose MPHL or FPHL. This is done by looking at the typical patterns on microscopic slides associated with hair loss. Similarly, bloodwork helps give clinicians an idea of whether hormones are involved in hair loss. Knowing this allows the disorder's underlying cause to be determined.

Actual Customer Success Stories

A Measure of Success

John had always been immersed in the rock and roll scene, and his hair was his signature look. He began to worry when he realized his once-thick ponytail was thinning, counting the increasing loops of the elastic band. The thought of leaving his band of twenty-seven years crossed his mind, as he couldn't fathom wearing a wig. On the recommendation of his sister-in-law, he mustered the courage to see a hair loss specialist. Using a scalp microscope, the expert revealed that John had lost nearly 40% of his hair. They suggested trying laser treatments. Documented through before-and-after photos, John saw significant improvement in just two months. His hair was denser and fuller. Reinvigorated, John rallied his band to shoot their debut music video.

CHAPTER 6
Hiding Hair Loss

"The hardest thing to hide is something that is not there."
— Eric Hoffer, Philosopher, 1982

Hiding Hair Loss: Exploring Strategies for Concealing Hair Loss

The issue of hair loss has led individuals to seek various methods for concealing this aesthetic concern. Wigs, extensions, weaves, hair coloring, scalp tattoos, and hair fibers have emerged as popular approaches to addressing hair loss. While these techniques offer potential solutions, it is essential to evaluate their advantages and disadvantages comprehensively. While there exists an extensive body of knowledge surrounding wigs, extensions, weaves, coloring, and scalp tattoos, hair fibers have garnered relatively less attention. Therefore, this discussion will begin with hair fibers and their potential role in concealing hair loss.

Hair Fibers

Hair fibers, comprised of positively charged keratin fibers, create a visual effect of thicker and fuller hair. Hair fibers have a similar effect as when children rub balloons on their hair and the balloons pick up static electricity when you rub them, making them temporarily stick to walls and surfaces. These fibers, typically made from wool keratin, rayon, or plant materials, are sprinkled over the hair, binding to the negatively charged hair shafts. The result is a significant increase in hair volume, making the scalp less visible and giving the appearance of denser hair coverage. This instant volumizing effect makes hair fibers an attractive option for individuals seeking a quick and temporary solution to their hair loss concerns.

Hair fibers are available in a range of colors, allowing individuals to select a shade that matches their natural hair color or closely resembles it. The application process involves sprinkling the fibers onto the thinning areas of the scalp using a specialized spray applicator. To enhance the longevity of the results, the use of a fiber holding spray is recommended in conjunction with the hair fiber treatment. It is important to note that hair fibers can be easily washed away with ordinary shampoo, and the use of conditioner should be avoided while utilizing these products.

Disadvantages of Fibers

While hair fibers offer a temporary and visually effective solution for concealing hair loss, it is important to recognize their limitations. Their effectiveness is dependent upon individual hair type, texture, and the extent of hair loss. Additionally, the temporary nature of hair fibers necessitates regular reapplication. They are made of a fine powder that tends to cover bathroom sinks and floors and find its way into every crack. Finally, the dyes or other chemicals used in hair fibers—FD&C, parabens, alcohols, fragrances—can cause skin allergies. Wearing a face mask would be highly advisable when applying hair fibers.

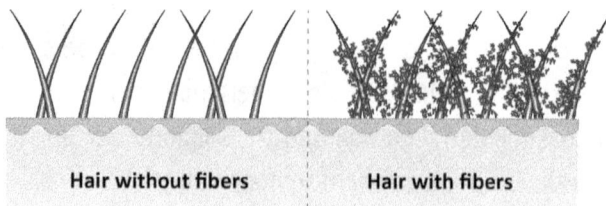

Hair without fibers   Hair with fibers

Figure 6.1. Hair Fibers. Hair is negatively charged. Sprinkling positively charged hair fibers on existing hair results in the appearance of a fuller hair head of hair.

Heavy winds and strong rains can wash away hair fibers, so hair spray is always recommended after applying hair fibers. Nevertheless, promising advancements in the form of newer, relatively water-resistant products are emerging, mitigating some of the issues associated with traditional hair fibers.

Additional limitations include their diminished effectiveness as hair loss advances, as they require existing hair strands to effectively bind to make them a temporary rather than long-term solution to cover hair loss.

Fibers in Conjunction with Other Treatments

Hair fibers can also be utilized in combination with other medical therapies for hair loss. Individuals with mild cases of AA have found hair fibers to be effective camouflage in concealing their hair loss. Moreover, when used in conjunction with Minoxidil (a popular medication for hair growth), the Minoxidil should be applied first, allowing the scalp to try before the hair fibers are sprinkled onto the treated areas. On the following days, the hair should be shampooed before reapplying both treatments.

Hair fiber can be used as soon as two weeks after undergoing a hair transplant procedure. This integration assists in concealing the effects of telogen effluvium, a temporary condition characterized by hair loss that often follows hair transplant surgery. However, for optimal results, it is advisable to employ a combination of low-level laser phototherapy (LPT) and hair fibers. As time progresses, the reliance on hair fibers is likely to diminish as LPT tends to facilitate the regeneration of new hair, thereby filling in the sparser areas.

Wigs, Extensions, and Weaves and LPT

Extensions and weaves are extremely popular with women (not so much with men) and are used to make the hair look fuller—but at a cost.

Disadvantages of Wigs, Extensions, and Weaves

Hair extensions, especially those that are attached using tight braiding or weaving techniques, can contribute to traction alopecia. The additional weight of the extensions, combined with the constant pulling and tension on the hair follicles, specifically the tiny muscle we covered in Chapter 3, the arrector pili, will be damaged and lead to hair loss over time. With repeated use of hair extensions, the hair follicles can become permanently damaged, resulting in permanent hair loss. To prevent traction alopecia from hair extensions, use extensions in moderation and choose attachment methods that are not too tight and do not cause discomfort or pain. Additionally, taking breaks between extensions can give the hair and scalp a chance to rest and recover from any potential damage.

Wigs, Extension, and Weaves in Conjunction with Other Treatments

The solution for preventing damage to the arrector pili and preventing traction alopecia is to minimize the use of weaves and extensions. Traction alopecia is very common in Black and African people. However, it is important to note that anyone can develop traction alopecia if they repeatedly use hair styling methods that put tension on the hair follicles, regardless of ethnicity or race. It is advisable to use them in moderation and opt for attachment methods that do not exert excessive tightness, discomfort, or pain. Incorporate breaks between extension applications to provide the hair and scalp an opportunity to rest and recover from potential damage. Most importantly of all, safeguard the health of the arrector pili muscles and prevent traction alopecia by utilizing laser phototherapy (LPT) to strengthen their hair follicles.

It is worth mentioning that LPT may have limited effect in treating traction alopecia if force and tension continue to be exerted on the hair follicles. LPT primarily targets active hair follicles, emphasizing the need to reduce the usage of weaves, extensions, and other practices that impose undue pressure on the follicles. It is essential to recognize that LPT has its limitations in addressing traction alopecia.

Scalp Tattoos and LPT

A scalp tattoo procedure, also known as scalp micropigmentation, is a non-invasive cosmetic treatment that involves using specialized techniques to deposit tiny ink dots onto the scalp. The procedure is typically performed by a skilled technician who uses a hand-held device to apply the ink, creating the appearance of hair follicles.

The procedure is often used to create the illusion of a full head of hair, even if the natural hairline has receded or is thinning. Unlike traditional tattooing, which penetrates deeper into the skin, scalp tattooing is more superficial and therefore less painful.

During the procedure, the technician will first create a customized design based on the client's natural hair color and skin tone. Then, using a series of small needles, the ink is gently deposited onto the scalp, mimicking the look of hair follicles.

While scalp tattooing and laser hair phototherapy are not even closely related, using LPT after a scalp tattoo can maintain any existing hair and reduce any need for further areas to be tattooed. The longer effects of getting a scalp tattoo have not been conducted on participants as they aged. Scalp tattoos are permanent so no one will know what this would look like in ten, twenty, or thirty years on their scalp. Many people have regretted their tattoos; what's more, unlike art tattoos, removing hundreds of tiny dots might be more difficult. Most scalp tattoo customers are younger and it would be interesting to see how these tattoos fare in older customers. These tattoos might work as a temporary hair loss coverup procedure, but I would recommend foregoing permanent ink and suggest using temporary inks like Henna.

In general, there are no conflicts in using LPT and scalp tattoos but I would not suggest getting them unless you are trying to hide HT scars or similar conditions. The only caution is that higher-powered LPT products (especially super-pulsed lasers) for pain or wound (not for hair LPT) management applications might generate heat and cause the ink to discolor over time. However, using an LPT hair device should not cause any issues as a well-designed LPT hair device does not generate excess heat. This gives you even more reason to select the right type of LPT device.

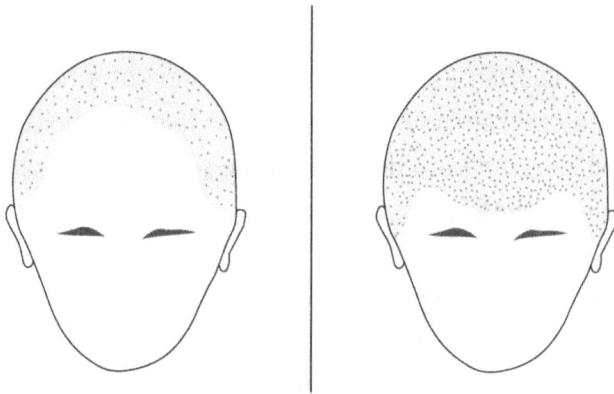

Figure 6.2. A Scalp Tattoo: The subject on the left has a classic advanced Androgenetic Alopecia pattern. After performing a scalp tattoo procedure with thousands of black ink-based tattoo dots to resemble, the hair line now appears like a shaven hairstyle.

After the procedure, clients may experience some minor discomfort or redness, but these symptoms usually subside within a few days. The final results of the scalp tattoo can last for several years, and clients may need occasional touch-ups to maintain the desired look.

One great application is to use scalp tattooing or micropigmentation to effectively camouflage hair transplant scars (e.g., FUT). The area most affected by FUT HT scars is the back of the head—scalp tattooing or micropigmentation would cover up the scars and provide an improved appearance. Overall, a scalp tattoo procedure is a safe and effective way to achieve the appearance of a fuller head of hair, without the need for surgery or other invasive treatments.

Concealing Agents

Like fibers, concealing agents come in various colors and forms (powder, cake, lotion, and spray). Powder and cake can be applied over dried, thinning hair with a wet sponge. These bind to the scalp as well as hairs. By reducing the contrast between the scalp and the hair it gives the illusion of thicker and fuller hair. These are ideal for thinning areas.

Camouflage spray is applied to hair and allowed to set for sixty seconds before the setting spray, which is basically hair spray, is applied. Although it's easy to put on, taking off camouflage spray can be tricky because it is water-resistant and sticky.

Hair crayons, which can be rubbed onto the thinning scalp, are also available. They're easier to apply and easier to wash off. More and more, these are being used by women with chronic telogen effluvium to cover visible scalp. However, they're not such a good idea when hair loss is advanced.

Some people use hair coloring to cleverly mask hair loss problems by making the hair look denser and fuller, helping to create the illusion of thicker hair. The issue is that harsh chemicals are used to open and help close the outer layer of the hair (the cuticle) to ensure the right color of hair is applied.

Well, the truth is LPT can close hair cuticles much better than chemicals, making the hairs last longer. In fact, there's nothing these methods offer that comes close to LPT. This new application for LPT, closing cuticles, is new and could help the hair coloring industry to achieve hair coloring that lasts much longer.

Of course, all these solutions just cover up hair loss and do nothing for continued hair loss. If you'd rather enjoy your own natural hair, LPT is the best alternative.

Actual Customer Success Stories

Hats Off

It never even occurred to Jose that his hair loss could be stopped. He thought it was a natural part of getting older, and that made him feel even worse about it. One day, a friend remarked on the sheer number of caps scattered throughout his apartment—over 200 in total. That's when it hit Jose: His affinity for hats wasn't about team loyalty or fashion; it was a shield against his insecurities. By chance, a YouTube ad introduced him to a laser helmet designed to combat hair loss. Finally, a piece of headgear that actually solved his problem. Within a few months, he felt much more comfortable crowned by nothing but his own hair, and he could give the hat collection to Goodwill.

CHAPTER 7

Over the Counter Hair Treatments

"Avoid a remedy that is worse than the disease" — Aesop, *Slave and Storyteller, circa 600 BCE*

Over the Counter

Hair follicles are living cells. Their activities lead to the growth or loss of hair. This means that follicle cells must be treated with the right ingredients if they're going to grow. All cells are sensitive to the compounds they take in, meaning there's a therapeutic window (a minimum beneficial dosage and a maximum tolerance).

Some of the snake-oil remedies out there are so concentrated they overwhelm or burn the cells. They can even include acids. When such industrial-strength compounds are applied to the hair follicles, they make the problem worse. They may even kill hair follicles and injure the scalp. Imagine rubbing acid on your struggling follicle cells and thinking it will help! Even if it helps a little, it can cause early graying or increased shedding because instead of being strengthened the follicles have been pushed to their limit.

If you're reading this book, you've probably already tried or are trying a hair loss product besides an LPT. In that case, I hope you're still OK! I'm writing this book to educate, but also to help you protect your money and health by persuading you never to buy those useless products again.

Shampoos

Shampoo is one of the most popular cosmetic products in the world. You probably have several bottles in your bathroom right now. The shampoo products we use today have been with us since 1927 and can be found in almost every household. Humans have, however, used hair-cleaning products for centuries. That's why shampoos make up the world's largest category of haircare cosmetics.

So how does shampoo work, and why does it make our hair look nice? Most people have no clue. I'm going to break down the science of shampoo so you can understand exactly what's happening to your follicles every time you wash your hair. More importantly, however, I'll tell you which shampoos are best for hair loss and hair growth.

Science of Shampoo

To start with, the science of shampoo hasn't changed in many years, and one of the things we can say with certainty is that very few shampoo ingredients are absorbed by the scalp. And if there's no scalp penetration, these ingredients usually can't help with hair loss.

The water in shampoo is absorbed by the scalp but, of course, has no effect on hair growth. Alcohol and menthol are also absorbed, but these ingredients cause dryness of the scalp and hair. They may also cause scalp irritation or tingling, but they don't put a stop to hair loss or help you grow new hair.

Many "hair growth" shampoos contain very expensive ingredients that, unfortunately, aren't taken in by the scalp and simply go down the drain.

This is good for the manufacturer (because you'll buy more product hoping more will help), but frustrating for you.

You will often see the term "antifungal" on a bottle of shampoo, but this is a bit of a misnomer since humans share from 30% to 50% of the same DNA as fungi (depending on specific species as fungi), and whatever we use to kill a fungus is often dangerous to humans as well. There's another issue, though. Shampoo only reaches the dead parts of the hair, not the important parts (the bulge and papilla). It can't wipe out a fungal infection completely because each time you shampoo the fungus retreats under the scalp. Then, two to three days later, the fungus reappears in the form of dandruff.

This means we can only control fungus rather than eradicate it. Once fungus takes hold in an area, even controlling it is very difficult. Remember, fungi love heat and moisture. So, if you keep your hair long, you'll be creating the perfect habitat for fungi. To control the fungus population on your scalp, you either have to use an antifungal shampoo often and keep the scalp dry, or you must cut your hair short since fungi don't do well with short hairstyles.

We need shampoos, of course, because our hair absorbs dirt and dust from the environment. Also, there are often remnants of other products in our hair, (hairspray, gel, mousse, etc.) and since some of them don't dissolve in water, they don't come out with water alone. Shampoo helps remove these sticky particles. After shampooing, our hair looks clean, shiny, and, often, healthier as well.

The secret to the cleaning power of shampoos is the surfactant. A surfactant dissolves the bonds that make oils and dirt cling to your hair and scalp. Ten to twenty percent of any given shampoo is composed of surfactants. The dirt is washed away into the water during shampooing, and any remaining shampoo can simply be rinsed off. After shampooing, the scalp is clean and oil-free. Hair hygiene is maintained, and itching, reddening, and unpleasant scalp odors are prevented. The use of shampoos also reduces the amount of dandruff in the hair.

Shampoo and Hair Regrowth

Telling you the story of shampoo's composition, use, and effects is helpful for what comes next. Yes, shampoo helps keep your scalp and hair healthy and makes your hair look nice, but nothing we've seen so far suggests that shampoo can help regrow hair. Nor is there any mention of an effect on the hair follicles themselves, which are deeply involved in hair growth phases.

During clinical trials for an LPT device all variables needed to be aligned for all participants to secure impartial results. The group conducting the trail opted in for a very popular All-American baby shampoo. Most hair trichologists recognize this baby shampoo as containing caustic surfactants which are toxic to the scalp. However, clinical blind trials are not conducted by trichologists or LPT specialists as it might taint the results. Trials are conducted by objective third parties to ensure unbiased results. The baby shampoo used is always touted as a clean and gentle shampoo, but reports from over 50% of the participants complained of itching, inflammation, flaking, and dry scalp. They were forced to stop using the baby shampoo, and the trial was rendered unusable for understanding the effectiveness of LPT devices.

To stimulate hair regrowth, a shampoo must act on the follicles. Just as a car wash only cleans the outside of a vehicle, the vast majority of shampoos only affect the exterior hair. Oil leaks, however, come from the engine. Similarly, shampoo may give hair a spectacular appearance, but hair loss is a deep-scalp condition. It is in the follicles.

You might be rolling your eyes and thinking, "Of course, shampoo doesn't regrow my hair." But if you look at the hair product market, you'll see that hundreds of shampoos claim to be a remedy for hair loss. Many promise incredible hair growth after just a few weeks of regular use! Despite the lack of evidence to back up these claims, these products have become extremely popular. The truth is that most shampoos making claims like these do more harm than good.

What you need to know is that the only shampoos with any clinical evidence at all to back up the potential of hair regrowth are the ones that contain ketoconazole, piroctone olamine, or zinc pyrithione. The others base their "success" on individual reports—usually unverified stories from anonymous people on social media or from friends who claim they're effective.

As we all know, when it comes to our health, it's not a good idea to rely on verbal reports. A product or substance must give consistent results in different settings to verify the results are not coincidental. For example, you might think your shampoo is helping you in your struggle against hair loss without realizing you've just finished your normal, seasonal shedding, and that's why you've stopped losing hair.

The truth is there are millions of shampoos on the global marketplace today, and most of them can damage the scalp and hair because they contain caustic ingredients. In fact, over 50% of the world's population is allergic to these harsh ingredients, which leave the scalp inflamed and in distress.

The good news is that there are some new topical products that are being introduced. Don't throw out those bottles just yet though—check your labels and we will show you how to look for the good ones! As I said earlier, shampoos can improve hair and scalp health. They keep your hair looking good and get the scalp ready for hair loss treatments that do work. In addition, medicated shampoos often include conditioners. These conditioners may improve scalp circulation. Although better scalp circulation doesn't necessarily mean hair growth, it's not a disadvantage when it comes to hair health.

One of the rare studies conducted on shampoos reported that the use of shampoos that contained antioxidants and anti-inflammatory agents improved hair growth. But was it the shampoo or the antioxidants or the anti-inflammatories or all three working together? We don't know because the study was done on only forty-five people. Studies like this are too small to allow us to make accurate generalizations.

Medicated Shampoos

Medicated shampoos treat dandruff as well as certain scalp diseases. Remember Malassezia furfur (MF), the fungus that plays such a key role in causing dandruff and hair loss? Well, here's the good news: Studies have shown that antifungal shampoos reduce MF (and other fungi), making an antifungal shampoo the best type of shampoo for treating hair loss.

Salicylic Acid

Salicylic acid is a naturally occurring molecule derived from the bark of willow trees and has been technically used for all types of ailments for over 1,500 years. The more common name today for salicylic acid is Aspirin. Though Aspirin today is synthetically produced, it has all of the attributes of salicylic acid. This powerful ingredient is excellent at reducing topical inflammation issues with the scalp. Many shampoos contain salicylic acid to primarily remove thick, scaly skin and scalp cells that have been damaged.

Sulfur

This is one of the most abundant ingredients that acts as an antifungal and has been added to shampoos since the mid-1900s. Its main job is to kill fungi. One of the negative aspects of sulfur is that it smells of rotten eggs, which is usually masked with fragrances. Sulfur is not to be confused with sulfates, which are covered later in this chapter. Sulfur is an element and sulfates are derivatives of sulfur. Sulfur has no side effects when used topically. Shampoos that use a combination of sulfur and salicylic acid are more effective than those that only use one or the other.

Selenium sulfide

Other medicated shampoos contain selenium sulfide, another fungus killer. Selenium sulfide also slows the growth of scalp cells and keeps the surface of the scalp healthy. Available over the counter, it's a very effective treatment for dandruff. So far, the only major side effect it causes is an oily scalp.

Steroids

Steroids sometimes also make it to the list of ingredients on the shampoo bottle. While they don't kill fungi, they do ease scalp inflammation. Using steroids in shampoos, however, is really overkill since steroid ingredients are expensive. Moreover, if you're going to use them, you're better off using a tube of steroids to treat your scalp. The best option of all is to skip the steroids and use LPT for inflammation of the scalp.

Coal tar

Coal tar shampoos work by shrinking groups of yeast. Yet, coal tar is problematic. For one thing, it's hard to find. For another, the smell is . . . well, it stinks! Coal tar is also unnecessarily controversial. As its name suggests, it's a byproduct of the coal industry, and that seems to have led to rumors that it can increase cancer risks even though it has been used for thousands of years and is one of the oldest treatments for dandruff. There's no evidence linking coal tar to cancer. This is an internet scare tactic to keep people from using coal tar shampoo. Unfortunately, these bogus cancer claims have prompted many countries to outlaw coal tar, which is frustrating since it's great for treating fungal infections, psoriasis, and many other causes of scalp inflammation. It's also interesting to note that another product made from coal tar is saccharin—yes, the sweetener! In the 1970s, researchers claimed that rats fed enormous quantities of saccharin developed bladder cancer, but they later discovered that this only happened to rats!

Tea Tree Oil and Honey

Some substances, such as tea tree oil and honey, can be used in their natural form to treat dandruff. Tea tree oil, which has fungus-killing properties, shows almost no side effects and can be used daily. Unfortunately, both are very weak antifungal treatments, so if you have a mild case of dandruff, these might work, but they're not a good idea if you have a moderate to severe case of dandruff.

Minoxidil

Some shampoo manufacturers include Minoxidil as their primary ingredient in their shampoo formulation and I can safely say that this is a terrible idea and concept. As you may know, Minoxidil is not cheap, and when someone washes their hair, the majority of the ingredients go down the drain. The amount of time the Minoxidil is on the scalp is so short that it is not worth the hassle or the extra cost. Minoxidil has been successful for hair loss for the past forty years but it should only be used as a leave-on product, not as a shampoo.

Zinc Pyrithione

If you're a fungus, another ingredient you don't want to meet is zinc pyrithione. Zinc pyrithione kills yeast, such as MF, and helps keep the surface of the scalp healthy. Shampoos made with either of these are very effective in controlling dandruff. Zinc pyrithione, however, has at least two drawbacks. One is that it can thin out the hair shaft. The other is that it makes the scalp produce too much sebum, making your hair look oily.

Ketoconazole

Ketoconazole, which kills yeast by punching holes in its cell walls, was originally used to treat dandruff and other scalp disorders. It also decreases the scalp irritation fungal infections cause, and that's important where male or female pattern hair loss is present. But there's more to this lethal adversary of yeast. In a small research study, six men were given ketoconazole lotion to treat hair loss. Three of them showed an increase in hair growth, which seems to indicate that ketoconazole is about 50% effective for males with pattern hair loss. A much larger study was done in 2000. A hundred men participated in the study, which was a double-blind. The men who volunteered for the study had dandruff that was somewhere between mild and moderate (their scalps were also somewhat oily). They were given a shampoo that contained either 1% ketoconazole or 1% zinc pyrithione and used it two or three times each week for six months.

Piroctone Olamine

As impressive as ketoconazole is, piroctone olamine is my favorite fungus killer. In addition to fighting dandruff by killing MF, which helps prevent hair loss, piroctone olamine cuts down on shedding. It also promotes hair growth and, like ketoconazole, increases the thickness of individual hairs. Basically, piroctone olamine does everything ketoconazole does but it performs better in two key categories: boosting hair shaft diameter and reducing shedding (see chart below). Finally, unlike many other shampoo additives, piroctone olamine is considered safe.

Comparing the Top Three Medicated Antifungals

We have taken the top three antifungals from above and compared piroctone olamine, ketoconazole, and zinc pyrithione to each other as related to hair loss, hair shaft diameter, and sebum production. All three have a positive effect on multiple aspects of hair growth. They have a similar effect on itch and dandruff. Piroctone olamine generally scores better when it comes to hair growth.

Thus, the study shows that there is a preference for the use of 1% piroctone olamine to achieve the greatest possible effect on hair growth.

Results Piroctone Olamine

Piroctone olamine, despite the recent upsurge in usage, has historically not been a hugely popular ingredient. It has been used in Europe and other Asian countries but the FDA has allowed it to be used at 1% without any issues.

Piroctone olamine is an excellent ingredient for combating dandruff due to its antifungal properties. Like other antifungals, it works by preventing the growth of the fungus Malassezia furfur. A recent trial compared 1% of piroctone olamine to ketoconazole at 2%, which makes piroctone olamine a much-desired product to combat MF. The table clearly shows that PO is a much better alternative than any other antifungal ingredient.

While no single ingredient like piroctone olamine alone may be a cure for hair loss, it can be a beneficial addition to an LPT regimen as it will assist the LPT device to work as intended.

By regulating the growth of this fungus, piroctone olamine can help reduce flakiness, itching, and inflammation of the scalp associated with dandruff. Additionally, removing sulfates, phthalates, parabens, and other caustic ingredients, a topical shampoo with PO will make a great addition to one's hair journey. It stimulates hair growth by decreasing hair loss, increasing the number of hairs in the growth phase, and increasing hair diameter.

Piroctone Olamine	Ketoconazole	Zinc Pyrithione
16.5% of hair loss was reduced among people who used piroctone olamine.	Ketoconazole reduced hair loss by 17.3%.	Zinc pyrithione managed to lessen hair loss by 10.1%.
People who used piroctone olamine saw a 7.7% improvement in their hair shaft diameter.	Hair shaft diameter increased by 5.4% among people who used ketoconazole.	Zinc pyrithione decreased hair diameter by 2.2%.
Piroctone olamine decreases sebum production in the scalp.	Sebum-oil volume falls after treatment with ketoconazole.	Zinc pyrithione does not affect sebum output in the scalp.

Table 7.1. A Comparison of Piroctone Olamine, Ketoconazole, and Zinc Pyrithione. Piroctone Olamine has been shown to be a great hair growth promoting ingredient.

Results Ketoconazole

The news for men suffering from hair loss was good, particularly for those who used ketoconazole (1%). They saw their hair get thicker, that is, the diameter of the hair shaft increased over those six months. Also, sebum production fell with ketoconazole shampoo. Ketoconazole cut down the number of hairs shed in a full day (twenty-four hours) and increased the percentage of hairs in the growth phase by 6.4%.

A study was also done on a shampoo containing 2% ketoconazole, which requires a prescription, and once again hair shaft diameter increased slightly. The results were comparable to the control group in a study in which participants used Minoxidil (2%) and a non-medicated shampoo.

Another experiment showed that, by preventing the growth of fungus, ketoconazole also prevented hair damage. This, in turn, helped prevent hair loss. But there's still another way ketoconazole fights hair loss. Recent studies show that ketoconazole also promotes hormone-free hair growth.

Another study was done by McNeil Pharmaceuticals, makers of Johnson & Johnson Nizoral® shampoo, which contains up to 2% ketoconazole. Most of the participants who used Nizoral® saw more stable sebum production, less shedding, and additional benefits the study wasn't looking for.

It is important to note that oral ketoconazole, which is a systemic anti-fungal treatment, has been associated with liver toxicity and has a higher potential to cause liver-related side effects. However, when one compares the risk of liver side effects from ketoconazole shampoo at a 1% concentration, it is extremely low due to its limited systemic absorption.

The problem with Nizoral® as a hair loss solution is that it contains sulfates, SLS, phthalates, dyes, and fragrances in such quantities that it had some benefits for the fungus, but was not very pleasant for patients who were sensitive to these caustic ingredients. We'll talk more about these ingredients below.

Results Pyrithione

Unfortunately, the diameter of the hair shaft shrank (by 2.28%) for men who used a zinc-pyrithione shampoo and bumped up sebum production by 8.2%. The zinc pyrithione reduced shedding, too, but only by 6.02%. Yet, the zinc pyrithione did a little better than the ketoconazole when it came to increasing the percentage of hairs in the growth phase. It saw an increase of 8.4%.

Even though pyrithione zinc is the least effective of the three we have compared in the table, it is likely to remain a valuable ingredient in the fight against scalp conditions and hair loss. This ingredient will remain the workhorse of Head & Shoulders unless restrictions or limitations on the use of pyrithione zinc in some countries prevent the use of this ingredient.

You should be aware that when you use a medicated shampoo the effects of any of the antifungals mentioned in the previous section will control the proliferation of Malassezia furfur for up to three or four days maximum and then the growth of MF will return. We don't encourage daily shampooing as this is excessive but you should monitor your scalp for dandruff and dry scalp. This is an indication that MF has returned.

MF will resurface and cause more havoc and inflammation between hair washing with antifungal products. It will take approximately forty days before pyrithione zinc has a noticeable effect in controlling MF. It takes that long for the antifungal ingredients to affect the MF population on your scalp, specifically, the MF lodged between the epidermis (the outer layer of skin) and the dermis, which is underneath it. MF will never be completely gone or killed. Contemporary anti-dandruff and antifungal shampoos contain stronger ingredients than previous versions and the costs of these new solutions are more expensive, but the results have been very encouraging for attaining a healthy scalp.

LPT devices are limited in controlling the effects of Malassezia furfur (MF), but using shampoos or scalp creams that contain piroctone olamine, ketoconazole, zinc pyrithione, sulfur, or coal tar will help control this yeast more effectively. These compounds reduce Malassezia populations, but again, none of these completely eliminate them outright, which means that if antifungal treatment is stopped, Malassezia return.

If you are a hair transplant patient, you should start a regular course of shampoos that contain one of these key ingredients but do *not* contain SLS, sulfates, phthalates, dyes, fragrances, or silicone. Remember that our theory is that the reason humans lose their hair is due to allergic reactions to MF and one must continue using medicated topicals for their scalp after an HT; in addition, those types of shampoos/conditioners must not have any caustic ingredients.

The less fungus there is on the scalp, the less scalp inflammation you'll experience. This will also make an LPT device more effective since reducing scalp inflammation will open up more hair growth opportunities.

Along with the apparent benefits of antifungal shampoos come a few minor side effects, including scalp irritation, dry hair and scalp, oiliness, discoloration, and changes in hair texture. Despite these undesirable reactions, antifungal shampoos are considered one of the best ways to treat hair loss.

Harmful Surfactants in Shampoos

Surfactants are necessary to make shampoo lather. They're the compounds that dissolve the oil in hair to make the hair clean and healthy. The use of surfactants, however, can lead to side effects. Surfactants are associated with skin dryness and irritation. People with these symptoms should look over the ingredients in their shampoo and avoid harsh surfactants. Hair loss is bad enough but adding more issues like caustic ingredients from topicals only makes things worse.

Sodium Lauryl Sulfate (SLS) in Shampoos

The surfactant some shampoos contain is sodium lauryl sulfate (SLS). Reports show that SLS used in very small amounts is safe, but SLS has been linked to an increased risk of developing several health conditions.

Many people don't know they need to wash SLS shampoos out of their hair immediately after use, so they may leave the shampoo in. This can harm their scalp and hair. Also, when SLS stays on hair for an extended time, there's an increased risk of skin irritation.

Propylene Glycol

This ingredient helps to mix water and oils so they can bind together (in other words, it is an emulsifier) and is used in over 90% of shampoos. This can cause an allergic reaction to the scalp, causing inflammation and dermatitis. Propylene glycol (PEG) is also used as an antifreeze for automobile engines, and in clinical studies, it is used to induce inflammation in test mice. All of which should tell you that this cannot be a good thing to put on your head!

Phthalates

Phthalates are another common additive in shampoos and conditioners. They do several things. Primarily, they help soften other shampoo ingredients and make them more spreadable. They also help fragrances last longer. Unfortunately, phthalates have been connected to numerous health issues including breast cancer, asthma, obesity, attention-deficit hyperactivity disorder, type 2 diabetes, allergies, hormonal problems in men and women, and even low IQ. Now, to be clear, there are numerous chemicals classified as phthalates, and although phthalates are connected to numerous health issues, we know that most of the population is using shampoos without these severe side effects. That is because many phthalates have not been studied for adverse effects on humans, and many are not found in shampoo.

Phthalates are also used in vinyl flooring, lubricating oils, children's toys, cosmetics, cleaners designed for home use, and even food. Yet, to be safe, it's best to avoid them when you can, and this means phthalate-free shampoos and conditioners.

Preservatives in Shampoos

Shampoo manufacturers use preservatives to prevent the growth of bacteria. A group of preservatives called parabens has been linked to an increase in the occurrence of breast cancer. Parabens imitate the action of estrogen and increase the growth of breast cancer cells. Another preservative in shampoos is formaldehyde, which has also been linked to an increased risk of cancer. Other preservatives in shampoos may cause allergic reactions after prolonged use.

Summing up Shampoos

Using certain shampoos can be devastating for people with allergies to caustic ingredients. The ingredients in shampoos are what separate the beneficial from the harmful. Shampoos are beneficial if they perform their primary task: cleaning the hair and scalp without causing harm. Side effects range from skin allergies to irritation, dryness, and increased risk of cancers. As for shampoos that claim to grow hair back, they should be approached with extreme caution. Only the ones that contain keto-conazole, piroctone olamine, or zinc pyrithione have any such potential at all and the positive results that have been seen so far have been limited and require more study. So, we recommend a shampoo with none of those sulfates/sulfides, phthalates, parabens, propylene glycol, or other caustic ingredients. A safe shampoo with one of the three antifungals would be the ideal product to use on your scalp.

The most problematic issue is that LPT devices in conjunction with bad shampoos will not work as effectively as intended because the scalp will be inflamed. Thus, the LPT device will have to work harder to stabilize the scalp. This will prevent progress for any hair loss or hair growth regimen while using LPT.

If a good shampoo is used, then the LPT device will be solely focused on hair regrowth and reducing hair loss.

Shampoos and Laser Phototherapy

Based on research, I would strongly recommend a medicated shampoo when using an LPT device. Just be careful not to use a low-quality shampoo with caustic ingredients that might cause inflammation. The LPT would have to work that much harder! Generally speaking, medicated shampoos support an LPT device in working more effectively. In fact, researchers at my company did a clinical study in which seventy-eight participants used a proprietary shampoo along with our LPT device. The shampoo had no SLS, sulfates, phthalates, dyes, parabens, silicones, or fake fragrances, and it contained piroctone olamine. The trial was an amazing success. All seventy-eight subjects concluded that using the device and the shampoo stopped their hair loss and resulted in the regrowth of hair in less than six months.

Shampoo and LPT were made for different things and, as you might expect, work differently. Laser phototherapy reaches down to the hair follicles and has been proven by countless studies to stimulate hair growth. No treatment is more effective against hair loss or grows hair back better than LPT. However, shampooing before an LPT session ensures that scalp gunk and build-up don't interfere with the laser. Also, a shampoo that contains piroctone olamine, ketoconazole, or zinc pyrithione, when used in combination with LPT, might produce still better results. Just don't expect a shampoo on its own to do the impossible.

Conditioners

After shampooing, many people apply conditioner. Shampoo removes the dirt, while conditioner helps improve the look of hair by making it softer and shinier. Some hair can be difficult to manage, especially curly hair, due to differences in hair texture and quality. A conditioner may help to maintain hair and "mold" it into the shape or style you want.

Why do we need conditioners at all? Primarily because of the shampoos we use. Hair has natural oils, but shampoos can strip these away. Also, the chemicals in shampoos can be tough on hair follicles, leaving hair dull, dry, and difficult to style. This makes using a conditioner after shampooing a necessity. It's worth noting that shampoos work on the scalp, while conditioners act on the hair itself.

Hair conditioners usually contain oils and fatty alcohols. These compounds are responsible for making hair more flexible and softer. In some cases, conditioners have additives that can temporarily close up split ends. Some conditioner manufacturers even add agents to "thicken" hair and create the feeling that it is fuller, but this is only an impression. There's nothing permanent or long-term about this effect. It's just a brief reaction to the chemicals in the conditioner.

In some cases, conditioners make brushing easier, which is helpful for people with tough hair. As marketers often say, conditioners give you the "silkiest" feel and appearance. This happens because the negative charge of hair is neutralized by the positive charge of the conditioners. These reactions reduce hair clumping, making it easier to comb and leaving a smooth appearance.

So far, conditioners sound great. The purpose of describing how conditioners work isn't to give them cheap advertising, though. Again, notice how nothing in their design addresses hair growth. Conditioners act on the scalp and the hair, that's true, but they have no effect on stimulating hair growth. The only function of conditioners is to improve hair appearance, make styling and combing easier, and improve texture. Any hair growth claims are hype from people who say their hair looks and feels better.

Many men and women can attest to the role conditioners play in improving the look and feel of their hair. Yet hair appearance isn't hair growth. While certain conditioners make hair appear fuller by binding split ends, it's an effect that lasts only a few hours. A split end, after all, is an actual separation of the tip of your hair, and a conditioner can't "glue" the breakage back together. The ends must be trimmed to be remedied. Also, remember that hair above the scalp is essentially dead, so there are no magic repairs going on at the tips. Nor is there any increase in the hair growth phase or any reduction in how long the resting phase lasts.

I should also point out that men use conditioners less often than women and that women use more conditioner than shampoo. I would strongly encourage both men and women to use shampoo as well as conditioner. Also, leave them on the scalp for at least five to ten minutes, especially a medicated shampoo or a medicated conditioner. Using medicated conditioners makes a big difference! Again, as with shampoo, look for a conditioner that has little or no impact on the scalp for the LPT device to work as effectively as possible.

Medicated Conditioners and Hair Regrowth

It is important to note that the primary focus of treating one's hair is to reduce Malassezia furfur activity on the scalp surface. By reducing the presence of MF, the primary source of excessive sebum production is reduced and the symptoms are kept in check. Advances in the hair product industry have brought new developments. One development includes conditioner antifungals said to improve scalp and hair health. Since conditioners work mostly on the hair, these antifungal ingredients are expected to further help with reduced fungal loads on the scalp. We've discussed some of these antifungal additives in previous chapters, but the concept of using a medicated conditioner is relatively new, especially for fighting against androgenetic alopecia. Since MF is an extremely fungal species, it is important to use all of the tools and strategies possible to reduce it on the scalp.

Are Conditioners Safe?

What about the safety of conditioners? Just like shampoos, they can cause adverse reactions. Reported side effects include eye irritation, scalp irritation, and even cases of increased acne (following facial contact). Be cautious before slathering on conditioner, especially if you're unsure what it contains.

Another substance in conditioners that causes a stir is silicones. Silicones are artificial compounds. Their purpose is to cover hair shafts to lock in moisture and reduce kinks. This is what produces a silky-smooth appearance. But the silicone layer interrupts the entry of nutrients into hair follicles when they need it most. In the same way, prolonged use of silicone causes a build-up on hair, which can cause dryness, leading to an unattractive look. Hairs can also be weakened, leading to breakage. And, as you know, breakage is to be avoided.

With these combined disadvantages, the use of silicones in conditioners is discouraged. Many hair product manufacturers are trying to avoid silicones, even advertising that they don't use them. Today it's common to find the word "silicone-free" on the packaging of many hair products. Double-check the ingredients before you buy, though, in case they're just using a new term for a nasty chemical.

Conditioners and Laser Phototherapy

While conditions may improve the look and feel of your hair, they have never been known to help with hair growth. Even newer conditioners, with added essential oils that are believed to improve scalp circulation, may not be effective because the results so far are limited. The effects of conditioners may also be impacted by other hair-enhancing products or drugs being used at the same time.

I highly recommend a medicated antifungal conditioner as part of your haircare routine particularly when using the LPT. Just make sure you use a high-quality conditioner free of sulfates (such as SLS), phthalates, silicones, parabens, dyes, and fake fragrances. These are the ones, especially those with silicones, that may cause unwanted side effects.

The antifungal ingredient in your conditioner should be different from the one in your shampoo. For example, if you use a piroctone olamine shampoo, the conditioner should contain zinc pyrithione, coal tar, or another antifungal. That way your shampoo and conditioner will attack the MF on your scalp differently. Using two antifungals also helps ensure that MF doesn't become immune to the antifungals you're using.

Laser phototherapy penetrates right to the hair follicles to regrow hair and there's no risk of adverse reactions from using LPT. Using a good shampoo, combined with a medicated conditioner and LPT will give you better odds when it comes to stopping and, ultimately, reversing hair loss.

Supplements

When people lose their hair, one of the first things they try is increasing the nutrients they take in. Often, there's a tendency to go overboard. The most effective treatments are those that are moderate but specific. In the case of hair growth, "less is more." This advice contradicts the widespread belief that doing more means getting better results, but it's better to do a few things right than to do many things wrong. Chasing after every available product could mean gaining small benefits at the price of doing your hair extensive harm. Not to mention the risk of canceling the advantages of the few good products out there.

One important fact to know is that male or female pattern hair loss is not strongly related to diet or nutrition. You might wonder how this can be—after all, it seems like every day that nutritionists and dieticians are recommending a new "super" supplement for hair growth. While it would be nice to be able to combat hair loss with a daily fish oil capsule, the truth is a little more complicated, and lies in the annals of history. It is either coincidence or altogether by accident that humans started to really develop after vitamins and minerals were entered into their diet, at the start of the Industrial Revolution in the beginning of the twentieth century. There is a minimum amount of necessary ingredients needed to sustain and optimize the body, but unfortunately no one knows exactly how much is needed for exactly what purposes.

The discovery of vitamins and minerals during the industrial age revolutionized human health. Deficiency-related diseases diminished as fortified foods became widespread. This newfound knowledge allowed for the development of balanced diets, boosting productivity and public health. Vitamins and minerals became integral to human well-being, shaping a healthier and more productive society. So, while ensuring your body receives proper nutrition is important for health overall, and presumably these effects rub off on scalp and hair health, there is as of yet no secret formula or supplement that will repair hair loss or promote growth more than a negligible amount.

In fact, there have been numerous studies conducted on malnourished people in India and the rate of hair loss for them is not substantial. Other studies came from prisoners during WWII concentration camps, who experienced severe starvation. Their hair loss had not increased in comparison to a normal population distribution. These are extreme examples, but they are worth noting.

Of course, certain vitamins and proteins are necessary for proper hair growth. A very low protein diet with just vegetables and fruit or some type of intentional starving can result in the appearance of limp or lifeless hair. We believe that a supplement that contains all of them in one pill (please never take a gummy vitamin—they are worthless!) with all the right ingredients is more than enough to maintain a healthy scalp. The fact is, the amount needed for just basic nutrition per day is miniscule and taking one "multi-vitamin" for hair loss and hair growth is more than enough, and in fact, should be enough to sustain other organs and organelles in the body.

Remember that hairs on top of your scalp are essentially dead and the action is below the scalp where the complex chemistry is occurring and being regulated by even more complex biochemical decisions.

In contrast to topical agents, which are applied directly to the hair, supplements are taken orally. Both may include nutrients or vitamins. Let's explore supplements and what works based on proven science.

Vitamin D

We talked about the "sunshine vitamin" at length in Chapter 3, so some of this will be familiar. As mentioned, various studies have shown that some hair conditions may be connected to vitamin D deficiency. These include telogen effluvium (a temporary hair loss due to three to four times more than normal that lasts for around two months following acute illness or stress) which gets worse. Alopecia areata, an autoimmune disorder that causes hair to fall out, has also been linked to low vitamin D levels. Female pattern hair loss (FPHL) is associated with low vitamin D levels as is hair loss in young people. This suggests a strong connection between vitamin D and hair loss.

No doubt your intuition is telling you that vitamin D supplements should be able to reverse these conditions since they're caused by a lack of vitamin D. Before we make that jump, though, let's check what scientific studies say about using vitamin D for hair regrowth.

In 2019, a study claimed that a diet supplemented with low doses of vitamin D could improve the symptoms of androgenetic alopecia and telogen effluvium (TE). That was great news! But the study also reported contradictory results about vitamin D levels in FPHL. As a result, further studies had to be done to determine the relationship between vitamin D and these conditions.

A more recent review in 2021 confirmed the role of vitamin D in the growth of hair follicles. It also supported the relationship between vitamin D deficiency and hair loss. It failed, however, to support the idea of taking vitamin D to correct hair loss. The bottom line is that there's no scientific consensus on using vitamin D supplements to improve hair growth. Instead, the results of completed studies are under review and more research is required.

Now, this doesn't mean vitamin D supplements don't play a role in preventing hair loss. While some dermatologists recommend vitamin D supplements for people experiencing hair loss and that seems like a good idea, the results can't be guaranteed.

Biotin

Biotin is part of the vitamin B family. Also called B7, it plays a vital role in the body by helping convert certain nutrients into proteins or energy. It has other roles that include hair, skin, and nail health. Although biotin supplements are said to be effective in improving hair growth, there isn't enough scientific evidence, nor enough personal reports to support that claim. While it may grow existing hairs longer, what it does not do is regrow or awaken new hairs.

The link between biotin and normal hair growth is the keratin cells in hair, skin, and nails. We know that biotin improves the structure of keratin, but that's all we know. Many of the studies conducted on the role of biotin in enhancing hair growth provided weak and inconclusive results. And even the studies that concluded that biotin supplements improved hair condition are problematic. This is because biotin is often packaged with other vitamins, and it may have been one of these that improved hair health.

The human body doesn't need a lot of biotin, so a healthy diet provides most of what we need daily. Not surprisingly, a biotin deficiency is very rare, so supplementing this vitamin when we already get enough in our daily diet is questionable. In fact, the Food and Drug Administration hasn't felt it necessary to recommend a dietary allowance for biotin. The medical professionals who suggest a biotin supplement are basing this suggestion on the popular opinion that it may be beneficial.

In conclusion, biotin provides minimal to no benefit for hair regrowth. Supplement manufacturers continue marketing biotin for hair health without clinical proof. You are better off avoiding biotin and saving your money unless you have a confirmed deficiency, which again, is extremely rare.

Methylsulfonylmethane (MSM)

MSM is a sulfur compound found in animals, plants, and humans, but it can also be made in a laboratory. MSM is a white, crystalline powder that is odorless and nearly tasteless.

Like DMSO (dimethyl sulfoxide—used to reduce inflammation and pain), MSM was originally used as an industrial solvent. It has only recently become popular as a nutritional supplement and topical application.

After doing a great deal of study on DMSO between the 1950s and 1970s, researchers found that it had several therapeutic uses, including as an anti-inflammatory agent. They also discovered that they could make MSM from DMSO.

Two chemists, Dr. Robert Herschler and Dr. Stanley Jacob, wondered whether MSM could also offer health benefits and began a long series of tests on MSM. As it turns out, they were on the right track. When taken as a dietary supplement, MSM proved to have the same health benefits as its parent compound, DMSO, without side effects such as bad breath, itchy skin, nasal congestion, and shortness of breath. Better still, MSM also seems to promote the growth of hair.

In a study performed on rats, researchers concluded that, when used with a magnesium ascorbyl phosphate (MAP) solution, MSM increases hair growth. The amount of growth seems to be dependent on the levels of MSM and MAP. Some scientists believe that MSM does this by strengthening keratin, the protein hair is made from. MSM may also help to strengthen hair bonds.

Few studies support hair growth claims when MSM and only MSM is being used. Nonetheless, based on what we know, I would strongly recommend MSM as a part of your daily hair growth supplements.

Curcumin

Curcumin occurs naturally in turmeric, a spice that comes from the turmeric plant (part of the ginger root family). Turmeric, which gives curry its yellowish color, has become one of the most extensively studied herbs in medicine. It's the curcumin in turmeric that is believed to help prevent hair loss. Curcumin is thought to work against hair loss by reducing the overproduction of DHT. DHT, as we already know, prevents the growth of new hair cells. Curcumin also has anti-inflammatory properties that help maintain a healthy scalp.

Does it work? One 2012 study reported positive effects for curcumin on hair growth. However, the study got these results by using Minoxidil and curcumin together. A study in 2017 showed similar results when curcumin was used in an essential oil formulation. Curcumin may help with hair loss, but the studies done so far have used curcumin in combination with other drugs or oils.

Quercetin

Quercetin is a natural substance found in leaves, flowers, and fruits. It is reported to be an anti-inflammatory as well as an antioxidant. Research on quercetin also reveals some other benefits. Firstly, quercetin is believed to improve cell activities, especially those that take place in the mitochondria. It also helps increase the production of essential factors for cell growth. In addition, when human hair follicles received quercetin, the improved hair shaft growth was comparable to the growth observed with Minoxidil. This all points to quercetin's potential to promote hair growth when used as a supplement. A word of caution: These results were obtained from studies performed outside the model of the human body. In other words, they used laboratory cultures.

In another study, mice were used to see how effective quercetin was against androgenetic alopecia. The results were similarly positive. More recently, a study showed that quercetin is effective against alopecia areata. Moreover, unlike corticosteroids, which have catastrophic side effects and can be used only for a short time, quercetin has several other documented benefits for human health. Since quercetin is available as a dietary supplement, it's more likely patients will take it regularly, which increases the odds of positive outcomes for the treatment of alopecia areata and androgenetic alopecia.

While these studies are promising, large-scale studies still need to be done with humans to see how effective quercetin is when it comes to human hair growth.

Saw Palmetto

Indigenous to the southeastern United States, saw palmetto has been used for centuries by Native Americans as both food and medicine. As an herbal supplement, saw palmetto is made from the small berries of the saw palmetto palm. The berries are thought to block the action of the enzyme (5-alpha reductase) that converts testosterone to DHT. Since DHT is well known for killing hair follicles and disrupting hair growth, preventing the body from producing DHT gives hair growth a boost.

For years many people assumed that saw palmetto was a "natural Propecia (Finasteride)." This was especially true of people who were concerned—rightfully so—about the ever-increasing number of side effects caused by Finasteride. This assumption, however, is overly simplistic and largely false. For one thing, saw palmetto doesn't work the same way as Propecia. Propecia promotes hair growth by lowering blood levels of DHT by about 65%, while, theoretically, saw palmetto may block a small percentage of DHT from binding to the scalp.

Again, there is limited research on the medicinal value of saw palmetto, but one study showed that up to half of the participants who used saw palmetto saw an increase of 11.9% in hair growth after four months. Although encouraging, more evidence is needed to prove that the effect came from the saw palmetto supplement and the results are repeatable in other groups.

Iron

Iron's connection to hair loss has to do with the production of hemoglobin, the compound that binds oxygen in the blood so that it can be carried to cells throughout the body. The body needs iron to make hemoglobin, so when iron levels are low, hemoglobin production drops. Since hair follicles need oxygen to survive, hair growth activity falls off when oxygen levels are low. This, in turn, leads to increased hair loss.

Iron deficiencies are common. Iron deficiency hair loss looks very much like male and female pattern hair loss. Anyone suffering from this condition will likely see a lot of hair being shed after washing and a larger amount of hair left behind in their brush. In more severe forms of iron deficiency hair loss, bare spots on the scalp may appear. The good news is that iron deficiency hair loss is easily treatable. Once you up your iron intake, it disappears.

A word of caution, however, before you start taking iron for your hair: too much iron can be harmful. Iron deficiency hair loss must be diagnosed by a ferritin level test. This test will tell a doctor whether your iron levels are low and whether iron supplements are necessary. If you've been diagnosed with anemia, then you should consider taking iron supplements. This is especially true if you are a woman and still menstruating. If you are still menstruating and anemic, you should not only take iron supplements, but you should also include high-iron foods in your diet. Include a daily vitamin C supplement for proper absorption of iron. Interestingly, copper is needed for proper iron absorption, so low copper levels can also make it harder for the body to use the iron it has.

There's no good reason to boost your iron intake to combat hair loss unless it's caused by an iron deficiency. Most clinics don't recommend giving iron supplements except in the case of iron deficiency anemia. This is because too much iron in your diet can result in an iron overload, leading to serious harm. Iron supplements aren't something to experiment with!

Folate

Folate (vitamin B9) is one of the nutrients that promotes healthy cell growth, particularly when it comes to the skin and nails. Folate also helps maintain a healthy population of red blood cells. Folate's twin benefits for cells and blood got some researchers thinking it might have similar benefits for hair. Research, however, hasn't found any solid evidence that links folate to hair growth. The evidence that the use of folate supplements promotes hair growth is sparse, so it's not likely to be the magic treatment many claim it is.

Astaxanthin

Astaxanthin is a recently discovered relative of beta carotene (found in carrots) and lycopene (found in carrots and tomatoes). It seems to be the most potent natural antioxidant identified so far. This is a new entry in the list of hair regrowth supplements, and I think it's one of the five best supplements to take for scalp and skin health.

Like beta carotene and lycopene, astaxanthin is a carotenoid. Carotenoids give foods such as watermelon, red beets, carrots, tomatoes, and cantaloupes their color. They are also involved in photosynthesis and protect plants and other organisms from ultraviolet light. Humans get the same benefit from eating carotenoids. Astaxanthin, however, is significantly stronger than other carotenoids and seems to protect all cells, including hair follicles, from the damage caused by oxidants. It's sixty-five times more potent than vitamin C, fifty-four times more potent than beta carotene, and fourteen times stronger than vitamin E.

Supplements and Laser Phototherapy

While conditioners and shampoos perform obvious functions on hair health, the same can't be said of supplements. Numerous supplements are touted as the solution to hair loss, but most of them have no verified benefits. Often, it's merely a case of unfounded hype.

Unfortunately, the first thing someone with hair loss does is look for a magic pill, and they will dump every supplement they can find into their bodies. This is where wasted time and money, along with ever-increasing frustration, come in. More importantly, most of these supplements can cause serious liver issues because the ingredients are of a poor quality, non-water soluble, or worse, contain harmful toxins.

After several months without any improvement, desperation sets in. Therefore, LPT should be the first line of defense against hair loss. Laser phototherapy has been scientifically tested, and its ability to promote hair growth under different conditions has been shown again and again. What's more, over a ten-year period, it's cheaper than taking vitamins or using expensive shampoos and conditioners.

That said, some supplements can be helpful. Vitamin D supplements may be somewhat beneficial. Curcumin, quercetin, and saw palmetto may also help promote hair growth. We need more evidence, though, to be certain.

Yet heed the warning: Certain supplements may result in an overload of nutrients in the body, which can lead to serious complications. This is the danger of using supplements that have no proven effect on hair growth.

Shampoos, Conditioners, Supplements, and LPT

When it comes to growing hair, shampoos, conditioners, and supplements might offer some benefits, but research is limited. What we do know from clinical testing is that by using them in combination with an FDA-cleared LPT helmet, hair loss can be slowed more efficiently and hair growth encouraged.

Actual Customer Success Stories

A Safe Solution For The Most Special Times

Navigating motherhood was challenging enough for Sandra, but losing her hair added an unexpected twist. Around three months postpartum, despite all of the distractions, Sandra couldn't ignore the alarming amount of hair collecting in her brush. Sandra had always taken pride in her hair, especially on days when she couldn't spare the time for makeup or a stylish outfit. But now, even her even her hair was letting her down. Hesitant to take hair loss medications while breastfeeding, she sought alternatives. Once her baby began eating solids, her physician recommended laser phototherapy. Conveniently, Sandra could use the wearable device while tending to her child. As her baby flourished, she rejoiced in seeing her hair regain its former thickness and vitality.

CHAPTER 8
FDA-Cleared Medications

"Medicine is the art of entertaining the patient while nature cures the disease." — Voltaire, Philosopher, 1768

Minoxidil

There are currently only three FDA-cleared solutions for hair loss on the market today: Minoxidil, Finasteride, and now, laser phototherapy (LPT).

Minoxidil is a popular FDA-cleared hair loss medication, originally developed in 1965 to treat high blood pressure by dilating blood vessels. Offered in concentrations of 2% or 5%, it can be taken orally or applied to the skin as a lotion or foam. As a cream, it's used to treat male and female pattern hair loss.

Since Minoxidil wasn't initially intended for hair loss, its ability to regrow hair is a little-understood side effect. Once someone starts using Minoxidil, they must keep using it to prevent the return of hair loss. Minoxidil shortens the resting phase of hair, pushing hair follicles into the growth phase. It also contains a compound called nitric oxide, which causes hair in the resting phase to shed. New hairs then replace the shed hairs during the growing phase.

However, there are concerns about how Minoxidil regrows hair. Minoxidil causes the scalp to shed hair in the resting phase. These hairs are replaced by new ones, but the question remains as to why resting hairs are shed in the first place. Some researchers believe this is an effect of the drug's nitric oxide content.

We know hair growth is a tiny portion of what Minoxidil does. What we don't know is what other changes it causes in the body and scalp. Minoxidil should therefore be used with an abundance of caution. The results of numerous Minoxidil trials average a 13.4% increase in hair count. In comparison, LPT averages 39% over a six-month period with no hair shedding.

Minoxidil vs. Laser Phototherapy

Minoxidil use has several limitations when it comes to hair growth. Minoxidil studies suggest that it doesn't regrow hair on all parts of the scalp; it can mostly regrow hair on the crown. This could be because they primarily focused on men with hair loss issues on the crown. Since hair loss patterns differ substantially, only those losing hair from their crown area benefit from Minoxidil. It can't help with hair loss at the temples or other parts of the scalp.

Conversely, laser phototherapy addresses all types of scalp hair loss. So, if you only want to stop your hairline from receding, Minoxidil won't work. LPT, on the other hand, can help restore your hairline.

Additionally, to prevent hair growth from recurring, Minoxidil must be a lifelong daily treatment. LPT, in contrast, can both prevent further loss and increase hair count—often in fewer than twenty minutes per treatment and only on certain days of the week. Plus, additional laser treatments are necessary only for maintenance once you've reached your target hair growth.

In addition, using Minoxidil as a liquid or a foam can be messy; the liquid version of Minoxidil can run down the face. Many customers have complained of hairs growing on the sides of their faces (skin on the side of the face is thinner than scalp). It's also known to cause scalp irritation in people with sensitive skin.

Laser phototherapy, on the other hand, is clean and convenient. A more elegant laser device like an LPT helmet can be used stress-free and mess-free anywhere, anytime, and is more cost-effective than purchasing Minoxidil on a regular monthly basis.

Another important difference between Minoxidil and LPT is that Minoxidil can cause additional hair loss at first. But even worse, if you stop using Minoxidil abruptly, the shedding will virtually eliminate all new hairs that were generated by it. LPT, however, prolongs the hair's growing phases without causing any hair loss, even if you slow down your use of LPT.

There's a type of Minoxidil that can be taken orally, but it can have serious side effects, such as sodium and fluid retention, and cause damage to the cardiovascular system. There have been reports of ischemic heart disease, pericardial effusion, and pulmonary hypertension when Minoxidil is taken regularly. As we saw in the previous chapter, LPT is a different story. The side effects are minimal—neither serious nor permanent. A small number of patients have reported mild itching of the scalp or a burning sensation just after LPT application. It is possible to get a rash on the treated area, but it quickly disappears if treated with the proper cream or lotion.

What about the Cost? Minoxidil may seem cheaper than many other hair loss treatments since a month's worth costs about $10. But once you start using it, you can never stop, or your hair loss will return. So Minoxidil treatment costs about $120 annually. Over the course of ten years, that's $1,200. LPT costs hundreds of dollars less and doesn't require daily use for sustained hair growth.

Finasteride

It was Hippocrates who first noticed that castrated men (eunuchs) did not have hair loss issues. In the mid-1970s, scientists then associated hormones (such as testosterone) with hair loss when they saw that men with small prostates had very little or no hair loss. This has led to the association of testosterone with the pathology behind hair loss. Therefore, it was assumed that a certain reduction of specific hormones could potentially treat hair loss.

Finasteride, commercially known as Propecia®, is another drug used to treat hair loss. Like Minoxidil, it wasn't originally developed as a hair loss treatment. It's an oral medication used to treat non-cancerous enlargement of the prostate gland. Later, it was found to help improve hair growth in patients. Finasteride is now an FDA-cleared treatment for an enlarged prostate as well as for androgenetic alopecia (male pattern hair loss). It's usually marketed in 1 mg tablets.

Remember DHT, the hair assassin? Finasteride attempts to reduce DHT levels. In a 0.01 mg dose, Finasteride didn't inhibit the production of DHT any better than did a placebo. But with a dose of 0.05 mg, there was a 60% decrease in DHT production. Finasteride improves hair growth and slows the rate of hair loss. Overall, Finasteride users reported close to 10% hair regrowth from the baseline hair count. Again, when comparing LPT to Finasteride, LPT boasts a 39% increase in hair count in only six months, and has no side effects.

Finasteride has also been used to treat hirsutism, the abnormal growth of hair on the face and body. Transgender women may take it along with estrogen as a testosterone blocker. It can also treat women suffering from an overgrowth of hair.

This popular hormone-targeted treatment is effective to an extent, but still leaves much to be desired. Like Minoxidil, Finasteride requires lifelong use to maintain hair growth.

Finasteride use is also linked with serious side effects, such as erectile dysfunction (2% to 4%), reduced sex drive, lower semen production, enlarged breasts in men, and ejaculation disorders. In some patients, persistent sexual dysfunction may lead to suicidal thoughts and other kinds of psychological distress. In these cases, counseling is called for. These side effects are predictable since the drug alters DHT levels. Although they may disappear if a person stops using Finasteride, this can take one to three years. Also, as mentioned, if one stops taking Finasteride, the hair that was gained while on the medication will most likely be lost again.

Finasteride can also cause hypotension, a type of low blood pressure that makes you feel lightheaded or dizzy when you stand up after sitting or lying down. This happens with about 9% of users, but that number jumps to 18% for people taking heart medications (e.g., alpha-blockers) along with Finasteride.

Finasteride vs. Laser Phototherapy

Finasteride treatment hasn't been used much for treating receding hairlines and their clinical results have not been strong as compared to LPT.

Another major drawback of Finasteride is that it really is not specifically designed to be used by women with hair loss even though Finasteride is an anti-androgen. As I explained, the benefits for women using Finasteride are not worthwhile due to the side effects. One major side effect is that if a woman gets pregnant while taking Finasteride it may have negative effects on the unborn baby and potentially cause a birth defect. Specifically, the unborn fetus could be born without any genitals. For this reason, pregnant women or women who are breastfeeding cannot even touch or handle the Finasteride pill. So, at the very least, only postmenopausal women should consider taking Finasteride and premenopausal women should consider taking birth control pills if considering Finasteride. Imagine starting a hair treatment that makes your problem worse!

Laser phototherapy, on the other hand, has the advantage of producing similar hair growth benefits in both men and women. Instead of removing DHT from the scalp, laser phototherapy focuses on restoring hair-cell health. It is an effective, 100% natural way to counter the toxic presence of DHT without removing it from the body. This way you don't suffer the side effects that come with lost hormones.

Finasteride costs $25 a month. That's about $300 a year. Since it requires continuous use, you could spend more than $3,000 on Finasteride over ten years. Compare that to laser phototherapy devices, which on average cost $800. That's a savings of $2,200 at the end of ten years.

The Ten-Year Cost: How Minoxidil, Finasteride, and LPT Compare

To better understand the overall cost of treatment and management over just ten years, let's compare the leading topicals with LPT. The prices of topical Minoxidil and oral Finasteride vary from store to store and brand to brand. So, to give a fair comparison, let's compare them to the available products on Amazon—the largest online retailer in the United States.

A three-month supply of 5% Minoxidil (Rogaine®) costs $61.99, while a one-month supply of generic Finasteride costs $114.00. This is equivalent to a yearly cost of $2,469.60 for 5% Minoxidil and $13,680 for Finasteride over ten years. These prices exclude the shipping costs on each order.

	Minoxidil	Finasteride	LPT
How It Works	• Prolongs the duration of the growth phase of the hair growth cycle	• Blocks the conversion of testosterone to Dihydrotestosterone by acting against the enzyme that catalyzes the process	• Affects the hair growth cycle in that it prolongs the growth phase, promotes the re-entry of hairs in the resting phase to the growth phase, and prevents the early transitioning of hair to the transitional phase
Hair Count from Published Studies	• 13% average hair count increase over baseline over one year at 2% solution	• 10% average hair count increase over baseline over one year at 1mg	• 39% average hair count increase over baseline over twenty-six weeks (two twenty-minute treatments per week) • Cessation of hair loss • Increased terminal hairs and less vellus hairs
Efficacy (the ability to produce a desired or intended result)	• 83.9% of patients reported good patient satisfaction but for 51.6%, hair loss was slightly increased • More effective compared to testing drug	• 57.5% of subjects reported major improvements after 18 months, 45% reported moderate improvements, while 7.5% showed none • Hair growth was exhibited by most of the subjects	• 59.7% of the subjects reported an overall improvement in hair loss • High patient satisfaction scores on the treated side • Marked improvement in patients with pattern hair loss over a six-month period
Side Effects	• Minoxidil causes shortening of resting phase, causing more hair to be shed • Skin irritation • Scaly scalp • Itchy scalp	• Finasteride also shortens resting phase, causing more hair to be shed • Loss of sex drive, erection problems, decreased volume of sexual fluids, enlargement of breasts in men • Fertility issues • Adverse effects continue to appear • Can't be used in children	• No reported side effects

Table 8.1. Comparison Table of Minoxidil, Finasteride, and LPT. In this table, LPT clearly is the winner in terms of safety, efficacy, and long term usage.

In comparison, FDA-cleared, at-home LPT devices like helmets cost around $695.00 to $995.00 on Amazon. The hair growth comb costs $385.00, depending on the number of lasers in the device. While they aren't cheap, they're a one-time buy.

Hair Transplants

As the name suggests, hair transplants (HT) involve surgery. This delicate procedure moves hair from one area of the scalp to another. The scalp may become tender after a hair transplant, and pain medication might be necessary and there are side effects to surgery. Most people can return to work two to five days after the transplant and, around two to five weeks after the surgery, the transplanted hair begins falling out. New hair growth becomes noticeable about six to nine months after the surgery, and up to 3,000 new donor hairs can be transplanted from either the back of the scalp or other places such as the chest, legs, and arms. Hair transplants have become extremely popular for advanced hair loss patients and are an excellent way to fill in areas where hair is completely void of active hair follicles.

Hair Transplants vs. Laser Phototherapy

Doctors in the United States started performing hair transplants in the 1950s, so LPT is a newer treatment in comparison. While transplants can produce satisfactory hair growth, they have serious limitations. Firstly, hair transplants are pretty pricey, and in years past they've been out of reach for many. One measure of the psychological pain caused by hair loss might be the millions of dollars we've cumulatively spent on getting it back. Fortunately, technological advances have resulted in a steady decline in the cost of hair transplantation. An increase in competition, including low-cost countries with cheap medical labor, has contributed to the price drop as well.

Although the cost per graft varies from one clinic to another, the average cost of each hair graft is $5.44 in the United States. By comparison, it's $7.00 per graft in Canada, one of the most expensive countries in which to get a hair transplant. On the other end of the scale, Turkey offers one of the cheapest hair transplant rates: $1.07 per graft.

There are three ways of going about a hair transplant. The first is called follicular unit extraction, or FUE. A doctor performing FUE surgery takes individual hair follicles, usually from the back of the head, and makes tiny incisions—punctures, really—in the scalp where the hair is thinning or gone. The follicles that were removed are now placed in these incisions. It's a lot of precise work, and the whole procedure can take more than ten hours. In some cases, the patient will have to undergo a second day of surgery.

The second method is called follicular unit transplantation (FUT for short). With this method, a surgeon cuts a large strip of scalp from the back of the head (this wound will require stitches to heal). The strip of scalp is cut into numerous tiny pieces—sometimes numbering in the thousands—and these tiny pieces are grafted onto the scalp areas where hair is needed. This usually takes from four to twelve hours.

The third method is a combination of these two.

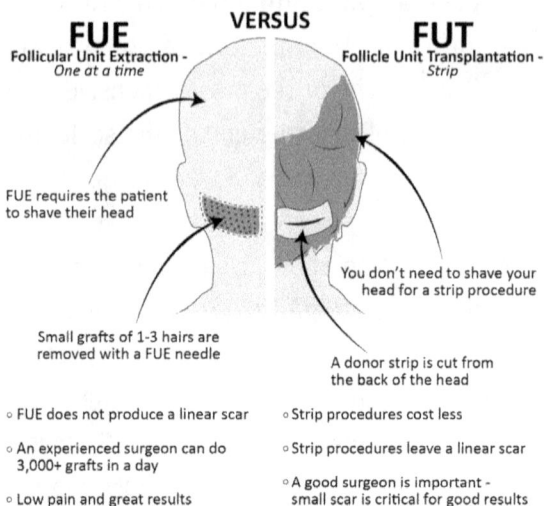

FUE VERSUS FUT

FUE
Follicular Unit Extraction -
One at a time

FUT
Follicle Unit Transplantation -
Strip

FUE requires the patient
to shave their head

You don't need to shave your
head for a strip procedure

Small grafts of 1-3 hairs are
removed with a FUE needle

A donor strip is cut from
the back of the head

○ FUE does not produce a linear scar

○ An experienced surgeon can do
3,000+ grafts in a day

○ Low pain and great results

○ Strip procedures cost less

○ Strip procedures leave a linear scar

○ A good surgeon is important -
small scar is critical for good results

Figure 8.2. Two Hair Transplant Methods. FUE is now the primary method used for hair transplants around the world. LPT plus FUE is a great solution for people with advanced hair loss.

An FUE is the most popular type of hair transplant (66%). Next in line is the FUT (29.8%). The combination of FUE and FUT is fairly rare. FUT is slowly being phased out due to better tools and techniques.

Once the surgery has been performed, the main difference between the first two is scarring. With an FUT there is a good deal of visible scarring, which means wearing your hair short would probably not be a good idea. The scarring from an FUE is fairly minor. Instead of a long scar at the back of the head, there may be tiny white dots where hairs were removed. Some HT physicians have created novel techniques to avoid these tiny white dots by filling it with excess tissue from donor sites.

Although the number of hairs transplanted will determine the cost of an HT, a hair transplant has a one-time cost of up to $15,000. That's almost twenty times the cost of an average LPT device and should, therefore, be a reason to justify investing in an LPT device before considering an HT procedure. Besides, laser phototherapy provides similar or even better hair growth without inflaming the hair follicles or the risk of infection. The effects of laser phototherapy occur much quicker, too, as much as the third month of use. A considerable difference in hair growth can be seen within six months with LPT. And there is *no* healing time or pain.

Another important point to consider is that at any given time about 30% of your hair is in the dormant (catagen) or resting (telogen) phase, but the surgeon has no way of knowing *which* 30% that is. This is a problem because if they take dormant or resting follicles, the grafted hair will probably not survive when placed back into the scalp.

Maximizing an HT also requires a combination of hair treatments. For example, doctors often encourage patients to use Minoxidil after an HT. Sometimes, laser phototherapy is even used to improve the success of the HT (see more on this below). So HTs often involve additional costs. Even worse, hair transplants can fail. Some of the transplanted follicles may lose their ability to grow new hairs, so transplanting these dead follicles may not provide any hair loss improvement. In other cases, thinning of the surrounding hair may follow transplant surgery. Finally, there is the risk of scarring.

Like LPT, hair transplant surgery can treat hair loss on every part of the scalp. Unlike hair loss medications, many hair surgeries can restore natural-looking hairlines. This makes an HT better than drugs like Minoxidil or Finasteride. But even if you endure the pain and everything goes well (so you need only one treatment), you've paid thousands of dollars for a 60% chance of success.

A well-made LPT device provides a 90% chance of extending the life of new hair transplants for a fraction of the price and should be used right before, right after an HT, and then never stop using the LPT device. Plus, LPT is painless and will reduce the necessity to have an HT in the future.

A Hair Transplant and the LPT Play Well Together

Even if a patient is determined to get a hair transplant, there are good reasons to use an LPT device. Depending on the type of transplant, thousands of punctures will be made in the scalp, which needs to be prepared for such a surgical assault. This event can be a shock not only to existing hairs but it can also irritate other parts of the scalp. Up to a month before the transplant, the patient can use LPT to boost scalp health.

Remember, most people who get hair transplants have been suffering from advanced cases of androgenetic alopecia. This means that DHT has been killing hair follicles in the areas consistent with male and female pattern hair loss. It also means scalp health, in general, is not good in those areas. Hair follicles have been miniaturized (making them thin and frail), sebum production is unstable, and the epidermal growth factor is increasing (this leads to new skin that will not grow hair). Applying lasers before transplants helps reverse these problems. It also increases mitochondrial activity, minimizes your scalp's distress, reduces swelling following surgery, and helps ensure that hair follicles damaged during the surgery will survive the transplantation.

Side effects of HT surgery: Because the red light of lasers reduces swelling and improves healing, using an LPT can assist in healing. Many patients who do not use LPT after an HT report a great deal of swelling. This is due to the surgery itself as well as the saline solution and local anesthetic used in the procedure. Severe swelling of the eyes is common for at least twenty-four to thirty-six hours. An LPT device will help reduce this inflammation. Remember, if you get an FUE and a surgeon places 2,500 grafts, that means a total of 5,000 punctures were made and this really is brutal for the scalp. Both the transplanted hair and the neighboring hair can be lost due to inflammation. Therefore, you should begin using the LPT device as soon as the bandages are removed, which is usually about forty-eight hours after a hair transplant.

Red lasers are already used for inflammatory conditions, such as arthritis, as well as for pain and wound management, so this is no different. Many clinics provide a simple headband device, which may be tight and a bit uncomfortable, to reduce swelling. Using an LPT device will ease or eliminate the need for these headbands. LPT also allows the anesthetic to drain out of the head, which, in turn, helps reduce swelling.

In short, LPT ensures better healing, and the area where new hairs were implanted will recover much faster. Surgical punctures will heal with little or no scarring. The trauma of numerous punctures can shorten the lives of non-grafted hairs. These hairs automatically go into the resting phase or, worse, die. The LPT device protects these neighboring hairs.

There is also the risk that a puncture might cut into the papilla or bulge due to the angle at which higher-density, non-HT hairs grow. In this does happen, LPT can help reverse the damage (depending on how bad it is). By charging up mitochondria, LPT helps the hair follicle try to repair itself.

Equally important, LPT gives relocated hairs a better chance to survive. The likelihood of a new hair graft being successful depends on many factors, but one of the most important is called angiogenesis. This is the medical term for the process a hair goes through to "reconnect" to the scalp in the five to ten days after an HT. It's important to wear the LPT device as much as possible during that time. It speeds up angiogenesis and prevents HT grafts from being rejected.

An LPT helmet helps both transplanted *and* existing hairs on the scalp. After a transplant, the scalp is like a boxer who's been battered and bruised after a tough fight. Many HT patients suffer from redness on the scalp for several weeks after the HT procedure. It can be reduced using an LPT device. The amount and length of time it stays on the scalp depends on the quantity and number of implanted HTs. At this time, there are no standard of care guidelines for LPT and HTs; as such, the quality of treatment now depends on the HT surgeon and their knowledge of LPT.

Some hair follicles will cycle out of the growth phase and be lost. So, it's vital to try to maintain them with aggressive laser therapy for the first several weeks after the surgery. It is important to note that LPT and HT should not be compared to each other as competitive options; rather, LPT should always be used when an HT is performed, and both have distinct advantages over each other.

The Cost of Hair Transplant Hair Loss

About 5% and up to 10% of all HTs fail after twelve to eighteen months, especially if the scalp is not properly managed by the patient. One key reason for this is that, as mentioned above, a surgeon doesn't know where a hair is in its cycle. Some hairs are at the beginning of the growth phase while others are at the end of it. If the hairs are at the end, they may be alive only for another few months and not recover after being transplanted. The other reason is because of the trauma caused by the HT and the failure of hairs to reconnect to the scalp (angiogenesis failure).

That said, an HT patient will still lose fifty to one hundred hairs per day, and this will happen faster where the scalp has been damaged. So, what's the cost involved? On average, the cost of an HT is about $7 per hair. At a loss of a hundred hairs per day, a typical scalp can lose about 3,000 hairs per month (thirty days). LPT slows down or stops hair loss for both non-grafted and grafted hairs. This means that if an HT is about $7 per graft, LPT saves about 50% to 75% of potential hair loss, which at the low end means 1,500 hairs. This results in a total savings of $10,500 ($7 x 1500) to $15,750 ($7 x 2,250 hairs saved). Since an LPT device costs anywhere from $695 to $995, it pays for itself.

Turkey is currently the leading place to get HTs, and for a while, it was so much cheaper to have the surgery done there that it was more than worth the airfare and hotel costs. However, it is still a tremendous time commitment to travel to Turkey and stay for the procedure and recovery, not to mention the trauma of the surgery itself.

On the other hand, no matter how cheap a hair transplant may be, patients will still lose new hairs if they do not use an LPT device to assist with their hair transplant process.

Patients want more of a guarantee that this very painful procedure will last more than a year or two. That's where the LPT comes in. It can ensure that 93% of the hairs will stay on their heads. We strongly encourage all patients who want to do an HT to begin using an LPT two months before their HT procedure and increase usage after the HT for two years at a daily rate. This will ensure a great HT result and keep the hairs that were not transplanted. It will keep the new HTs as well as make the donor sites heal properly.

All things considered, if you have a hair transplant, you should definitely consider purchasing an LPT device. It's a good idea for both patients and clinicians. I envision that once everyone sees the benefits of LPT, all HT surgeons will make using an LPT device a requirement for all HT procedures. LPT offers clear benefits to HT patients, and happier patients will recommend clinicians who have given them a great experience and great results.

Actual Customer Success Stories

Last, Best Hope

Joshua's hair loss seemed to happen suddenly. He tried every potion and pill under the sun, all of which ended in disappointment or worse—side effects like breast growth and withering libido. Lured by the affordability of hair transplants in Turkey and the persuasive marketing of a particular clinic, he overlooked the unverified reviews and the conspicuous absence of the practitioner's credentials. He was devastated when the surgery left him worse off than before—his head looking like a wheat field, with visible scarring from cheap but botched Procedures. How could he have wasted so much time and pain, only to move backwards! He gave up, accepting hair loss and scars. Worried for him, his girlfriend bought him a wearable laser device. Within weeks, his mood and hair showed recovery. Soon he could no longer see his scars, and his bare patch disappeared altogether.

CHAPTER 9
Off-Label Treatments

"The greatest enemy of knowledge is not ignorance, it is the illusion of knowledge." — Daniel J. Boorstin, 1995

Platelet-Rich Plasma in Hair Treatment

Platelet-rich plasma (PRP) cells contain growth factors that help heal inflammatory diseases. Platelet-rich plasma is made from a patient's own blood. After blood is drawn, it is spun in a centrifuge which separates blood components by their densities. It's then injected into the area of the scalp showing hair loss. PRP can be used to heal injured parts of the body and was first used at the end of the 1980s on an open-heart surgery patient. Today, it's used in orthopedics, sports medicine, neurosurgery, ophthalmology, dermatology, and cosmetic surgery. Because of its restorative properties, PRP is becoming a popular way to naturally promote quick healing. However, since the FDA has not cleared PRP, physicians use this as an "off-label" treatment. Performing PRP in a clinic is simple and the cost to the doctor is low. A nurse or technician can draw the blood and prepare for the PRP treatment.

However, PRP for patients with hair loss is not only a costly option but also lacks conclusive scientific evidence and FDA clearance to support its efficacy. Some patients do also complain that PRP is a somewhat painful procedure.

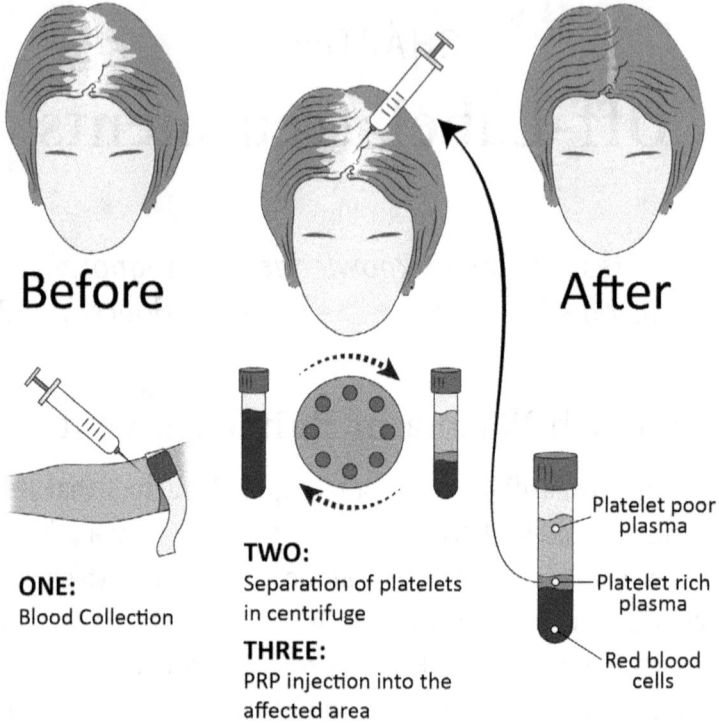

PRP Therapy
for Hair Loss

Before

After

ONE:
Blood Collection

TWO:
Separation of platelets
in centrifuge

THREE:
PRP injection into the
affected area

Platelet poor
plasma

Platelet rich
plasma

Red blood
cells

Figure 9.1. PRP Therapy: "Before" vs. "After". This technique is primarily
done by physicians in clinic settings. The results are quite ambiguous,
and this is not an FDA-cleared procedure.

Injecting PRP into patients' scalps has been shown in some cases to improve hair follicle function and promote new hair growth. A significant reduction in hair loss accompanied by improved density has been observed as well. PRP is a simple, feasible, and natural therapeutic tool for fighting hair loss in men and women. It has high overall patient satisfaction without any serious side effects.

Results of PRP injections aren't instantaneous, though. It takes around six months before they are noticeable. This translates to several sessions, typically two or three, spaced four to six weeks apart.

Because PRP works only by affecting the hair growth cycle and doesn't address the genetic aspect of hair loss, several maintenance treatments are needed for the results to last. Typically, this means treatment sessions once or twice a year.

Since PRP is taken from the patient's own blood the risk of contracting communicable diseases or allergic reactions is low. The only potential side effects come from the injections. These include pain, bruising, swelling, and redness. Nerve and tissue injuries can also occur although this is related to the skill of the healthcare professional administering the PRP.

Studies and Results on PRP

The main concern with PRP as a hair growth option is the costs, time, maintenance, and contradictions in outcome. Despite the excitement over PRP as a hair loss treatment, studies are ambiguous. One study showed clinical improvement using PRP to correct hair loss. The average number of hairs was 33.6 in the target area, and there was an increase in hair density of 45.9 hairs per square centimeter after three treatments. However, a different study found that PRP was not effective against hair loss as there was only a slight increase in the number of hairs.

This disagreement in the scientific community regarding results stems from a lack of standardization within platelet-rich plasma hair transplants. There is still no agreed-upon way of preparing and administering PRP. Further studies are needed to ascertain its benefits.

The price of PRP treatments for hair growth varies per clinic, but one "set of injections" is typically priced at $400. It would, therefore, cost around $1,200 or more to see initial results. Often more treatments are required, depending on how much hair has been lost. Then there are the annual maintenance treatments that must be added in. All this costs time and money.

Platelet-rich plasma treatment is comparable to other hair loss treatments with minimal side effects.

In contrast, patients who take oral Finasteride show a drop in sex drive, and those using Minoxidil as a lotion or cream show an increase in hair loss within four to six weeks of application.

The main concern with PRP as a hair growth option is the costs, time, maintenance, and contradictions in the outcome.

Platelet-Rich Plasma and Laser Phototherapy

However, just like HT, many clinical doctors report positive results when combining PRP injections with an LPT treatment schedule. LPT reduces inflammation, which can affect patients who receive PRP injections. Clinics often offer LPT because PRP is often not enough on its own for treating hair regrowth.

It's no surprise that more and more dermatologists are recommending PRP and LPT as combined treatments. Partnering with PRP vendors and clinics to put the LPT devices into the hands of more clinicians should be a required process, especially since PRP is not FDA-cleared for hair loss and having LPT alongside PRP will improve a clinician's chances that their treatment will satisfy their patients.

Just as HT and LPT make a great team, so do PRP injections and LPT. Combined, they make a powerful tool for fighting hair loss. They increase hair density, minimize shedding, and promote new hair growth. In fact, the regenerative capabilities of platelet-rich plasma and laser phototherapy mean that PRP-LPT hair restoration treatments are becoming the most effective way to fight hair loss. They are also natural medical alternatives without harmful side effects.

Platelet-Rich Plasma Drawbacks

As mentioned, PRP is new and the effectiveness of PRP is still under study. Since so few studies have been conducted, our knowledge is limited compared to how well LPT works. Although LPT can help in the efficacy of PRP, PRP as a standalone treatment is still under scrutiny with most critics of PRP coming primarily from European doctors.

Mesotherapy

Mesotherapy for hair loss involves a series of injections into the upper part and sides of the scalp. These injections contain hormones, hyaluronic acid, minerals, medicines, proteins, and plant extracts. The clinician decides the frequency of treatment, but it's usually intensive—weekly procedures for one to two months. After that, sessions become monthly.

Although mesotherapy may help improve hair loss, there's little scientific evidence to back it up.

The field of mesotherapy was founded by French physician Dr. Michel Pistor in 1952. At first, Pistor and other physicians used mesotherapy injections to treat pain, injuries, infections, and vascular diseases. Later, mesotherapy was found to be effective in treating skin conditions, such as wrinkles, fat deposits, stretch marks, and acne. This discovery led to research on the benefits of mesotherapy, including its effects on hair loss. Since vitamins, minerals, medicines, and plant extracts help prevent hair loss, mesotherapy seemed promising.

Supporters of mesotherapy claim it's beneficial in treating hair loss because it enhances blood circulation to the scalp, delivers nutrients to the hair, reduces inflammation, improves scalp immunity, and strengthens hair.

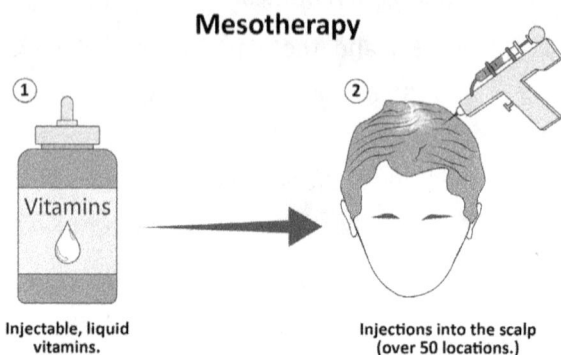

Mesotherapy

① Vitamins — Injectable, liquid vitamins.

② Injections into the scalp (over 50 locations.)

Figure 9.2. Mesotherapy. Multiple injections are delivered to the scalp to stimulate and prevent hair loss. Results vary and mesotherapy is not FDA-cleared.

Studies and Results on Mesotherapy

Some studies claim Mesotherapy helps prevent hair loss, but these results are controversial, since no proper measure of hair loss was documented before-hand. Currently, there's no objective proof that mesotherapy regrows hair.

Yet, despite the lack of evidence, some clinicians still use mesotherapy to prevent hair loss.

What is certain is that the treatment generates a profit for clinicians—an average treatment for hair loss costs between $1,000 and $2,000. And like PRP, this is an off-label treatment since it hasn't been cleared by the FDA.

Mesotherapy and LPT

Again, LPT can help in mesotherapy treatments. The series of injections during a session of mesotherapy can inflame the scalp. Using LPT after a mesotherapy treatment reduces discomfort and inflammation. Because LPT is a proven technique for treating hair loss and growing new hair, it should be used along with mesotherapy to minimize hair loss and ensure hair regrowth. LPT and mesotherapy are not, however, comparable treatments since LPT is an FDA-cleared medical device proven to regrow and retain scalp hair. And considering that an LPT device is much less expensive than mesotherapy treatments, we recommend opting for LPT only!

Dermaroller

A dermaroller is a roller with a few hundred sharp needles (each needle is about 1 mm to 3 mm long) that is rolled back and forth to induce an injury site. Now this is great for superficial wrinkles and to revive old skin for the face, but for hair loss and hair growth, inducing injury sites into the scalp is a futile exercise. The procedure can be somewhat painful and a topical anesthetic can be used to reduce the pain. One advantage is that dermarollers do help ingredients penetrate deeper into the skin. There are presently no ingredients that can be used to stimulate hair growth or stop hair loss, so this procedure is not ideal for the scalp at this time. Unfortunately, there are no clinical studies or evidence that this procedure works for hair loss or hair growth. These devices are sold mostly on the internet and users usually apply this procedure to themselves.

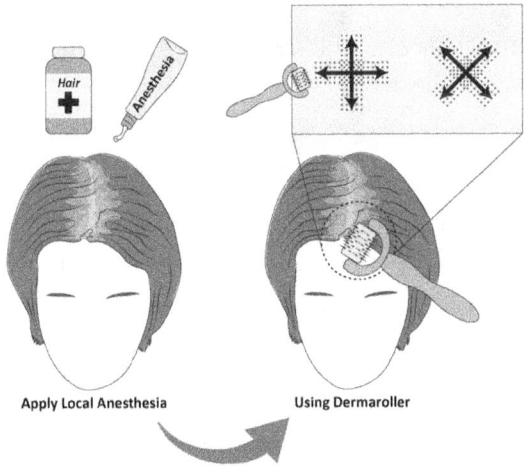

Apply Local Anesthesia   Using Dermaroller

Figure 9.3. Dermaroller. This technique has been popularized by DIY type of users and very few medical clinics offer this service. There are no published studies on the results of a dermaroller procedure for hair growth.

Dermaroller and LPT

We do not recommend dermarolling for hair growth or to prevent hair loss. If you have already chosen this route, LPT can help to reduce the unnecessary inflammation that was created by the dermaroller process. In that process, LPT can generate hair regrowth.

We strongly recommend opting for LPT only!

Hair Cloning: A Future Treatment

There is a very exciting potential hair treatment which is called hair cloning or hair multiplication which has been shown to make some progress. The concept behind hair cloning is simple: It consists of a physician collecting some of your actively growing hair follicles (with stem cells), replicating them in a lab setting, and then reinserting your new active hair follicles (now multiplied) into the parts of your scalp that need more growing hair. Theoretically, this process can generate thousands of identical hair follicles that are technically your hair but without the need to extract them from other parts of your body.

However, this procedure is still very far away from being available to consumers.

The biggest hurdle is growing hair in a lab; this just hasn't been successfully done—yet. There have been some limited successes in mice as recently as 2020 and researchers are still trying to determine the exact scenario in which hair will grow and what is needed for hair to multiply in a petri dish. However, translating these findings into a consistently effective and commercially viable treatment remains a challenge, as researchers continue to grapple with issues such as ensuring the cloned follicles retain their hair-generating properties and the successful integration of these follicles into a patient's scalp. Other potential issues include maintaining proper growth direction, achieving natural density, ensuring consistent results, and addressing potential side effects, as these new hair follicles would constitute a new type of man-made tissue and need plenty of testing.

Once hair cloning is proven viable, the addition of LPT and hair cloning will be a great combination.

Actual Customer Success Stories

A Bang For Your Buck

Claire always made smart choices with her money. When she noticed the beginning of hair loss, her salon suggested she try mesotherapy, the injection of vitamins into the scalp to prevent further hair loss. She trusted her salon and was hopeful. She paid a lot for this procedure over the new few months, but saw no improvement. Hair was still falling out, and now she started to see a bigger gap in her part line. This made her sad, and the thought of the money she was wasting made her even sadder. She finally invested in a wearable laser device, a fraction of the cost of her mesotherapy treatments, and backed by science. The device stopped her hair loss within just three weeks and within three months her part line started to fill back in, making her confident that at last she'd gotten her money's worth.

CHAPTER 10

Debunked Treatment Choices

*"Pessimism: A valuable protection against quackery." —
John Ralston Saul, Writer, 2001*

Home Remedies

Hair loss has been with us since the beginning of human life, so it makes sense that people have devised home remedies. We've all tried home remedies for various ailments. Perhaps you've used parsley to treat a stomachache or vinegar for hiccups with some success. Unfortunately, though, many home cures do not work. And some might be dangerous.

These are not to be confused with health and nutrition (including supplements). A healthy body goes a long way in producing healthy hair. As has already been mentioned, the body will cast off hair as unnecessary when it perceives a need for putting its energy and nutrients elsewhere. So, supplements used correctly, can and are beneficial see Shampoos, Conditioners, Supplements, and LPT.

Let's drill down into some of the more popular home remedies for hair loss.

Concoctions

Concoctions are different mixtures thought to be beneficial for hair. Their successes, however, are based on unfounded theories or personal stories, not clinical trials. Also, concoctions have no standard dosage. Correct drug dosage is vital to getting the results you want without serious side effects. That's why concoctions pose a risk to users. Concoctions used for hair growth may even contain unsafe ingredients. For example, some include compounds that affect the size of blood vessels, which can cause blood pressure to rise or fall suddenly.

The effects of concoctions can be unpredictable. Their safety can't be guaranteed, especially for people with a history of medical conditions. Nor is there any way of telling which concoctions work and which don't as they are not accompanied by any standardized testing.

It's possible that some natural compounds increase hair health, but since there has been no standardization, the therapeutic window is a guess at best. Using a concoction at a lower-than-required concentration could have no effect at all. People who claim success with concoctions often use other hair growth products, like Minoxidil, at the same time. This makes it even more difficult to know whether the concoctions actually work.

Finally, accounts of adverse reactions to concoctions are common. A sore scalp, irritation, inflammation, dryness, and headaches are often reported. Some concoctions may even result in further hair loss.

While only you can weigh the pros and cons of using concoctions for hair loss, it's usually not worth the risk since there are better, safer hair growth options, such as LPT, that have been clinically tested. And some, like our helmet, have FDA clearance. Why risk a bad reaction when you can read documented studies proving the effectiveness and safety of LPT?

Herbal Hair Oils and Plant and Food Extracts

Some claim that herbal agents are effective at treating hair loss. Since herbal solutions are often tested on animals, their effectiveness on human hair loss remains unclear. At the same time, though, we can't ignore the possibility that they may help.

Natural hair loss treatments include apple cider vinegar, rainwater, crude oil, castor oil, rice water, onion brew, garlic, egg yolk, beer, vodka, peppermint and cayenne pepper. Rainwater in a list of hair loss remedies may seem like a joke, yet some people believe that rainwater, along with the other products on the list, is a viable hair loss treatment. One possible advantage of using rainwater is that most rainwater has higher concentrations of ozone (O3), which, as an oxidizer might help cleanse the scalp. In the early 1900s, Nichola Tesla proposed ozone as a treatment for all types of ailments. But no viable product for hair loss or growth ever came out of it.

Since the benefits of these treatments remain unproven, we don't recommend them. You can experiment with drinking rainwater if you want, or you can rely on proven science to fix your hair loss issue.

Headstands or Inversion Tables

Headstands or inversion tables are sometimes proposed for treating hair loss. This is a preposterous idea! Imagine standing on your head or being tied to a table that is upside down to regrow hair. Nevertheless, believers in this method say it increases blood flow to the scalp, but we already know hair loss is not a blood flow issue. They also claim it can grow hair by an inch or two per month.

Apart from the risk of breaking your neck, standing on your head or being strapped to an inversion table are unsuitable methods for people with high blood pressure, heart disease, vertigo, or any other medical issue. And pregnant women should NEVER consider this method.

Inversion tables do seem to be beneficial for back issues, especially if discs in the spine are compressed, in which case they can help relieve some of the pressure. Using an inversion table for backaches makes a lot of sense, since this is an attempt to resolve a mechanical solution but, using an inversion table in hopes of improving hair growth while soothing a backache might not be so effective.

Most importantly, no research has ever been conducted to study the effects of headstands or inversion tables on hair growth.

Ultraviolet (UV) Light Contraptions

Another unfounded belief is that shining UV light on the scalp can improve hair growth. Rife systems use UV light with a high-voltage source: a kind of wand held above the scalp to regrow hair. UV light may improve scalp circulation due to the heat it produces, but hair growth is not dependent on heat (or electricity or electromagnetic fields) reaching the scalp. So, UV light doesn't guarantee hair growth. UV is best used to kill bacteria and other pathogens. In fact, dermatologists use a UV light-emitting device called a Woods lamp to detect fungus on the scalp. Fungal overgrowth is harmful to hair growth and treating the fungus can help your hair.

However, to the best of our knowledge, detecting fungus on the scalp is as far as UV light can go to support hair health.

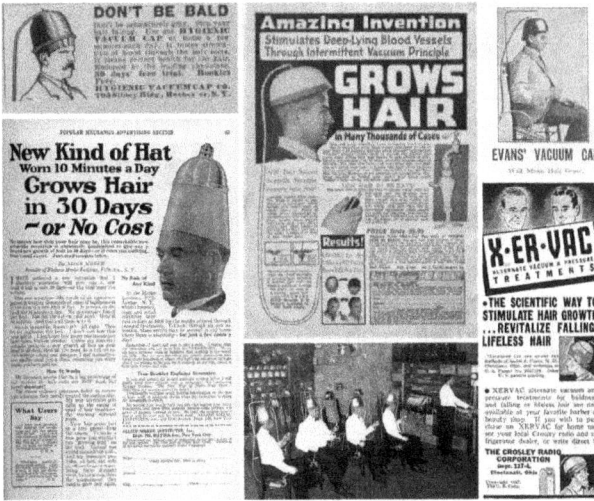

Figure 10.1. Many Early 1900s Solutions for Hair Growth: Of course, none of them worked as this was before there was an FDA overseeing these bogus claims.

In the vast majority of other cases, exposing the scalp to UV light can hurt hair. A 2008 study showed that excessive UVB radiation from the sun can cause the loss of hair protein. So rather than cause hair growth, too much UVB radiation can damage hair cells. Another study revealed that UV exposure can lead to an early hair-shedding phase, promoting telogen effluvium. The research also showed that UV light made pattern hair loss worse.

Overall, UV light is not good for hair. It's even worse than those fake LEDs. You might have heard claims that UV-based devices regrow hair. This is not only scientifically impossible but comes from sellers with absolutely no background in the science of light.

Lasers are the real deal!

Science has come a long way since the Middle Ages, from draining blood out of patients, or even the early 20th century, when hair loss sufferers were encouraged to wear vacuums on their heads. In every society, however, there are scammers out to deceive an uninformed public. That's as true of those selling vacuum caps as of those peddling RIFE systems.

Bioelectrical and RF (Radio Frequency) Gadgets

There have been multiple new attempts to use different technologies to stimulate the hair follicles, which I will collectively summarize here. One of these new technologies is RF frequency, which has been attempted for a variety of aesthetic applications like skin tightening and rejuvenation. Almost all of these devices, however, failed to show any real results. Some companies are trying to apply the same concept to hair loss and hair growth. Unfortunately, the basis of the technology and the effectiveness is still unproven.

Another type of gadget on the market now are bioelectric stem cell devices, which target the stem cells of the hair follicles. Unfortunately, bioelectrical signals are different stimulation types than light is being marketed to stimulate stem cells. The scientific fact is that is our body's stem cells have been proven to be stimulated with light and at different wavelengths. There is no research that has shown that stem cells react to electrical stimulation. The amount of electrical signals (whether RF or bioelectric) has never been shown to work specifically for certain human structures, let alone hair follicles. Stem cell stimulation has been around for nearly sixty years, and very little has been produced in terms of FDA-cleared solutions in the marketplace—in fact, there have been zero bioelectric stem cell devices to date cleared by the FDA. The fact is that these RF or bioelectrical devices are very far from receiving FDA clearances, as there is absolutely no clinical proof that they work. My advice is to always stick with FDA-cleared laser-based solutions.

Actual Customer Success Stories

The Secret

When Frank's wife, running her hand through his hair, suggested he'd developed a thin patch, he wasn't laughing. He wasn't ready to get old. But he hated going to the doctor—why should he, there was nothing wrong with him! Nevertheless, he tried unlikely cures—an ultraviolet wand he found online, an inversion table to channel blood to his head. The failure of these made him feel worse about himself than ever. His friend noticed Frank was down and asked him what was wrong. Frank told him, and his friend laughed. He said he had the same problem before and told Frank about a laser treatment for hair. Frank tried it for himself, with great results. Now Frank loves it when his wife touches his hair. .

CHAPTER 11

And the Undisputed Champion Is . . .

"I don't ask for much in the world—only the best, and there's so little of that." — Michael Arlen, Essayist, 1939

. . . The Four-Pronged Approach

Ultimately, the solution to hair growth revolves around minimizing hair loss and maximizing hair growth. Conditions such as pattern hair loss, telogen effluvium, and alopecia areata have one thing in common: They all promote hair loss and reduce hair growth. Once there's a tilt toward hair loss, more hair shedding, and loss follow. To promote sustained hair growth, I propose a four-pronged approach involving LPT to maximize hair growth, the right hair care to minimize hair loss, and the *effective* use of supplements.

The truth is that not one single thing is the magic bullet, as various factors, such as genetics, fungus, hormones, and medical conditions can contribute to hair loss. We have discovered that having a system-based solution is needed to regrow hair successfully.

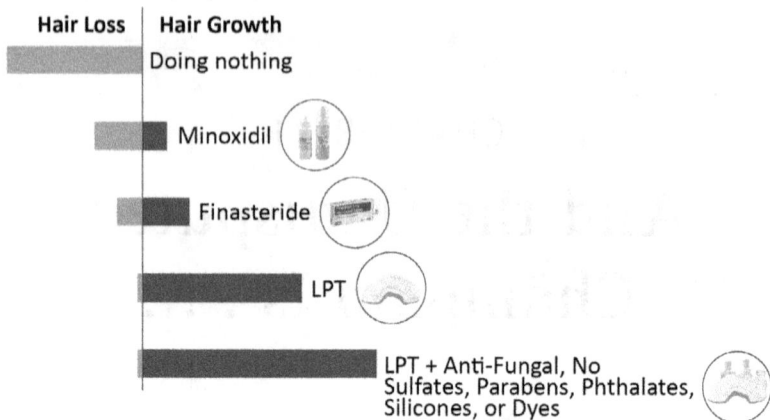

Figure 11.1. Factors That Can Affect Hair Loss and Hair Growth: Doing nothing just increases hair loss and using Minoxidil and Finasteride is not as effective as LPT plus medicated topicals and supplements.

1. Maximizing Hair Growth with the Right Kind of Lasers

Since we already know the best approach to increasing hair growth is the use of LPT, the real question is what kind of lasers work *best*? As not all lasers are created the same. Once our researchers felt they knew the answer, we crafted an LPT device to provide the perfect depth and coverage. We also used cold lasers to minimize any possible safety issues.

Allowing a device that pumps trillions of photons per treatment, we had to be very cautious about where the lasers were sourced and where they were manufactured. The lasers must be engineered to penetrate the scalp to a depth of 3–5 mm and deliver the right amount of energy to the base of the hair follicles. This allows hair cells to absorb the energy they need to grow into healthy follicles. With a wavelength optimized for hair growth, the helmet also ensures that new hair is born with a healthier, longer hair growth cycle.

We then moved on to prove their helmet was the best. Two studies compared our LPT laser helmet with other hair growth devices that claimed to regrow hair. The results showed that the laser hair loss helmet was proven to regrow hair in the majority of users. In addition, researchers reported a substantial increase in hair thickness, volume, and density after twenty-six weeks. The other devices, however, produced negligible results.

The downside of any LPT device is that it's bound by a single rule we can't break: You must be losing hair to regrow it. In cases where hair follicles are already lost due to terminal-stage male and female pattern hair loss, LPT shows reduced effects. So, if you are losing hair but not suffering from a terminal stage of male and female pattern hair loss, ask yourself: Would I be interested in a device that offers regrowth of hair follicles and more thickness, volume, and density in just six months?

It's not much of a gamble, especially when LPT is backed by more clinical proof than any other medical device or drug to date. And it's the first device to receive FDA clearance for in-home use for hair rejuvenation. It's so safe and effective you can sit on your couch watching TV and regrow your hair in just six months through the power of laser technology.

Welcome to the future!

2. Minimizing Hair Loss with Proper Hair Care

There are things you can do (and avoid doing) to keep your hair healthy and minimize hair loss. When it comes to shampoos and conditioners, for example, the best ones can improve hair health without harming your hair. But it's up to you to choose the ones with the right ingredients. Shampoo can control dandruff as well as wash away dirt and oils, making it easier for nutrients to filter into the scalp. Similarly, conditioners, especially those without sulfur, silicones, or preservatives, can help maintain hair health. They can untangle your hair, making brushing easier and giving hair a smooth, silky look.

Actions, especially habitual ones, play a key role in hair loss. Playing with, brushing, pulling, ruffling, or merely touching hair can weaken it if it's already struggling. Hairstyling practices, especially those involving heat, can damage hair too. Extreme caution should be taken when performing these activities. Being extra careful with your hair can prevent further loss. Lastly, something we haven't addressed yet is using high-quality water sources. It's essential for maintaining healthy hair and preventing further hair loss, as impurities and harsh chemicals found in poor water sources can damage hair follicles, weaken hair strands, and disrupt the scalp's natural balance.

3. Effective Use of Supplements

Using supplements is most effective when a medical professional identifies a deficiency. The use of clinically unproven supplements, however, is not recommended. For instance, research doesn't support the use of biotin to improve hair growth.

Similarly, certain well-known drugs, when taken regularly, can promote hair health. Vitamin D, curcumin, quercetin, and saw palmetto may also help promote healthy hair and maybe even hair growth, but we need more evidence to be certain.

4. LPT – Laser Phototherapy

The consistent use of the right LPT device, as discussed thoroughly below, is your best bet for both improving hair growth and slowing hair loss! Continue to Chapter 12 to learn all about the most effective LPT therapy for your hair.

Use the Best—Ignore the Rest

We all know we should pick the right tool for the right job, but to do that we need to know what jobs need to be done and which tools are most effective. When it comes to hair, you need to maximize growth, minimize loss, and avoid making things worse. The four-pronged approach outlined above is the best way to ensure hair growth because it emphasizes LPT, which maximizes hair growth, includes guidance to minimize hair loss and discourages the use of ineffective supplements.

Actual Customer Success Stories

Simply Special

Ella felt that at thirty-nine years old, she was too young to accept hair loss. She didn't know women her age could have this problem and didn't want to believe it. Methodically, she explored various solutions, from over-the-counter potions to potent prescriptions. Her hair loss slowed, but she didn't like the idea of taking pills forever. With mixed feelings, she decided not to pay for any more pills, and to try laser therapy and less damaging shampoos and conditioners, avoiding SLS and sulfates. She started to take nutrients like Curcumin and Quercetin that boosted her from the inside out. Soon she saw new baby hairs growing. Within months friends and family were commenting on the change. She wished she had taken a more natural and holistic approach from the start.

CHAPTER 12

Laser Phototherapy and Laser Phototherapy Devices

"Excellence is never an accident. It is always the result of high intention, sincere effort, and intelligent execution; it represents the wise choice of many alternatives."
— Aristotle, Philosopher, 4th Century BCE.

Laser Phototherapy and Laser Phototherapy Devices

Understanding LPT Devices

By now you understand how LPT can stop hair loss and promote hair growth. You've also learned about the characteristics of light and how it can target hair cells and bring about hair growth. Yet this book won't fully achieve its purpose if it fails to do one crucial thing: provide you with the information you need to make the best choice in selecting a laser phototherapy device and how to use laser phototherapy for maximum benefit.

You should not only have the right knowledge, but you should also be motivated to use LPT to improve your hair growth and to stop or slow hair loss. In this chapter, I'll show you how to select the most suitable LPT device for you, what to expect, and how to ensure it's working. LPT is based on physics, but don't let that scare you. This chapter is dedicated to teaching you what you need to know about laser devices without a single math equation!

The Consumer Buying Curve for Laser Phototherapy

Let's start with the three categories into which consumers can be divided when faced with new technologies in the marketplace (there are really five, but we can condense them into three for the sake of simplicity).

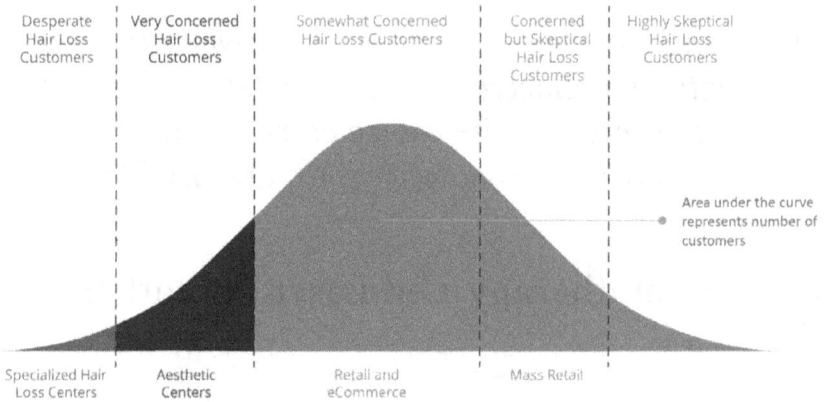

Figure 12.1. Customers Worried about Hair Loss and Where They Go to Look for Solutions. As LPT is introduced into the mainstream marketplace, more awareness and more people will adopt this solution in the near future.

If one looks at this as a graph, consumers look like a standard curve graph. The figure above is based on the evolution of LPT and hair loss—you will see that desperate hair loss customers will try almost anything with potential promise for stopping hair loss and regrowing hair. They try new devices/technologies. The next group is very concerned. The somewhat concerned group of hair loss customers represents the bulk of the customers. The concerned and highly skeptical customers will be the last to try any new devices or drugs without either doing a lot of research or consulting with a hair professional.

The category made up of people who are somewhat curious won't get their feet wet, so to speak, until they get more proof. They'll wait until others have gone first before they invest their hard-earned dollars in new innovations. They're a little more skeptical and a bit behind the other adopters. These folks will think about how a technology might improve their lives but, for various reasons, won't act on those thoughts. They prefer to watch what's going on from a distance.

In the third category are the doubters. They're overwhelmed by risks and are unwilling to change their minds. Doubters are too busy playing it safe to see the possibilities in anything new and dislike change of any kind. They rarely get what they're after since they miss out on the benefits that come with the latest innovations. They won't try something new until they see everyone else is doing it, and even then, they might still be apprehensive. Their entry point into the market is usually when the device is offered at a great price—they won't buy it based on its merits alone.

Most consumers fall into the mid and late majority groups. That is why it takes so long for an innovation to be fully integrated into the marketplace—that is, for consumers in all three categories to become regular customers. A good example is the way the smartphone entered the marketplace. Many people didn't switch from their outdated cell phones to smartphones until the right features and plans were offered.

LPT, although not new (remember our conversation about the history of LPT in Chapter 1), it is still considered "revolutionary," yet it is the right treatment for the scalp when hair loss is involved. We've proven that in the previous chapters. Remember, the goal of LPT is to stimulate the two most important areas deep in your scalp, the bulge and the papilla. Only a laser with the right wavelength and dosage can accomplish this. Don't let anyone convince you otherwise. However, emitting energy in the form of photons into the scalp is not something that should be undertaken lightly since living tissue is very complex. The light must be absorbed by the scalp, referred to as the First Law of Photochemistry. Without getting into any physics, all this law says is that a cell must receive the right type of light in order to get stimulated. A good analogy is that one must receive money to spend money. So, if a cell does not receive any light, it won't be affected, and harder to reach areas deep into the scalp require the strongest type of light possible. This is an important concept to understand as we discuss this section.

Selecting the Right Product

Since laser phototherapy is delivered by a device, it must be the right one. This is the sticking point for many potential customers. Which device should you choose?

The "right" laser device depends on many factors, some of which are obvious. Not all lasers for LPT devices are created equal. The laser must have the right amount of power to stimulate hair growth. The lasers must have the right wavelength. The right amount of energy must be delivered over the right length of time. The laser must be positioned properly in relation to the scalp; it must have appropriate divergence angle and heat production.

There are also less obvious factors that must be considered including where the device was made and who made it.

Let's discuss all these nuances so you can understand them and make an informed decision to choose the best device.

Clinical Studies and LPT Devices

To avoid buying a laser device that doesn't work, it's a good idea to look at the available evidence, especially evidence that comes from scientific trials. Unfortunately, many laser devices aren't tested on humans, or if they are, the results aren't readily available. This makes it difficult to tell whether the device serves the purpose for which it has been designed. Manufacturers often use the FDA 510k process to submit their devices so they can get cleared for selling, but never test them to prove they work so the general public will fully understand the capabilities and limitations of a product.

To fully understand the benefit of a product, clinical trials must be randomized (e.g., picking truly random patients), multi-centered (e.g., not relying on one clinic or physician), double-blinded (e.g., no one knows which devices are given to patients), and sham-controlled (e.g., need to have a sham (placebo) to fully test device). This helps ensure that all the test centers get the same results from the trial. Otherwise, manufacturers can skew results to their benefit and it can be hard to tell whether the device serves the intended purpose. There's nothing worse than spending money on something that doesn't work or worse yet, on something that was not properly clinically-tested.

Make sure the LPT device you choose has performed a clinical trial on human subjects, and that the results are published and available online. In the clinical studies, it will be revealed whether all participants benefited from using an LPT device and if they experienced either a slowing of hair loss, a doubling of hair follicle size, or new hair growth. Make sure you do your due diligence and pay attention to the information that is available.

We've conducted clinical trials on our LPT helmets and the results of the studies occurred in three phases. In the first phase, which occurred between the fourth and the eighteenth week, the helmet slowed the rate of hair loss. In the second phase, from week eighteen to twenty-six, existing hair was thickened. In the final phase, between weeks twenty-six and fifty-two, our LPT device use resulted in new hair growth.

As with most studies, individual results can vary and are based on several original components. These can include the initial stage of someone's hair loss, their present health and/or underlying medical conditions, and genetics. The bottom line is that 100% of all the participants in the trial experienced renewed hair growth when compared to a sham (LED based device). That's something to brag about!

The Internet of Misinformation

Surf the internet a bit, and you'll see there are countless websites and articles on LLLT or LPT and hair loss and hair growth. The issue is that no one has been regulating the misinformation about LPT, LEDs and red light in general—not even the FDA! That's why I wrote this book. There is so much content about LPT online that this book is attempting to be the gold standard for differentiating between science and misinformation.

Unfortunately, as I've shown you, websites that come from unscrupulous manufacturers or uninformed marketers provide information that is not only wrong but can actually make things worse for someone suffering from hair loss.

There are many myths and false claims associated with LLLT/LED manufacturers and the false information does not only stop with these light-based devices; it continues with shampoos, conditioners, and supplements. This misinformation further affects one's ability to combat hair loss. Over the years, the number of hair loss cures and miracle treatments has been marred by dubious claims, ineffective products, and false promises, often leaving those seeking genuine solutions with very little hope. That is why it is so important to have trials and protocols in place.

The FDA Process and Clinical Trial Protocols for LPT

Getting a new medical product cleared by the FDA requires passing a series of scientific trials under strictly ethical supervision. Human trials receive the highest level of attention to ensure the safety of every volunteer. Tests include double-blind studies.

In double-blind studies, the method is very simple: nobody knows who is getting which device, real or fake. Not even the physician giving the patient the device knows which device they are giving the patient.

The patients who participate in these trials might be wearing a device that uses laser light, or a device that simply doesn't work. These fake devices are called sham devices, just like the placebos (e.g., sugar pills) used by the pharma industry. These sham devices are usually helmet devices, but are outfitted with red LEDs so neither the clinical investigators conducting the trial nor the patient can differentiate between a real LPT device and a sham device. To claim that something works, testing should include as many of each type of participants as possible, ensuring that an equal number of participants are receiving either a real device or a sham device.

In 2017, a systematic review examined the use of low-level light therapy in treating androgenetic alopecia. The researchers conducted eleven randomized control trials on 680 patients (444 men and 236 women). Most of the patients experienced increased hair growth and thickness. They were also happier about the way they looked. We've proven this time and again in another 160 experiments.

Since Dr. Endre Mester first observed that low-intensity lasers could generate hair growth in mice, lasers have significantly improved. Today, many laser hair growth devices are available. You can erase lingering doubts you may have by looking at the proof of the effectiveness of laser phototherapy. The research is freely available online and I have provided every reference in the Bibliography and Appendix in the back of this book. You can search the papers and read as much as you'd like.

Clinical trials of laser phototherapy (LPT) show clear improvement in hair growth. Researchers believe LPT stimulates cells in the bulge and induces hair follicles to enter their growth phase.

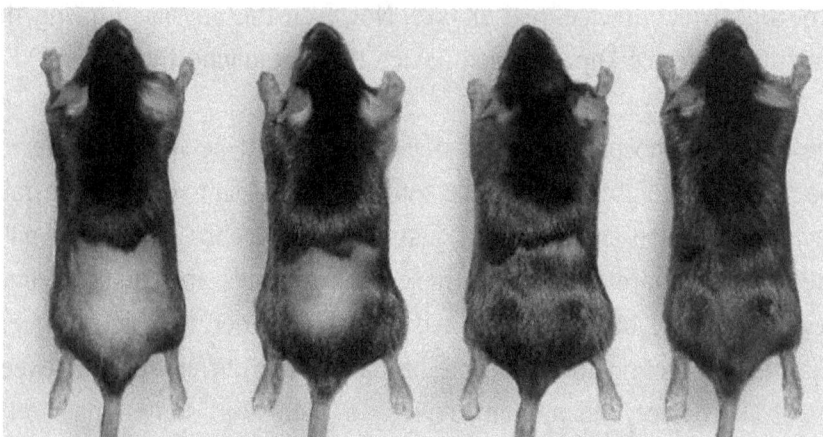

Figure 12.2. Laser Hair Growth in Mice. Dr. Mester's mice photos show from left to right the progression of hair growth when laser phototherapy is applied on their shaven backs.

FDA Clearance vs. FDA Approval

People often mistakenly interchange the words "FDA-cleared" with "FDA-approved." And guess what? The term "FDA-approved" isn't even correct!

To clear up any confusion, let's time travel back to 1976 and examine the Medical Device Amendments to the Federal Food, Drug, and Cosmetic Act (FDA). Three classes of medical devices were created based on their potential risk level to an individual's health. While Class I devices pose a minimal threat, Class II and Class III devices are capable of posing moderate to serious health risks to their users. Regardless of their classes, all medical devices, such as hair growth laser helmets, need to be registered with the FDA. How a manufacturer chooses to do so depends on the purposes of their device, or whether similar equipment already exists on the market.

Class I devices, such as examination gloves, and Class II devices, such as laser hair restoration devices, all require a 510(k)-submission form before they can be legally marketed. The FDA does not "approve" medical devices 510(k) submissions but clears them. It is, therefore, illegal to market any 510(k)-cleared device, like a hair growth laser phototherapy device as "FDA-approved," especially since this terminology is completely erroneous.

So, what about Class III devices? Since these have the potential to harm a person's health with serious impact (such as life-sustaining technology or physiological implants), a PMA (Premarket Approval Application) must be submitted before marketing a Class III device. Adequate and well-controlled clinical trials need to be performed to demonstrate that it is 1) safe and 2) effective. Brand new or significantly modified medical devices that are considered high risk require an approved PMA to demonstrate safety and effectiveness. To quote the FDA, "An approved Premarket Approval Application (PMA) is, in effect, a private license granted to the applicant for marketing a particular medical device." In other words, this device can now be legally marketed as "PMA-approved," although this terminology is not really used.

Notice how we just said "PMA-approved" and not "FDA-approved?" That's because once again, there is no such thing as "FDA approval." There is only a PMA form that won't be approved without a series of successful clinical trials.

There was so much confusion about FDA-cleared vs. FDA-approved that this subject was presented to the Federal Supreme Court. The final ruling was that FDA clearance does indicate a medical device is regarded as safe and effective.

Hopefully, you are now informed well enough that you can win any round of trivia having to do with the FDA, medical devices, and laser hair restoration helmets. So next time you hear a friend, relative, or even a stranger in the street toss around FDA terminology inaccurately, please feel free to interject and correct them with your newfound knowledge!

How Does FDA Clearance Affect Me?

To protect people from false claims and dangerous medical equipment, the United States requires rigorous testing, which includes laboratory and clinical trials to prove both safety and effectiveness. Data derived from these studies must meet specific requirements and be submitted to the FDA for review. Only after gaining clearance—the acknowledgment that the device is safe and effective for public sale—is an FDA clearance granted to the manufacturers of a medical device. This clearance allows consumers to distinguish between true and false claims about a product's safety and effectiveness.

The majority of the countries abroad, follow the guidelines of FDA clearance and use this as their basis to allow medical devices into their country. Therefore, getting FDA clearance is the first step in the process, and if one wants to go to other countries to market their devices, they will need at a minimum FDA clearance and whatever additional documentation those countries require.

It's very important that any device you consider buying is FDA-cleared. I advise you to visit the FDA.gov website to check for a product's FDA-compliance status before reaching a decision.

FDA clearance letters for any LPT product can be found on the FDA website.

Five Factors for Finding the Perfect Fit: Selecting a Device

This is the most important part of the book, understanding why and how each of these attributes is critical. So, let's dig deep and look at the five factors you should consider when selecting a device.

The best way to represent these five important design factors is called a radar chart (see Figure 12.3 below). This is a simple graphic that clearly shows each of them. This type of graphic and technique is used in the automotive industry, for example, when a supercar manufacturer like Ferrari designs their next generation of models. In car design, the five key attributes the engineering team might need to consider when aiming to build the best car in the world might be handling, chassis, suspension, powertrain, and aerodynamics. In an LPT device, they are wavelength, heat management, beam width, dosage, and scalp penetration, as shown in the chart below.

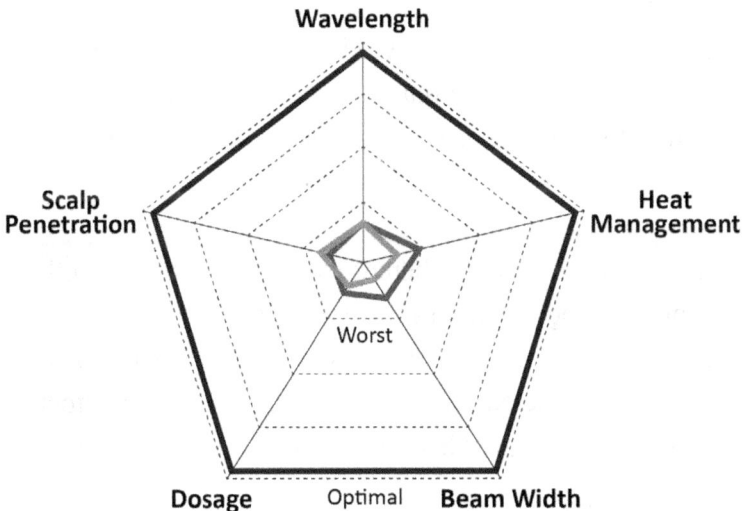

Figure 12.3. These are the five most important attributes of an LPT device. This chart is a great tool for designing a perfect device. The goal is to maximize each of the attributes so the device will be optimal.

I'll go over each factor and explain why it's crucial in selecting the right LPT product. The goal of this radar chart is to put the key attributes on the furthest outermost point for each of the five points—this is considered optimal design. The center of the pentagon is the worst place to have the attribute.

1. Wavelength

Let's start with the most important attribute: wavelength. Laser treatments must have the capacity to penetrate the scalp all the way to the hair follicle. This involves using the correct type of device, at the right wavelength, and with enough power. It's so important to know the quality of hair growth lasers. It is far more important than "how many" lasers are in a device. For example, our VL680 lasers, are made in the US and have a wavelength of 680 nm (nanometers). This stimulates the hair follicles 2.5 times more than lasers with a wavelength of 650 nm. That's only thirty more nanometers but it makes a huge difference. In the Bibliography at the end, there is a reference to a paper from T. Karu (the most cited LPT researcher), which explains why 680 nm has more absorption into human tissue than 650 nm. This means faster and much better results for keeping hair and growing it back. Remember—quality over quantity.

Lasers emit monochromatic coherent light, meaning a perfectly aligned single-color wavelength. It makes them ideal for many medical treatments including hair follicles which only respond to particular wavelengths of light. Because the coherence of laser light keeps the energy focused and the beam narrow, they are ideal for stimulating hair growth.

However, many laser devices and low-level light therapy devices don't use 680 nm because they use cheap lasers made for the consumer electronics industry. Consequently, they have very little effect on stimulating hair growth. What is worse is that when the wrong wavelength is used, 635 nm–655 nm, hair shedding will occur. That is the wavelength of LLLT devices and one of their side effects, especially at the beginning!

I can't stress enough how important it is for you to be aware of wavelength and not be duped into an ineffective or inferior product.

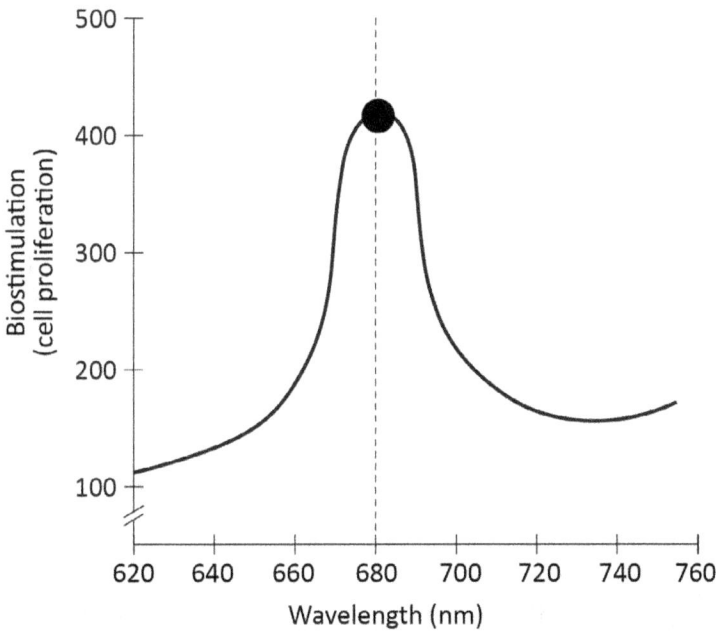

Figure 12.4. The Importance of Laser Wavelength on Biostimulation. The wavelength of 680 nm has been scientifically proven to be the perfect color for hair growth. Any other wavelength used does not have the same type of results.

Some LLLT devices combine LEDs with consumer grade lasers, and some LLLT devices only use LEDs and not lasers of any kind. The fact is that LEDs are simply not powerful enough to have a therapeutic effect on hair growth. LEDs are neither monochromatic nor coherent. They cannot target the very specific wavelength needed to reach hair follicles. LEDs' wavelengths are very wide, and even though some vendors suggest a 680 nm LED is the same as a 680 nm laser, this is not true or accurate. LEDs range from 600 nm to nearly 690 nm, which means very low light will reach the scalp, if any. This makes them useless when it comes to hair restoration. You may as well use a flashlight for all the benefits you'll get.

It must be strictly lasers with a specific dosage, as close to 680 nm as possible. This wavelength will penetrate the scalp and deliver measurable energy 5 mm below the scalp where the hair follicle resides. The scalp is like a sponge and, like a sponge absorbing water, the laser starts out very strong—but, by the time it reaches the bulge at 5 mm, there is only a tiny fraction of penetration. Therefore, it is important that the light is coherent and has the right strength. The longer the wavelength, the deeper the penetration, and deeper penetration is necessary to stop hair loss and stimulate hair growth. Less than 680 nm will not produce the desired result.

2. Scalp Penetration

The concept of scalp penetration is centered around how to get photons down to the papilla and bulge of the hair follicle. This depends on the wavelength and amount of laser energy applied to the scalp. When laser light hits the scalp, three things might happen: It might be reflected, absorbed, or transmitted.

The amount of reflection is based on how shiny the scalp is, so avoiding lotions, creams, and other topicals that make the scalp more reflective is key here. The ability for the laser light to be absorbed is based on the wavelength, laser energy, skin color, and beam width of the laser light. Considering these factors in designing, selecting, and using an LPT device is crucial. In Chapter 1, we discussed how laser light is similar to a syringe and the needle of the syringe is essentially the laser light. Nothing else can penetrate the scalp like laser light, or syringe in this example.

The optimum distance light must travel into the scalp is between 3 mm and 5 mm as hair follicles are located at various depths throughout the scalp. The terminal hairs are the deepest in the scalp, sometimes reaching beyond 5 mm. By the time laser light reaches 5 mm, the level of light is a fraction of what it was above the scalp. The deeper the light penetrates human tissue, the less light will reach the deepest part of the dermis. An LPT device has to have a lot of power on top of the scalp by the time it reaches the hair follicle since over 99% of the power will be lost in the dermis. Therefore, it is critical to get the maximum wavelength, maximum dosage, and the smallest beam width so light will reach the furthest possible point without causing heat buildup. This concept is pure science.

3. Dosage

Laser phototherapy only works if an optimal dosage of energy is absorbed by the base of the hair follicles. Any laser phototherapy device that fails to do this isn't worth your time or money. The trick is not to use too much or too little. The dosage needs to meet the therapeutic window. For hair loss, we already know the dosage. It's based on the Arndt-Schultz graph (Figure 12.5). Every drug company in the world bases its medication dosage on this graph. Laser phototherapy is medicine for the hair.

Every ailment has a recommended dosage; for example, the amount of acetaminophen recommended for minor aches and pain is 325 mg–500 mg, sufficient for common ailments occurring every four hours. For more serious ailments, physicians can recommend up to 1,000 mg. Usually, more than 6,500 mg in a day is not recommended, just like it is not recommended to get more than 10 joules/cm of LPT treatments.

The same applies to laser phototherapy. We measure dosage for light as joules per square centimeter. The optimum dosage for hair is 7 j/cm^2. Please note that unlike acetaminophen or other medications, which automatically target aches and pains or reduce fever anywhere in the body when ingested, LPT does not automatically reach hair follicles. It is necessary to directly point to the area of concern.

As I mentioned previously, the Arndt-Schulz graph (below) is used for all types of dosage-based applications in pharmaceutical industries as well as laser phototherapy. This graph shows, in the area labeled A, that if nothing is given (for example, no aspirin), then nothing will happen in terms of biological reaction. As one increases the dosage to B, a biological reaction begins. Maximum recommended dosage is reached at point C (1,000 mg for aspirin for example or 10 joules/cm^2 for LPT). At point D, when too much dosage is taken, a negative reaction starts to occur. Dosage beyond E will cause damage to biological tissue.

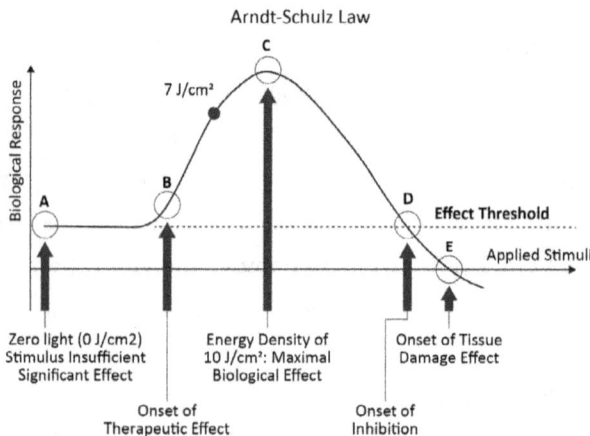

Figure 12.5. The Arndt-Schulz Graph. This graph shows how tissue are affected with different doses of light to better understand the relationship. Seven J/cm^2 is the ideal dosage for hair growth.

Hair follicles are deep below the surface and, therefore, restoring them requires the right penetration and a precise dose of energy. A fascinating thing happens when an optimal dosage of energy is absorbed by the mitochondria of hair cells—light energy changes into chemical energy by a process called biostimulation. Once hair cells are revived, the scalp retains the hair, and new hair can grow. That's why we need to know the energy dosage of an LPT device. Without it, we can't ensure biostimulation is taking place, and the goal of LPT is biostimulation.

Yet, what does this dosage mean in regard to time? When laser light is applied for about twenty minutes, the mitochondria are revived. Picture a shrinking hair follicle that has no energy and is dying. Zoom in with an imaginary microscope, and you'll see that it's the mitochondria, which make up a cell's powerhouse, that are no longer working properly.

In about twenty minutes, light energy is converted into chemical energy (biostimulation/the medicine), which reverses hair miniaturization (when weakened hair follicles produce shorter and more delicate strands of hair).

The reason twenty minutes is important, and not four seconds, ninety seconds, six minutes or even thirty minutes, is because twenty minutes is how long it takes for trillions of photons to stimulate all of the structures from the surface of the scalp to the very bottom of each hair follicle. Too little time will not be useful and too long of a time will cause over-stimulation which will not be useful for hair restoration.

Although low doses can still provide minimal benefits, higher doses are needed for hair restoration. You need between six joules per cm^2 and 9 joules per cm^2 to see hair growth with laser phototherapy. When the energy dosage goes above this range, it becomes harmful to the hair follicles. Knowing and obtaining a device with the correct dosage is essential for regrowing hair. Since we've covered wavelength and dosage, let's move on to power density.

4. Beam Width

The width of a laser is critical since the smaller the beam width, the deeper a laser can penetrate the scalp. Lasers have coherence, which means that the photons are all aligned—unlike other light sources, like LEDs, flashlights, and even the sun.

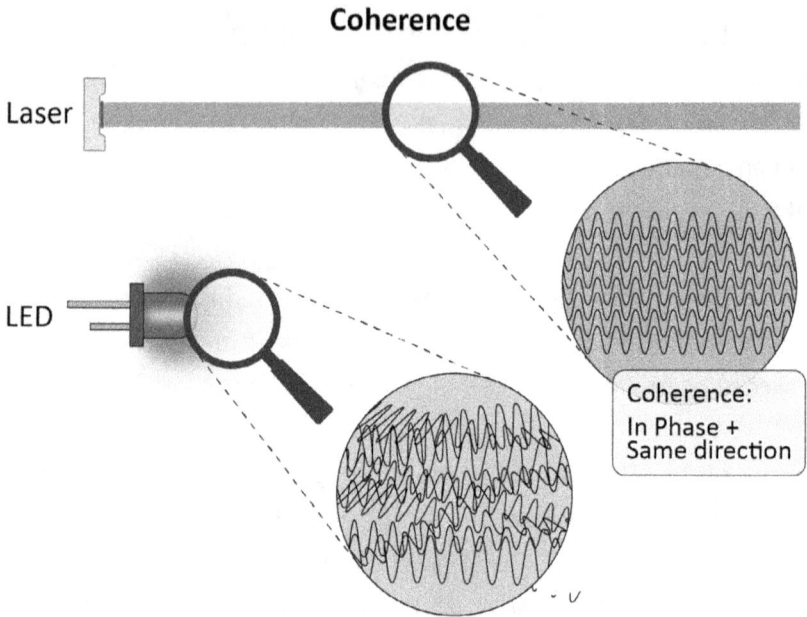

Coherence

Laser

LED

Coherence:
In Phase +
Same direction

Figure 12.6. Coherence vs. Non-Coherence. Lasers have beams of light that go in the same direction and that are necessary to enter thick tissue like scalp. LEDs cannot focus due to being non-coherent and not used for hair growth.

If someone wants to dig a hole for a fence post, which is usually about twelve inches wide and two feet deep, a post-hole digger designed to dig small deep holes in dirt would be the best tool to choose. Choosing a three-foot-wide snow shovel with a flat end wouldn't be very productive. Using a wide beam with no ability to get below the scalp's surface will not produce any hair rejuvenation results either. The goal is to get as deep as possible in the scalp using a narrow beam to provide the right amount of dosage and introduce the right wavelength to the hair follicles.

We use the term power density, which means the amount of power produced by a laser beam over a 1 cm^2 area. So, the smaller the beam the greater the dosage. The wider the beam the lower the power density.

The power density used for laser phototherapy varies for each device. A laser device should treat all scalp areas during one convenient session. As we know, the optimal time for this treatment is twenty minutes to guarantee an optimal dosage of energy is absorbed by the hair follicles.

Another term for LPT is energy density or fluence, which is the product of power and time. So, the longer you can keep a laser on a spot, the higher the energy delivered to that particular area. Therefore, a powerful laser produces higher energy in a short amount of time. Powerful lasers are effective and deliver the required results in less time. Only a few of the different types of laser devices available meet these criteria.

5. Heat Management

An overlooked factor that can affect the results of LPT is the physical design of the laser device and how this affects heat management. The device must cover the entire scalp area affected by hair loss to get the best outcome. The issue is that lasers love cool ambient temperatures. Their favorite environment would be working inside of a cold refrigerator since lasers normally run very hot internally. The top of the human head is already at 98.6 °F, which is way too warm for lasers. A properly designed LPT device must have cooling to reduce the heat generated from the dozens and dozens of laser diodes all running at the same time.

Electronics use different techniques to cool their components, and the challenge is to avoid using a cooling fan which would consume energy as well as be tricky to implement in a small space such as a helmet design. In addition, fans sometimes get a bit noisy over time.

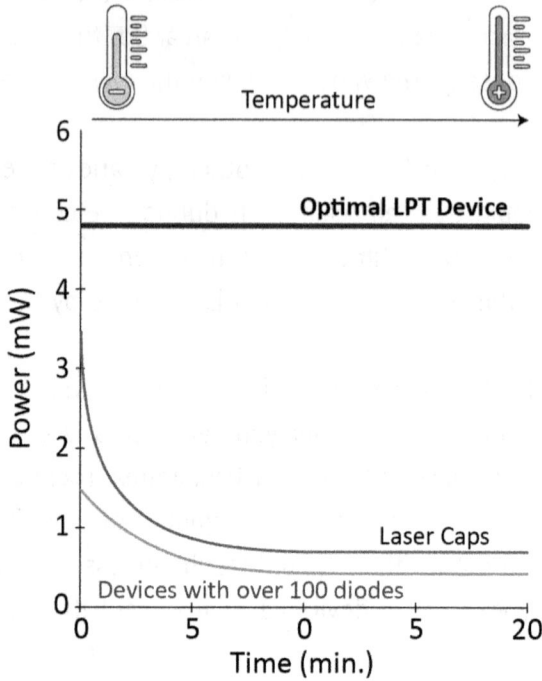

Figure 12.7. Heat output during a twenty-minute treatment session shows that the laser output drops significantly within the first twenty minutes with laser caps that trap heat inside.

Remember, lasers create heat and heat is the enemy of electronics as well as the hair and scalp. In addition, each laser diode must have a heat sink to help cool the laser diodes. Without heat sinks and ventilation, these devices can increase the scalp temperature considerably and burn scalps or cause telogen effluvium. We certainly don't want to use a product that is going to cause even more hair loss.

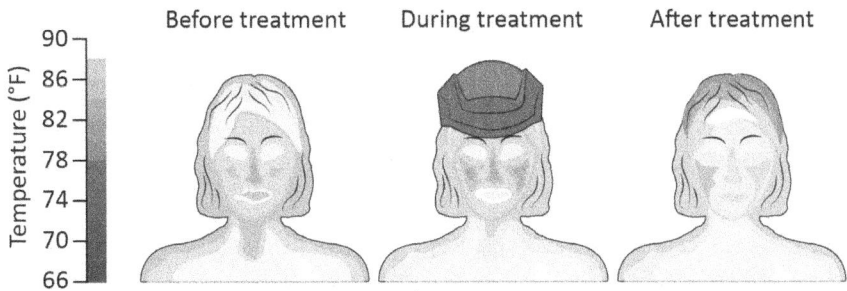

Figure 12.8. Thermal imaging shows that wearing an LPT device before treatment and after treatment results in minimal heat levels on the scalp after a twenty-minute treatment.

As the law of phototherapy tells us, light must be absorbed by the scalp before you get the results you're after. So, a laser device that doesn't jumpstart the hair follicles won't be helpful. Yet, we don't want to harm or burn your scalp!

Laser Sources and FDA-Registered Facilities

Knowing the quality of the hair growth lasers, as I've mentioned, is far more important than knowing how many lasers are in a given device. For example, VL680 lasers, are made in the US and are specifically designed for LPT hair applications. Other lasers and LEDs sourced by all other competitors are used for consumer applications such as DVDs, CDs, and laser pointer applications.

Where laser devices are manufactured impacts their quality and how well they work. Some laser-device producers outsource the production process to places where quality is not assured, workers aren't skilled, and conditions do not assure that quality is implemented into the manufacturing process. This can lead to the use of substandard components. For example, many laser device manufacturing companies don't have staff who know enough about physics to understand the light parameters that produce hair growth. In this case, the device's power, energy, and wavelength may be inappropriate. In other cases, cheap parts are used to make laser devices to increase profit margins, which may put users in harm's way. This is why many of the devices that are sourced from abroad have warnings about excessive hair loss due to massive tolerances not being optimal for hair applications.

Our LPT device is made in the United States with proprietary and customized lasers that penetrate the scalp for maximum follicle stimulation. The laser helmet operates at the proven wavelength for regrowing hair, 680 nm, no other LPT device in the world operates at 680 nm. This is more than any other at-home laser hair growth device. We are the only laser hair growth company that produces its devices in Silicon Valley, California. Other companies buy their lasers from Asia using Edge Emitting Lasers (EEL, which are laser pointer class gadgets). There are no US manufacturers of EEL's in the United States or Europe. The only wavelength Asia makes available is 630 nm to 650 nm. This limitation causes many issues with hair loss and hair growth damaging the reputation of LPT and giving it a bad name. The longer 680 nm wavelength has been clinically proven to produce deeper penetration of red light to the papilla and the bulge, the two areas crucial for hair growth.

Do you want a laser that is specifically designed for stopping and regrowing your hair? Or do you want to use just any light source that was never even designed for the human body and medical applications? All laser-device manufacturers have different production standards, and these standards affect the quality of the LPT outcome.

You took your time to consider what type of hair regrowth to pursue. You've studied the benefits of LPT, its history, and its alternatives. Now, the LPT device's production and manufacturer must be considered before you choose to make a purchase for something as important to you as hair growth.

Which Type of LPT Device is Right for Me?

At the time of this writing, there are four main types of LLLT/LPT devices in the market today:

1. Combs/bands
2. Helmets
3. Baseball caps
4. Stand-alone devices

Although we've touched on these devices before, let's go through each one of these in detail so you can understand the benefits and draw-backs of each type of device. What we have learned so far is that not all lasers have the same properties or effects, and this section explains why selecting a well-designed LPT device is crucial.

1. Laser Combs and Bands

The laser combs were the first FDA-cleared devices to hit the market and these were instrumental in getting people's attention about laser phototherapy. The technology consists of a brush-like device that claims from six to twelve (or sometimes more) laser beams. These laser combs are mostly just one laser but, for the sake of cost, use a fiber optic cable to create up to six to twelve different beams. The user has to act like they are brushing their hair, but they have to wait a few seconds at each spot for a beep to advance to the next spot. This must be repeated until the full scalp has been covered which can take anywhere from fifteen to thirty minutes per session.

Laser combs target different areas of the scalp while combing for an average of four seconds, and because of the generic power density of a comb, (there's an energy dosage of 0.02 j/cm^2), combs won't stimulate hair follicles.

Bands are derived from the same concept as combs and have the same concept of moving a band outfitted with laser diodes and moved around every few seconds. Laser bands are typically used for around thirty seconds. Their FDA clearance was based on combs, so the bands are technically the same product.

Assuming a generic power density of typical laser bands, (there's an energy dosage of 0.15 j/cm^2), they also fail to achieve biostimulation.

Disadvantages: The major drawback is that using combs and bands is a very laborious process and compliance is very difficult to maintain. These devices are cumbersome to use. A laser that is split into different beams is not as good as six or twelve individual laser diodes. Also, some combs have anywhere from two to four seconds per spot, which is nowhere near enough to penetrate the scalp and its most important parts deep within the scalp. We are grateful that they started the whole LPT process, but unfortunately, these will be phased out in the very near future and will be in a museum at some point in time.

2. Helmets

An LPT helmet is the most logical and best design for being able to cover male and female pattern hair loss. A laser helmet like ours was designed to be convenient, cordless, hands-free device that provides full scalp coverage, and users can relax and do other things, like watch TV, play video games, or read a book. A laser helmet that can deliver 680 nm and penetrate deep into the scalp to reach the base of the hair follicles is the ultimate solution. They also deposit an energy dosage optimal for a twenty-minute, laser hair growth treatment. The cold lasers penetrate up to 5 mm into the scalp and deliver the right dosage throughout each twenty-minute treatment session. The helmets are also 427 times more powerful than the laser comb or brush and fifty-seven times more powerful than a laser band. And it won't heat up your scalp.

A laser helmet provides full-scalp coverage and is worn on the head for twenty minutes without having to move the helmet around. This provides an energy dosage of 7 j/cm^2 (assuming the same generic power density). This is the optimal amount of energy dosage needed to trigger the effective biostimulation of hair follicles. It should be pretty clear that a laser helmet is the best option when it comes to dosage, time, and biostimulation. Combs, bands, and caps just don't compare and you won't get the results you desire.

The most common question for helmets is why eighty lasers is better than 200 or 300 lasers. This is explained in Dispelling Myth #2: More Lasers Are Better. It has to do with designing a device that has maximum optical output and low heat output. Eighty is the perfect number of laser diodes, as this amount is effective for hair loss and hair growth, but won't produce excess heat.

Disadvantages: Helmets that contain consumer grade laser diodes (e.g., EELs) and LEDs or LEDs alone should be avoided at all costs. Although some vendors claim that LEDs provide more coverage, this is not accurate. LED light cannot enter past even the first layer out of the seven layers of the scalp. Only helmets with 100% lasers at 680 nm work well, and over time, they will stop your hair loss and will regrow your hair. The only drawback might be that it is slightly more difficult to have lasers penetrate a full head of hair. As long as a small percentage of lasers hit the scalp, there should be no issues. Therefore, it is important to do treatments right after a shower and towel dry your hair before styling, comb your hair, and expose the scalp so the laser helmet can focus on the problem spots.

3. Baseball Caps

As of 2023, there are over twenty makers of baseball laser caps in the marketplace today. This is due to the flood of Asian manufacturers that supply these to US companies that resell the product as their own. These laser baseball caps all use the exact same EEL (edge emitting lasers) which are used for consumer applications (e.g., DVDs, CDs, and laser pointers).

Laser caps operate with pulsed lasers instead of emitting continuous light, meaning there are "on" and "off" periods during treatment sessions. This cuts the treatment time by half. In other words, if a cap is used for thirty minutes, only fifteen minutes will deliver energy to the scalp. The majority of laser caps have an energy dosage of less than 0.1 j/cm^2, which isn't enough for biostimulation.

Disadvantages: A baseball hat gets connected to the plastic bowl-type case which contains all of the lasers without any ventilation. The addition of the cloth baseball hat substantially increases the heat which tends to cause more cases of telogen effluvium to its customers and further damage can be done to the scalp. In addition, the baseball cap design is not optimal for male and female pattern hair loss, and the vendors market these baseball caps as if customers will wear these in public, which is a bit of an exaggeration.

These laser caps are designed to output at 5 mW per laser diode but after all of the heat has been accumulated, the resulting optical output of each laser diode drops from 5 mW within the first few seconds to less than 0.5 mW, making them very inefficient. The more laser diodes that are used in these laser caps the less optical output that comes from them. The output of the lasers (in-vivo) will drop well below the claims made by the manufacturer.

In-vivo testing studies mean that the correct way these LPT devices are tested should be using temperature and laser measurement sensors while wearing the device on the head. This is in contrast to ex-vivo testing which measures these devices on a laboratory bench and not on the head. We learned from previous sections that the top of the head gets warm, and that this will affect the laser diodes' performance, as lasers hate hot places. These laser caps were not designed by an engineer or scientist, and we highly recommend another solution.

4. Stand-Alone LPT Devices

These are panels with a stand that are placed behind a chair or couch where the patient sits. These are usually placed about six inches to eight inches away from the scalp and the person remains with their head fixed in one location for fifteen to thirty minutes per session.

Disadvantages: As you can imagine, these fixed panels are just not designed for convenience nor optimized for hair growth. The laser head is way too far from the scalp and these laser panels emit too much heat for the scalp; even though it is an open panel design, it still emits too much heat onto the scalp.

Now that you have an understanding of the different devices to make a wise and educated choice, it's time to understand how to use laser phototherapy devices.

Actual Customer Success Stories

The Helmet To End The War

Alex was proud of his wavy curly blond hair, which had made him school heartthrob. When it began to thin, he worked his way through OTC treatments, alternative remedies, and everything his physician could prescribe. His bathroom cabinet was cluttered with hair loss products, but he saw few results. At last, frustration led to discovery. He ordered a laser comb he'd seen on an infomercial late one night, and, before long, could see his thin patch subtly shrinking. It helped, but it took a lot of time and effort. He didn't want to devote time to combing and combating hair loss for the rest of his life. The solution was a wearable laser helmet. Soon everyone commented on his great-looking hair. The best part was he could just wear the helmet and not worry about his hair. He could focus on other things in his life.

CHAPTER 13

Show Me the Science: An Evidence-Based Guide to LPT

"Light is the physician of nature; it has the power to heal and restore balance." — Paracelsus, Physician and Philosopher, 1536

The Benefits of Laser Phototherapy

Despite sounding like science fiction, laser phototherapy is real. What began as an accidental discovery in the 1960s has spawned an entire industry. More importantly, hundreds of studies confirm lasers can regrow hair.

How Lasers Work and What They Do

It all begins with the First Law of Photochemistry, which states: "Light must be absorbed by a compound for a photochemical reaction to take place." In other words, light-sensitive molecules in our cells must take in enough light—in this case, laser light—for the light to have an effect. For lasers to trigger a photochemical reaction that affects your hair's roots, the chromophores in the dermis (the skin's second layer) must absorb light (you may recall from the first chapter that chromophores are light-absorbing pigments similar to chlorophyll). And for that to happen, light must penetrate the skin as well as the tissue beneath. Only lasers penetrate deeply enough to do this. It means faster and much better results for keeping hair and growing it back.

Penetration, as we will see, is a key point. To be effective, laser light must reach the bulge and the papilla, which is located at a depth of up to 5 mm. Getting to this depth requires the laser to have a single wavelength as well as waves of a specific phase and direction.

Here's where "scalp optics" come in. Optics refer to the behavior of light when it interacts with objects. It may stay intact, or it might scatter. Through optics, we can predict and understand the effects of light on the scalp and direct the right amount of light onto it. This means both coverage and depth. Picture the process as being like buttering toast. You need to use enough butter to give you the right coverage and depth. Too much or too little gives you a less satisfying experience than you want. You've got to get it just right. The same holds true for lasers on your scalp.

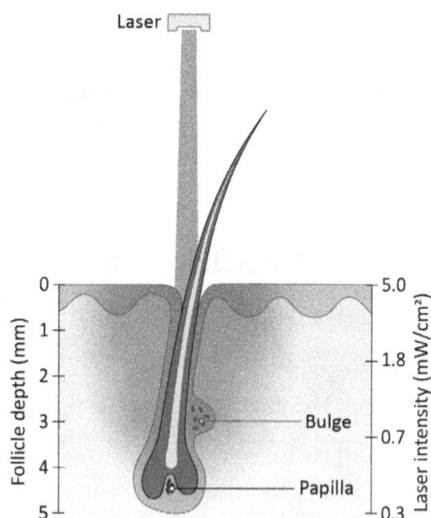

Figure 13.1. A Laser Penetrating to the Papilla. Laser applied to the bulge and papilla stimulates them to extend the hair cycle so it stays on the scalp for up to eight years and stimulating the papilla will make the hair grow faster.

When a laser beam hits your scalp, the chromophores located around each cell take in the light and kick-start hair growth. This process is called laser phototherapy. The way it works is similar to the way plants work. Plant cells change the light they receive into chemical energy to make food. Similarly, human skin cells convert light energy into chemical energy that is then used to regrow hair.

Let's explore for a moment the similarities between how humans and plants use light to their advantage. Humans are from the kingdom Animalia, while plants are from the kingdom Plantae. They're almost always separated based on their ability to photosynthesize. In other words, what separates plants from animals is that plants can convert light energy into chemical energy.

But hold on. Is it really that simple? Maybe not. Studies now show that mammals can also derive energy directly from sunlight. After all, their diet is often rich in chlorophyll, which makes photosynthesis possible. Chlorophyll builds up in plant-eating mammals, enabling their mitochondria to capture sunlight and convert it into chemical energy (in the form of a chemical called ATP). Since humans are also mammals, this raises the possibility that they too can accumulate chlorophyll.

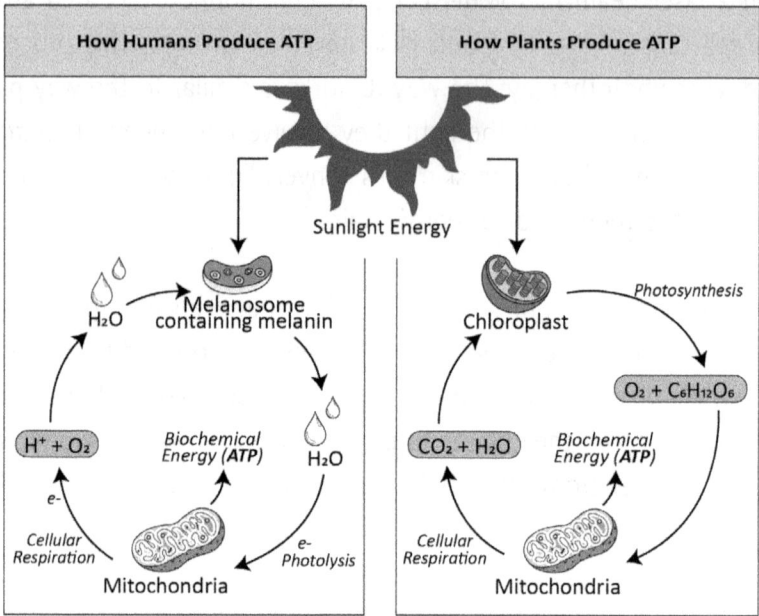

Figure 13.2. Sunlight Effects on Animals vs. Plants: Mitochondria are being stimulated by sunlight. This chart shows that light is instrumental in stimulating the mitochondria of both plants and animals.

We already know that chromophores, which are found in our skin, can capture light. Research also suggests that chromophores have the potential to be used as sunscreen. Thanks to their ability to absorb ultraviolet radiation, they may be able to protect against sunburn and skin cancer. Moreover, melanin, which gives our skin and hair their color, can set in motion the same reactions as chlorophyll. This means humans are also capable of converting light energy from the sun into chemical energy, a reaction that involves splitting water into hydrogen and oxygen. Lasers allow us to take advantage of this process to regrow hair.

When talking about lasers, it's useful to know a few terms, which we have explained previously.

- **Wavelength** determines a laser's penetrating power; in other words, how deeply it can go into tissue. These are monochromatic, which means containing one color.
- **Coherence** is how the light holds together. If it holds together well, it will not scatter on a smooth surface. Lasers are highly coherent. Together, intensity and coherence, which depend on wavelength, play a key role in how well a laser penetrates and is absorbed by human tissue.
- **Beam Divergence** relates to the width of a beam. A narrower beam generally means a lower divergence and provides a deeper penetration, which is what we want with LPT.
- **Energy Density** is the dosage or intensity of the laser beam, and we are always striving for the perfect dosage (measured as joules/cm^2). If you're not familiar with the joule as a unit of energy, think of a 100-watt light bulb. A watt is the rate of delivery of energy, so a 100-watt bulb is dissipating 100 j/sec of energy.
- **Continuous Wave** is a method of delivering light energy in the form of a laser continuously over a certain amount of time. This type of light delivery is very efficient and is ideal for LPT, since it does not accumulate or generate heat into the tissue. Other types of lasers for hair applications have to pulse (turn their lasers on and off) to reduce the heat generated by their lasers—these types of devices should be avoided at all costs.

Lasers are designed to deliver just the right amount of light at the correct depth and coverage to optimize hair regrowth. Part of the benefit of laser phototherapy is that it stimulates stem cells in the bulge and papilla.

A stem cell is a generic cell that can turn into a highly specialized cell. Stem cells enable the body to produce new cells. As we have seen, bulge stem cells in hair follicles are responsible for growing new follicles. These follicles produce hair shafts during the growth phase of the hair cycle.

In the scalp, bulge stem cells allow the hair strands that are shed every day to be replaced by new hair strands.

How LPT Works

LPT aims low-power lasers of a specific wavelength at certain areas of the body to get the body to produce certain nutrients and chemicals. The goal is also to activate the body's defenses and its powers of regeneration. When cells are exposed to laser phototherapy, they respond through a process called photobiomodulation, an idea introduced in the first chapter. Laser light sets in motion a chain of chemical reactions that produce energy in the cells. In other words, cells are converting light into chemical energy. The chemical reactions increase the metabolism of cells, speeding up cellular repair and stimulating the hair follicle.

For instance, hair cells go from being miniaturized—miniaturized hair cells make thinner, weaker hairs—to fully functioning terminal hairs. The result seen in clinical trials is a regrowth of hair. There is also less shedding.

When a "laser beam" shines onto the scalp the laser beam is in the shape of a cylinder or a cone. This is a common shape that we can determine its area. But once this beam hits the scalp, the red light will spread out and will be converted from a beam to a volume, meaning that the laser light will spread immediately as it hits the scalp and layers of skin. This is called scattering and is one of the properties of lasers. Fog is perhaps the simplest and most obvious example of scattering. If you can't see through it, light can't get through it. A laser is not going to penetrate fog any better than the light you're trying to see.

The best analogy for how lasers enter the scalp is very similar to someone taking a brand new sponge and putting it under the faucet and the water will do four things: 1) Hit the sponge and some of the water will be bounce off, 2) Once the water enters the sponge it will quickly scatter,

3) after it scatters, then the water will get absorbed by the sponge, and 4) when the sponge is full of water, the water pressure from the faucet will transmit through the sponge at a very low pressure on the diametrically opposite underside of the sponge. The same thing happens in the scalp—laser light hits the scalp and then spreads down, while the light spreads around where the light was placed.

Laser light is different from other types of light because all the waves are the same color and travel together in a straight line (this is called coherence). This means that the light doesn't spread out or scatter like regular light, which makes it easier for the laser to go deep into human tissue. The coherence of the laser light also allows it to stay focused as it travels through different layers of skin and tissue, which is why it can be used to penetrate the most important parts of the scalp, and the hair follicle. As the light travels through the scalp, every part of the hair follicle—hair structure, sebum, sweat, muscle, and more gets flooded with red light energy. Photons enter the cell, using the cell's chromophores to enter through the cell's walls and charge up the mitochondria, which energize the cell.

Some of this energy gets converted into ATP (adenosine triphosphate) which is the currency that measures energy in a cell, and which can be stored or used as energy within the cell. DHT renders hair dormant by closing the normal doors (chemical pathways) to each cell.

Photons now perform an essential role in healing through LPT. With LPT, we can enter the cell using a very old entryway—the optical gateway (chromophores). Using it is like attempting to move a huge cruise ship with a small outboard engine: It will eventually move the ship but will take much longer. Since the chemical pathways are usually closed off, the optical pathway will be the only way to stimulate the mitochondria in each cell. This is why when there is a lot of stress, or hormonal activity in the body, an LPT device should be used a lot more than usual, like when a cruise liner facing rougher seas and conditions.

The process photons set in motion in the cell is called the Krebs cycle, a name for how cells produce energy (ATP). Creating ATP, along with nitric oxide (NO), is the key to rejuvenating human cells.

LPT works by increasing ATP production in the mitochondria of the cell. Research has documented a significant increase in ATP, and up to seven times the amount of Nitric Oxide (NO) produced using LPT.

ATP is the product of all energy metabolism within a cell; the cell will die without it. With more energy available, the cell is free to spend it on "frills" not essential for survival and which the body quickly discards when ill or severely stressed—frills like hair.

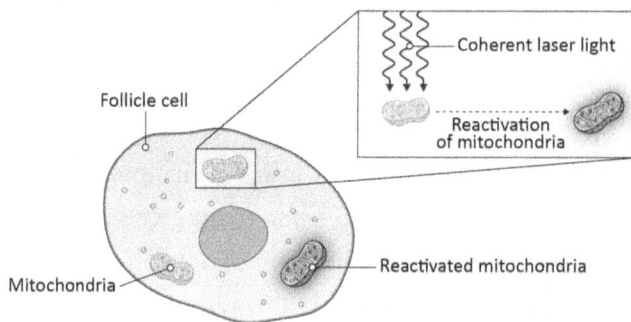

Figure 13.3. Laser Stimulating the Cell and Mitochondria. Human cells have many mitochondria in each cell and hair cells can be regenerated by providing the right type of wavelength and dosage so mitochondria be reactivated.

Not only does LPT increase ATP, but researchers have also shown that it stimulates the cell's enzymes and activates the immune system. The laser speeds up cellular reproduction, growth, and its ability to regenerate. It also stimulates hair follicles in their entirety, especially the bulge, which contains the cells that produce new hair follicles, and papilla, which determine how long hair will grow. As we observed in Chapter 2, the two key areas of the hair follicles, the bulge and the (dermal) papilla have the highest concentration of mitochondria. With that many mitochondria to stimulate, it takes trillions of photons of laser light energy to stimulate trillions of mitochondria in each hair follicle. Only a highly focused laser that has the wavelength to penetrate and apply the right dosage will be able to perform such a function.

How Does LPT Help with Hair Loss?

When your scalp is treated with laser phototherapy, the hairs in the resting phase are triggered to enter the growth phase and hair follicles are encouraged to prolong the growth phase. Lasers prevent hair from making an early entry into the dormant phase of no growth. Finally, lasers can turn hairs that were miniaturized back into terminal hairs.

All of this means that LPT encourages hair to continue growing instead of resting or falling out. Hairs thicken as well, allowing for a fuller head of hair, and thicker strands strengthen the follicles which prevent the hairs from breaking or falling out. Overall, hair grows better, and the scalp gets healthier with regular laser treatment.

No other known method even comes close to the myriad changes achieved with LPT without causing serious side effects. LPT works so well that users may see decreased hair loss or shedding in as few as three to six weeks because LPT activates the hair follicle's growth phase. During this phase, hair cells develop rapidly, and the hair shaft grows within the follicle. The duration of the growth phase determines how long hair will grow and may range from three to eight years.

Significant hair loss reduction, thickening, and changes to the color of existing hair can be seen within sixty to ninety days. Over the course of three to six months, hair continues thickening, and areas of the scalp that had been visible become noticeably less so. After sixteen to eighteen months of regular treatment, improvement peaks during the growth phase.

Laser light offers additional benefits to the immune system and reduces inflammation caused by fungal or bacterial infections on the scalp. The light also speeds up the hair cycles, normalizes the production of sebum (the fatty substance that builds up around hair follicles on the scalp), increases keratin required to produce hair, and strengthens the arrector pili, the muscle that moves hair.

Furthermore, LPT speeds up protein synthesis as well as DNA and RNA formation. LPT also increases blood and lymph circulation to the hair roots, removing blockages around the hair follicle. This process energizes cells and the hair papillae so that they absorb nutrients faster, allowing the hair to grow thicker and stronger. Clinical studies have suggested that all this activity at the cellular and even sub-cellular level breaks down the collection of DHT and flushes it into the lymphatic system.

LPT accelerates hair growth by reducing excessive levels of 5-alpha reductase, the enzyme that converts testosterone into DHT, that notorious hair assassin.

LPT is anti-inflammatory, so it improves scalp conditions such as psoriasis, dandruff, and itchy or scaling scalp. By normalizing sebum (oil) production in the scalp tissue, LPT reduces scaling, crusting, and blockage, and is an additional therapy for both before and after hair transplantation procedures. This is the most evident difference between low-level light therapy (LLLT) and laser phototherapy (LPT). There's some debate as to whether LLLT stops hair loss or merely slows it down. LLLT promotes hair growth by increasing hair growth periods while hair loss continues. LPT, on the other hand, solves both sides of the problem by preventing further hair loss and encouraging new and better growth.

The results of several clinical trials and systematic reviews show that LPT works on different types of hair loss in men and women, including androgenetic alopecia, telogen effluvium, and alopecia areata. A healthier scalp and stronger hairs stimulated by lasers help overcome several issues that could not otherwise be resolved.

What is the Right Dosage for Hair Growth?

Just as doctors adjust drug prescriptions to match specific medical conditions, every condition or disease that responds well to photobio-modulation requires a particular course of treatment.

A prescription for laser phototherapy would have to include the required wavelength of light, the number of points that should be treated on the scalp, the energy density (measured as j/cm^2), the power density (measured as mW/cm^2), and the length of time for each treatment and wavelength. There is not yet a standard for the dosage needed to stop or regrow hair by any one group. The dosages that have been used by FDA-cleared devices and manufacturers are low enough to cause no harm and are effective enough to show satisfactory results.

Hair growth, which takes at least four months to grow back, is very difficult to measure with the tools and techniques we have today. The best and ideal solution to measure LPT progress would be a set of identical twins with mild to moderate hair loss to test. Identical twins occur when one egg and one sperm split into two eggs. These identical twins have almost the same genes. Since identical twins have the same genes, a set of identical triplets would be even better, where one can be a control (no LPT), one can have the maximum dosage, and the third one can have a lower dosage of LPT. This would be a great study to measure dosage.

Today's animal laboratory testing for drugs has been done primarily using clones, which has worked well, but is quite controversial, and LPT is too far along to go back to animal testing. So, we should try to find as many human identical twins as possible, as this is the perfect model for measuring the right LPT dosage and testing all sorts of conditions as well as physiological and environmental impacts.

We do need an organization that would officially publish recommended treatment doses for different hair-related conditions. LPT device companies would then be able to provide guidance in their instruction manuals to direct users and clinicians. For example, instead of users wearing their LPT device every day versus twice per week, the recommended guidelines would instruct someone on the time needed to treat androgenetic alopecia with a specific Hamilton-Norwood pattern.

In most cases, LPT should be applied a minimum of two to four times a week for a person's lifetime. In the near future, the usage of devices containing just LEDs or LEDs in conjunction with laser diodes will be completely phased away due to the fact that science will prevail. Lasers are considerably superior to LEDs because laser light is coherent, meaning more photons are packed into a single narrow beam. Lasers are better at treating deeper structures such as hair follicles (e.g., bulge and papilla) than LEDs. LEDs work well in smoothing fine wrinkles or superficial scalp lesions. The most important thing to note, however, is that dosage matters.

Because the scalp has the second-thickest skin on the human body, it takes a lot of photons to penetrate it. Lasers affect how the scalp chooses to grow or release hairs and which hairs become tiny. Lasers stimulate hair growth in either case, and LPT strengthens existing follicles. By penetrating to the correct depth during the optimal time window, lasers help make the scalp healthier, encouraging hair growth. The red laser light enters an area and fills it with energy that hijacks the body's natural methods for regrowing hair.

Direct benefits are visible sometimes within the first week. Users experience a 54% increase in blood supply to the scalp after only one treatment. However, it's not the increased blood flow that stimulates hair growth; it's the stimulation of everything in the path of the laser's beam, including skin cells, blood vessels, muscles, and hair. Treatment also increases hair strength and elasticity, improves curl retention, and reinstates pigments. Furthermore, lasers enhance the lasting effects of hair color and perms by closing the cuticle (the hair's protective outer sheath), leading to longer-lasting color with less fading and oxidation.

Since the mid-1960s, many debates have raged about the ideal amount of light for stimulating hair follicles. The key questions are: "What's the perfect dose of laser phototherapy?" and "How much does your scalp need?" All LPT devices are preset with the exact dosage to provide the precise amount of coverage and penetration without going overboard, which could either deliver poor results or harm the scalp. It should be noted that other LPT devices for muscle or wound management require a much lower dosage, since we learned in Chapter 2 that muscle and other structures contain a lower concentration of mitochondria. Therefore, stimulating hair versus other organs should be considered.

Is it Possible to Disprove LPT's Efficacy?

New medical treatments and methods have not always been well received over the centuries. Take for example Dr. Semmelweis from Budapest, Hungary back in 1847. Before the microscope, Dr. Semmelweis theorized that there were invisible creatures on our hands that caused 90% of patients to die from infections by moving from surgeons' hands into patients during surgery. He suggested that doctors and surgeons wash their hands before surgery to reduce patient deaths. The medical community laughed at Dr. Semmelweis. His medical license was revoked. Dr. Semmelweis was so distraught that he ended up in a psychiatric facility where he died several years later.

It wasn't until thirty years after Semmelweis died, when researchers suggested that all physicians that researchers suggested that all physicians should wash their hands before performing surgeries. In tribute, they named the hospital after Dr. Semmelweis. Coincidentally, this hospital is where Dr. Endre Mester conducted the first LPT studies at the Semmelweis Hospital in Budapest, Hungary.

Firstly, to prove that LPT does not work, one would need to use a different light source, a normal light (non-laser).

There have been numerous clinical studies on humans and animals (five blind studies in humans) that compared the effects of LEDs vs. Lasers which conclusively showed lasers attained more hair count by a substantial margin in the reduction of hair loss. So, either the investigators of all of the 160 studies on cold lasers were mistaken, or the effects favored laser light.

Secondly, coherence is the difference between lasers and non-coherent light sources, which are only effective for superficial skin structures. Normal light is non-coherent so it cannot penetrate deep enough to get to where the hair follicles reside. Laser light maintains its coherence throughout the human tissue and speckles are found deep inside the human tissue.

Thirdly, no light source in the world resembles laser light. Laser light is a man-made phenomenon and does not occur in nature. If a light similar to lasers existed, it would produce the same results as a laser light. It is a narrow, cold, controllable, penetrating light. No other similar laser light exists.

Finally, the penetration of laser light into human tissue is not the minimal, useless amount of other lights. Laser light is highly penetrative, especially if the proper wavelength is utilized.

Clinical Proof Laser Phototherapy Works!

No one questions the efficacy of hot lasers (e.g., for hair removal or cutting tissue) because their results are instantaneous. This is not the case for cold lasers. Time, patience, and replicating treatment with exact parameters are necessary to achieve positive stimulatory effects in human cells with the use of laser phototherapy. Thousands of LPT studies have been published in scientific and medical journals. However, since LPT is a fairly new treatment modality, numerous studies conducted in earlier years lack the methodology and information needed to impact the medical community. The overall quality of research in the LPT field is still under constant criticism. A lack of experimental quality control produces negative results and creates doubt among positive studies. As a result, a lack of general acceptance of LPT still lingers amongst physicians, clinicians, hair experts, and of course, the end consumer. Improving experimental protocol and regulating methods for the publication of LPT clinical studies is a step in the right direction.

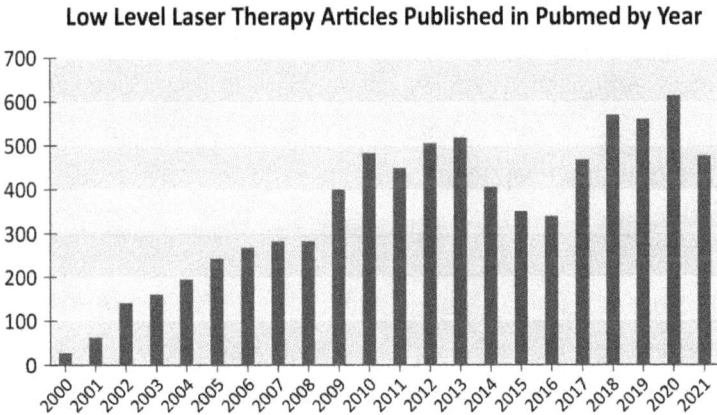

Figure 13.4. Laser Phototherapy Articles Published in PubMed® by Year. Every year more and more researchers are publishing their new findings on LPT and the human body.

Numerous LPT studies have been conducted on female and male patients diagnosed with androgenetic alopecia and alopecia areata. Overall, clinical studies report an impressive list of benefits to hair treated with Laser Phototherapy. These include:

- An average of 35% to 39% hair count increase after a few months of treatment.
- A decrease in the number of vellus hairs, an increase in the number of terminal hairs, and a larger shaft diameter.
- A shift of hair follicles into the growing anagen phase.
- Positive changes in the quality and texture of hair.
- Augmented mean hair diameter and greater hair density.
- Increased hair density and tensile strength. More specifically, five double-blinded randomized clinical trials (RCTs) are of particular interest when it comes to treating androgenetic alopecia with laser phototherapy.

With so many positive results found in the scientific literature, it can be puzzling to think that LPT is still viewed with skepticism in the medical and scientific community but it is still a new modality. There are numerous reasons behind why this is the case, including the omission of important parameters in published studies, the inability to reproduce experiments, the complexity of technical parameters needed in an experiment—which opens the door to cheap manufacturers—and the way LPT is still viewed in scientific fields, amongst other factors.

In 2016, a clinical trial was conducted, called "Efficacy and Safety of LPT with Theradome PRO LH80 for Promoting Hair Growth in Males with Androgenetic Alopecia: a multicenter, randomized, sham device-controlled, double-blind study and approved by an IRB (Institutional Review Board)" and submitted to clinicaltrials.gov. This is the first-of-its-kind study that clearly shows that using our LPT helmet versus a sham (placebo) helmet will regrow your hair and make it thicker as well as stop your hair loss. This type of study was designed to be the gold standard for evaluating devices to assure that the results are pristine and eliminate subjective data.

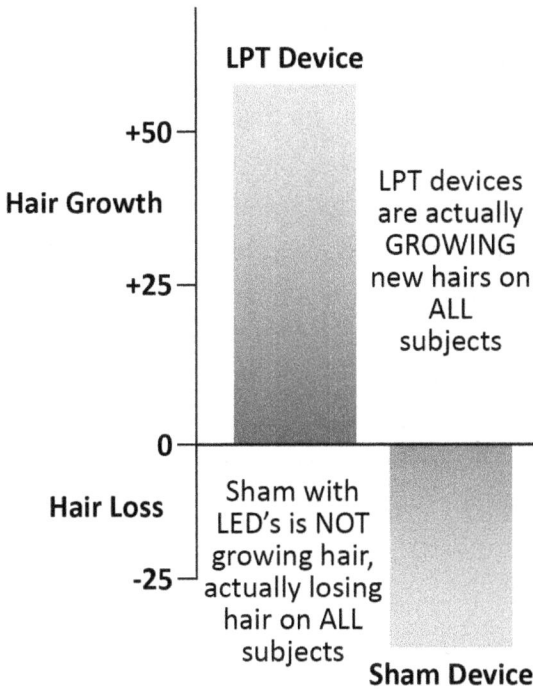

Figure 13.5. Total Changes in Hair Count and Vellus Width in Test vs. Sham Treatments. This graph clearly shows that laser light increases hair growth and stops hair loss compared to a sham device (LED), in which all subjects lost hair.

The results of this study were very clear: Patients who wore the helmet all regrew hair and/or kept their hair while the patients who wore the sham (LED) device experienced no hair growth whatsoever. One observation from the study was that younger patients resulted in better outcomes, which makes sense, given that just like treating any disease, the faster one can start treatment, the more likely a positive outcome. This is probably the most conclusive study for showing how LPT can stop and regrow hair while doing nothing or using LEDs will do absolutely nothing or, even worse, make hair condition deteriorate.

Actual Customer Success Stories

Science To The Rescue

Jenny was the go-to person for online product research, from TVs to shampoos. When she faced hair loss, she believed she'd find an answer. She first looked at Minoxidil and Finasteride, both FDA-cleared treatments. But Minoxidil wasn't ideal for women, and Finasteride wasn't right for her age. Then she found another new FDA-cleared method: LPT. It seemed safe and science backed. Now, she uses laser therapy after her showers. Her friends, who once teased her for her research, now ask for her hair care secret.

CHAPTER 14

Dispelling Myths About Laser Phototherapy

"The job is not to ridicule the myths, but to show the difference between myth and reality." — Norman Davies, Historian, 2002

Dispelling Myths about Laser Phototherapy

Because LPT is an unusual and cutting-edge type of medical therapy, there are misconceptions and myths about hair loss prevention and especially regrowth. When it comes to new and pioneering treatments, especially when they involve heavy physics, people understandably have questions that need to be answered to their satisfaction. Like other medical treatments, experts must dispel myths with scientific information, to curb disinformation.

Dispelling Myth #1: LED Lights Are the Same as Lasers

This is one of the most frustrating misconceptions when it comes to stimulating hair to grow or to grow back. This incorrect notion is based on several false assumptions and false equivalencies. For example, there's a wide range of LLLT (low-level light therapy) devices that use LEDs (light-emitting diodes) in their products but are marketed as laser-phototherapy (LPT) hair growth devices. LLLT and LPT, however, are not identical. Some of the manufacturers even have "laser" in their name, yet they use 90% LED technology to reduce costs. Other manufacturers claim that LEDs are just as effective as lasers and that since all focused light is the same, the scalp just needs plenty of direct light.

Numerous studies comparing the biological effects of lasers versus LEDs concluded that laser light is effective while LED is not because LEDs lack the key properties of lasers. Without these properties, there is no way to reach the hair follicles buried deep in the scalp.

LEDs generate only about 5% of the light energy needed to stimulate hair regrowth. They are too weak to have a coherent, focused beam and cannot be set at the specific wavelength needed to regrow hair. A proper laser, on the other hand, puts out 100% of the energy required to stimulate hair regrowth. In fact, a laser delivers about 150 times more energy than an LED!

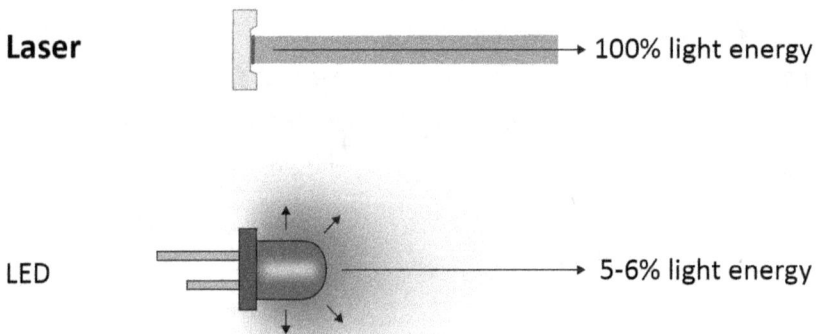

Laser   ➝ 100% light energy

LED   ➝ 5-6% light energy

Figure 14.1. Light Energy Being Focused. The difference between Lasers and LED is not comparable and lasers are superior for hair growth applications.

If you took a 100-watt LED light and stood about twenty feet away on a sunny day, you might not be able to tell whether the LED was on or off because so much of the energy would be lost in divergence (spreading out). Because LEDs don't produce coherent light, their energy is spread over a wider width of wavelengths.

If you stand twenty feet away from a 100-watt monochromatic laser and look right at it, you will be in danger of losing your eye! A 100-watt monochromatic laser is much stronger than the laser pointers we mentioned earlier or the lasers used for hair growth.

Lasers focus all their energy where they are aimed. Conversely, LEDs and other non-coherent light sources, like direct sunlight, scatter their energy. Only the coherent beam of a laser provides the penetration depth needed for therapeutic purposes.

Laser light is generally monochromatic (a single color) and its wavelength allows for the best penetration into tissue. Since light must be absorbed by a chromophore to have a biological impact, the depth of light penetration into tissue is critical. If the light doesn't penetrate the scalp deeply enough, the beam won't reach the hair follicle, and the follicle will not be stimulated to regrow hair.

Why, then, do some companies promote LEDs for hair restoration, despite knowing that they are useless? The answer is that LEDs are much cheaper than lasers. Therefore, it's easy for manufacturers to put out their own "LPT hair loss" unit on the market and make a quick buck using LEDs. What is interesting is that the very few papers that are published on LEDs are ironically funded by interested parties, such as the boards of LED phototherapy device companies, giving rise to some pretty major conflicts of interest. Nonetheless, the goal is to stick to the scientific facts.

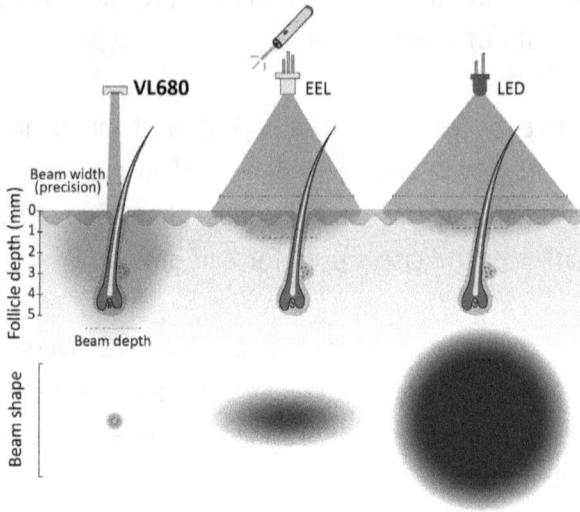

Figure 14.2. Beam Shapes Reaching Follicles. Comparison of LED, consumer grade laser diodes (EELs) and a customized laser specifically designed for hair follicles show deep penetration hitting the hair follicles.

Here's what to remember about comparisons between LEDs and lasers:

1. LEDs and lasers are not the same. LEDs lack the key elements that allow lasers to regrow hair. Tricks by LLLT manufacturers involve adding lenses to LEDs to disguise them as laser diodes or splitting the light of a single laser diode into multiple beams with the use of fiber optics.

2. LEDs deliver only a small amount of energy to the scalp compared to a true laser. Marketing statements that claim that LEDs deliver the amounts of energy necessary to grow hair qualify as myths. If potential customers base decisions upon such unequivocally false claims, they become victims.

3. LEDs don't regrow hair. Statements claiming or clearly implying that LEDs do regrow hair are myths. A plethora of clinical studies prove that

LEDs don't have the power to trigger the numerous benefits of LPT on human tissue.

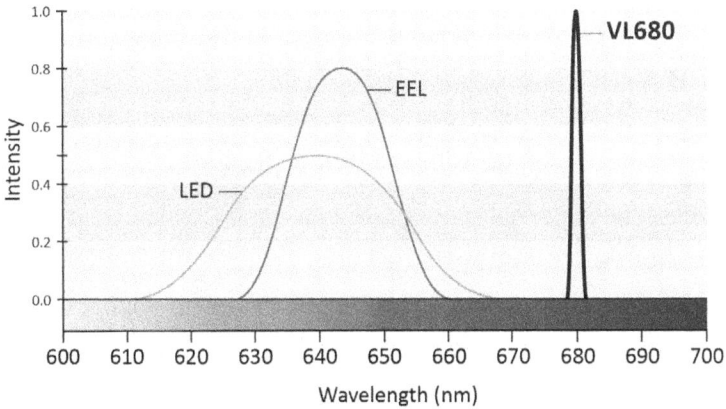

Figure 14.3. Laser Wavelength vs. Intensity. A specialized laser such as the VL680 is perfectly tuned to provide the correct wavelength versus other light sources which have wide variances.

4. One very good test to see if a light source is a laser source or not is via the phenomena of speckling. Only lasers speckle, whereas LED lights are a very flat light source. See the figure below for a comparison of LED versus a laser source.

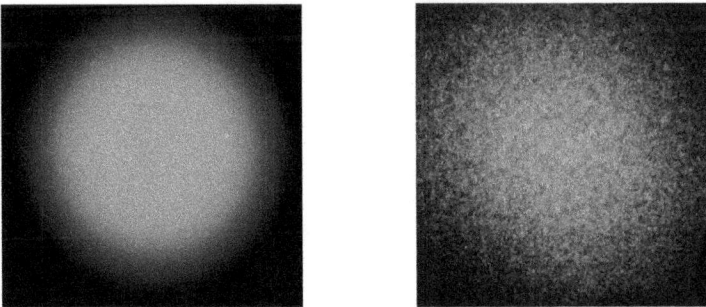

Figure 14.4. Speckling vs. Non-Speckling. Only laser light (right image) contains speckling, unlike the smoother illumination of non-speckling LEDs (left image).

Dispelling Myth #2: More Lasers Are Better

Companies that boast high numbers of lasers in their hair growth light devices are ignoring the drawbacks of having too many lasers. A 300-laser baseball cap might seem more effective than one with only eighty lasers, but devices containing a high number of lasers lose a considerable amount of their intensity due to overheating.

Ventilation is a critical component missing in many laser-packed devices, such as baseball caps, hairbrushes, or hair bands, which claim that more lasers are better. The fact is that all lasers exposed to extreme heat will not perform as intended and, therefore, will have no impact on hair loss and, in some cases, can even cause more hair shedding. Without proper ventilation, the quantity of lasers in any laser device is meaningless.

When lasers are applied, especially 100–300 lasers or more, it adds another ten to twenty degrees of heat to the scalp. Many people have complained of high temperatures from laser baseball caps. Adding heat to a molecule will change its state, and we certainly don't want to change anything in the hair follicles. We only want to stimulate the mitochondria inside each hair follicle.

The top of the head is already one of the warmest places on your body; that's why we check our temperature on the forehead, so putting a lot of lasers on will cause more hair loss as explained in Chapter 2. Heat and moisture cause more fungus and more fungus causes more inflammation and more inflammation causes more hair loss.

Heat and lasers do not mix; the more lasers, the more heat there is, which causes hair loss known as telogen effluvium. If the laser heat is not managed well, you may end up damaging your hair follicles. A product that can provide maximum dosage with minimal heat output is the ideal LPT. Our propriety lasers were designed and tested to emit less than 1° centigrade in one twenty-minute usage cycle. Do not ever think more lasers will be better. Yes, a device should have a decent amount of dosage, but unfortunately more lasers only bring more heat—and heat is not good for your scalp!

A device that provides maximum dosage with a low heat output is the best guideline for laser applications.

Dispelling Myth #3: More Power or a Higher Dose Is Better

Again, as with so many other features of laser phototherapy for hair growth, more isn't always better. This rule clearly applies to the myth that raising the laser's gross power output will improve results. Such tampering might create safety concerns. It's far preferable to focus on using safe levels of power more effectively.

Too many photons can inhibit hair growth. The ideal is to provide up to a maximum of ten joules per cm^2 for twenty minutes and to take a break of several hours (we recommend about twelve hours) before the next treatment.

The myth that more power is better is widespread because many man- ufacturers claim that the greater the total milliwatts of their lasers, the more effective their device will be. Some claim, for example, that since they have two hundred lasers and each laser uses 5 mW (theoretically!), their product has a total output of 1,000 mW (200 x 5 mW = 1,000 mW).

They use these numbers in advertising campaigns because numbers and sample calculations that resemble scientific data often impress customers who are looking for quick results. The scientific fact, however, is that photo biomodulation isn't measured by the power output of a laser diode. It's measured by power density, the amount of optical energy delivered *beneath* the scalp.

Fluence—the optimal energy delivered per square centimeter or inch—is fundamental. A combination of the right wavelength, coherence, beam-area width, and power density results in maximum fluence.

Otherwise, to use an absurd comparison, you could put two hundred 100-watt light bulbs inside a baseball cap or helmet. None of the light would be absorbed by the scalp or do what is intended—namely, to regrow your hair. But your head would surely be burnt.

Dispelling Myth #4: Treatment Time Does Not Matter

According to the Swedish Medical Society, which has been testing laser dosage and optimal durations for stimulating tissue since 1976, a full twenty minutes is necessary for the ideal dosage. The claim that effective results can be achieved in as little as ninety seconds or up to just six minutes daily is simply untrue—one among several myths. Lasers need to be absorbed by the scalp, and, depending on wavelength, beam diameter, energy delivered per square centimeter, and distance, that process takes twenty minutes.

Because the scalp is one of the thickest areas of skin on the human body, the lasers and the device they're housed in must be perfectly designed for the greatest penetration to reach the hair follicle, especially the bulge and papilla, to ensure optimal effectiveness.

Human tissue is highly receptive to red light and absorbs it quickly, but it takes some time for all available hair follicle cells to fully absorb the photons. Unlike hot lasers, which either burn or cauterize tissue, LPT is a very low-power laser application, requiring more time for the hair follicles to absorb photons and charge up the mitochondria in the bulge and papilla.

Dispelling Myth #5: Wavelengths Don't Make a Difference

The claim that the number of wavelengths a given laser contains doesn't make a difference when it comes to promoting and growing hair is an egregiously misleading myth. Lasers exist along a spectrum of different wavelengths, each of which is best for specific applications. With hair regrowth, the longer the wavelength, the more deeply it penetrates the scalp. The optimal wavelength for growing hair is 680 nm. Lasers that reach a wavelength of 680 nm have been proven to penetrate deeply enough into thick scalp tissue to target the papilla and bulge, which is necessary to stimulate growth. If a device doesn't reach 680 nm, it's not optimal for hair regrowth. Some wavelengths penetrate very poorly into human tissue and anything below 680 nm is not optimal for human tissue.

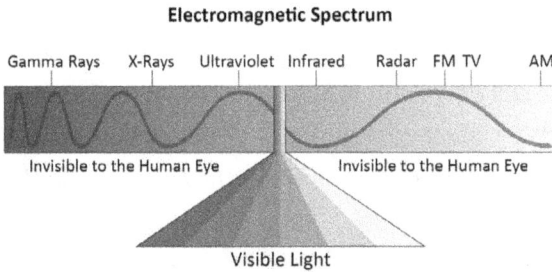

Figure 14.5. Visible Light on the Electromagnetic Spectrum. This chart shows that lasers in the visible light spectrum especially closest to the infrared region can easily penetrate human tissue.

Many scientific papers analyze which wavelengths have the most impact on specific parts of the body. A microwave oven provides an example of the importance of wavelength. The oven's wavelength is set to affect only water molecules. If you put an object without water in it, such as a rock, it won't get hot. Wavelength matters.

It's the same with 680 nm. Because this wavelength primarily stimulates melanin in hair, this wavelength is optimal for preventing hair loss and stimulating growth. This is critical information. If, for example, you were to use a laser with a wavelength of 650 nm, such as numerous lasers manufactured in Asia, it would not be nearly as effective. To be precise, tissue takes in about 2.5 times more light with a wavelength of 680 nm as compared to light whose wavelength is 650 nm. The impact of that 30 nm difference is significant—this is just so important.

Some observers of lasers have wondered why companies would promote lasers with inferior capabilities for hair growth. There are companies fitting devices with lasers whose wavelengths are used for DVDs, CDs, and laser pointers—consumer-grade lasers that are not meant to be used for hair growth. They have significant flaws. Not only are they the wrong wavelength, but they also generate too much heat. But they *are* cheap and easy to obtain.

As we've seen, longer wavelengths penetrate more deeply into the scalp. However, once the wavelength goes above 700 nm, it's no longer visible to the human eye. Furthermore, the FDA will not clear at-home medical devices of more than 680 nm because they are deemed unsafe.

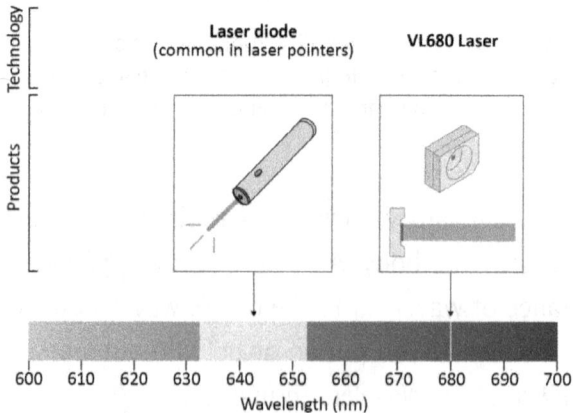

Figure 14.6. Different Laser Devices and Their Wavelengths. All devices use red-pointer laser diodes and only one device in the world uses the 680 nm proprietary type of laser diode which is effective for hair growth.

Dispelling Myth #6: UV Light or Other Non-Red Light Will Grow Hair

Ultraviolet (UV) Light and Wavelength: The ideal 680 nm wavelength represents a balance between the light's energy transference and its penetrative ability. The shorter the wavelength, the more energy can be transferred; however, the shorter wavelengths (UV) get absorbed too readily, while the longer wavelengths (LPT) are effective in stimulating deep structures like hair follicles, probably because the wavelengths at 680 nm and beyond are readily absorbed by the red blood cells.

The fact is that light near the blue end of the visible light spectrum penetrates less than 0.5 mm into the scalp. Light at the red end of the visible light spectrum penetrates about 8 to 10 mm into the scalp, and farther out, near-infrared light penetrates about 20 to 100 mm into the scalp. Near-infrared light is more energetic than visible light and is less resistant to reflection and absorption; therefore, it penetrates soft tissue to a deeper level. But unfortunately, attaining FDA clearance for a near-infrared light, which is invisible and no longer red, would be very difficult for over-the-counter products. So even though dosage can be achieved by using different types of light, staying on the visible light spectrum will achieve the best results.

A great test to see if blue or green or even yellow light can enter human tissue is to take a laser pointer in those colors and place them over your fingers. What you will see is that only the red laser pointer light will penetrate through your fingers; the blue, green and even yellow lights will not. If you take a flashlight, say from your cell phone, and shine it through your finger, only the red portion of the white light (which is visible light) will penetrate through your fingers.

Because the well-known standard known as the Arndt-Schultz Law (see Figure 12.5) determines what doses are beneficial or harmful, the best way to measure dosage is to create the Arndt-Schultz dosage response curve for LPT and hair growth. Research has shown that low dosage levels have a stimulating effect on our hair follicles' cells, but at higher levels, the same wavelengths of light can do more harm than good. Knowing the right dosage is therefore critically important for optimal results with no harm.

Dispelling Myth #7: Pulsing Lasers Are More Efficient than Continuous Lasers

Some vendors of laser devices falsely claim that pulsing lasers are more efficient than continuous lasers. But in fact, pulsing lasers turn on and off to prevent overheating. Unfortunately, the use of pulsing lasers requires manufacturers to compromise the dosage.

In sharp contrast, a continuous laser emits four to ten times more energy than a pulsing laser. A steady, continuous laser is far more effective than one that stops and starts during treatment.

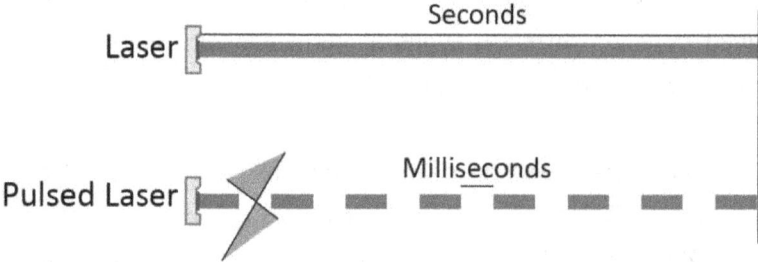

Figure 14.7. Non-Pulsed Lasers vs. Pulsed Lasers. Continuous lasers (top) have much higher power-absorption levels than pulsed lasers, since turning the laser on and off is not efficient.

The reason these laser caps pulse their lasers is that their lasers generate so much heat without any ventilation, especially when they pack hundreds of lasers under a couple of layers of plastic in a baseball cap. Lasers resist heat, and as the temperature rises (even with pulsing), the optical output of the lasers falls dramatically—typically by as much as 80% to 90%.

We have studied many of these baseball-cap-type devices, which often claim that they use 5-milliwatt lasers. Objective tests have confirmed that the measurements were made with temperature sensors while test subjects were wearing the baseball caps. A few seconds after turning on the helmet, the lasers dropped from 5 mW to less than 1 mW. By the time the twenty- to thirty-minute treatment session concluded, the actual optical output was near zero.

Dispelling Myth #8: Scalp Coverage Is More Important than Penetration

Some devices claim to offer greater scalp coverage with either more light sources or an increased spread of light throughout the device. While this may seem impressive to someone who doesn't understand lasers, it's misleading. As explained earlier in this chapter, laser penetration is similar to water hitting a sponge. Once the water hits the sponge, four things happen: Water is reflected, absorbed, scattered, and transmitted. A true laser behaves the same way when hitting the scalp. The laser itself provides optimal coverage only if it's used at the correct wavelength and given the right amount of power. This kind of saturation treats more follicles than does focusing on scalp coverage. The best way for lasers to penetrate the scalp is by having a greater number of lasers with smaller beams since these types of lasers will not heat up the scalp. One large laser beam will heat up the scalp, cause other issues, and will not provide the results being sought.

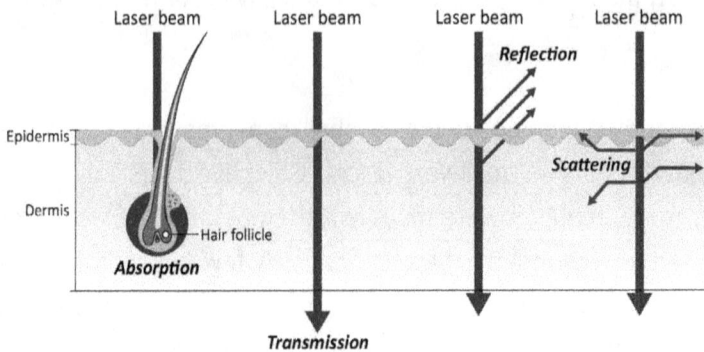

Figure 14.8. Transmission of Laser Beams. Lasers have a very specific behavior in human tissue. The right type of laser light is crucial for stimulating hair follicles. Absorption is key for optimal dosage.

Scalp LLLT devices using commercially available LED and EEL (Edge Emitting Lasers) diodes may offer greater coverage with more lights. They are, however, significantly less effective at delivering energy when compared to lasers. Four significant factors affect energy delivery: inconsistent power, a more divergent (spreading) beam, less-than-ideal wavelength, and a tendency to degrade due to heat. Research shows that using the correct lasers is fundamental, not optional, as the key to success is not total coverage provided by the device itself. The major injustice with these devices extends far beyond the false claims. The injustice is that users are paying extra for light sources that will not grow their hair.

Dispelling Myth #9: Improved Blood Flow Matters for Hair Growth

The head has the best blood flow in the body. This makes sense because it contains the most important organ in the body: the brain. Without proper blood flow, our brains wouldn't work. The head also contains our sense organs—eyes, ears, tongue, and nose. For these organs to work properly, they have to get nutrients through the blood.

You might be thinking, "Okay, but what about the scalp? Is that getting enough blood?" The brain gets a lot of blood directly from the heart through two sets of blood vessels. It receives around 700 ml to 800 ml or 15% to 20% of all our blood in one heartbeat. This blood goes to the brain, the sense organs, and the scalp. So, rest assured, the scalp and the rest of the head are well supplied with blood.

The amount of blood flow is irrelevant because the ultimate goal of all cells in the body is to activate mitochondria, which comprise the powerhouse of each cell. LPT focuses on preventing inflammation and getting cells to normalize their metabolism. That process leads to more ATP power cell activity, which is the key to rejuvenating human cells.

An LPT device can do this without causing heat or side effects.

Dispelling Myth #10: Laser Phototherapy Causes Shedding

Laser hair phototherapy does not promote shedding. The issue is that some LLLT or LPT vendors use the wrong dosage or wavelength thus causing shedding. A properly designed LPT for hair loss should not make things worse. The majority of these LPT/LLLT vendors have warnings that their device might cause hair to shed which is a mind-boggling concept. When the wavelength, dosage, and other design parameters are set perfectly, there will be absolutely no more hair shedding caused by the LPT device. There are instances where some users come off Minoxidil or Finasteride too quickly and this does cause shock loss.

In addition, hair shedding usually occurs from people who use LLLT/LPT devices during shedding in the winter months, when hair naturally sheds. They mistakenly attribute this hair loss to lasers.

The right laser will stimulate growth. A serious error in the choice of wavelength, however, can become the source of serious ongoing problems with shedding. The wrong wavelength, 635 nm to 655 nm, will cause excessive shedding because these wavelengths are not true red light and are better suited for applications such as DVD's, CD-ROMs and laser pointers. It is vital to stay with the wavelength that has been proven to stop hair loss and regrow hair, and that wavelength is 680 nm!

Dispelling Myth #11: Laser Phototherapy and Hormones

Since laser phototherapy doesn't affect hormones, it can't affect what DHT and other hormones do in the body. Most hormones are controlled deep inside the brain by the pituitary glands or other organs. Applying LPT on the scalp will not produce or decrease hormonal levels. This is one fact we need to make sure is accurate and that misinformation about LPT and hormones is not spread. This is one factor we need to overcome rather than correct. Stimulation with lasers helps in 98% of hair loss cases, so it can also help overcome problems associated with DHT.

By improving mitochondrial function in the hair follicles, laser phototherapy can boost cellular energy production and support hair follicles, but the power of hormones outmatches LPT. Excessive hormone secretions will require more LPT treatment sessions until both hormonal levels go back to normal.

The good news is that LPT does stimulate hair follicles and help in the majority of hair loss cases. LPT can try to help overcome problems associated with hormonal fluctuations. The bad news is that LPT cannot control hormone levels and will always be beholden to the secretions of hormones from various organs. It is always a good idea to have one's blood work done routinely to check hormonal levels if there is excessive hair loss happening in a given amount of time.

Dispelling Myth #12: LPT Works Best with Certain Hair Colors

Laser phototherapy produces beneficial results regardless of hair color or type of hair. In the case of dyed hair, new growth triggered by the laser will be in the hair's natural color. LPT can, however, speed up the coloring process and make it more effective. This leads to longer-lasting color.

There are some myths out there that only certain types of hair colors are compatible with LPT; this is not accurate. LPT focuses on the scalp and not on the hair or hair color. Therefore, any color hair can be treated with LPT. Although hair color doesn't affect lasers directly, hair color reduces the scalp's absorption of laser light. Darker hair can affect light transmission, and black hair allows the lowest passage of light. Patients should remove wigs, extensions, and weaves while LPT is applied. LPT can also interfere with tattoo inks, making it unsuitable for people with scalp tattoos.

When it comes to gray hair, LPT can work in a few different ways. LPT can help stop hair loss and maintain the health of already gray hair, but will mostly encourage the growth of new hair of the natural hair color (rather than regrowing new gray hairs).

Dispelling Myth #13: Darker-Skinned People Are Not Suitable for LPT

The darker the skin the more the dosage one receives—this is a fact of physics. Darker skin often accompanies darker hair. Just as wearing a dark shirt when going outdoors will make someone feel warmer, the darker the skin the higher the dosage. Darker-skinned individuals have better results than lighter-skinned individuals. The key consideration is that if no heat is generated from darker-skinned individuals using an LPT device, the product will be safe to use.

The FDA always associated hair removal lasers with heating tissue as these laser diodes cause a real burning sensation necessary to remove the hair. Unfortunately, darker-skinned individuals were not good candidates for laser hair removal treatments, but since LPT is not based on heat, darker individuals are fine to use LPT for hair loss and hair growth.

Since LPT products are available in many different countries, here are two lists that show where, geographically, the most dark-skinned and light-skinned people derive.

Top Five Type VI Fitzpatrick (Darkest) Groups of Skin Tone, Geographically:
1. Southwestern Pacific – The Bougainville Islanders
2. Nilo-Saharan Pastoralist of East Africa – The Mursi/The Surma/Dinka of South Sudan
3. West Africa – Senegal
4. Micronesia – Islands of Micronesia
5. Australia and islands of Tasmania – Aboriginal Australians

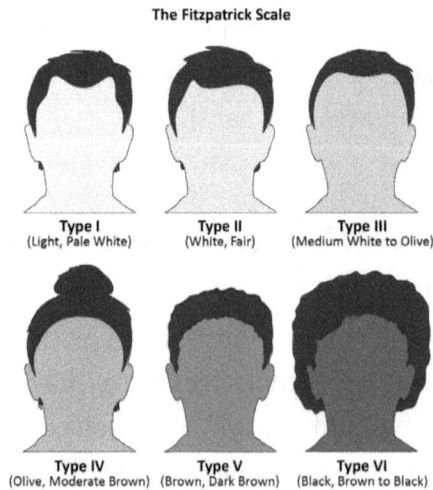

The Fitzpatrick Scale

Type I (Light, Pale White)   Type II (White, Fair)   Type III (Medium White to Olive)

Type IV (Olive, Moderate Brown)   Type V (Brown, Dark Brown)   Type VI (Black, Brown to Black)

Figure 14.9. The Fitzpatrick Scale. Anyone can use LPT for hair growth and hair loss. Lighter skinned individuals need more treatments versus darker individuals require fewer treatments. There are absolutely no side effects for dark or light skinned individuals.

Top Five Type I Fitzpatrick (Lightest) Groups of Skin Tone, Geographically:
1. The British Islanders
2. Scandinavians and Finns
3. Balts
4. Japanese
5. Ashkenazi Jews

The fact is that LPT works on every type of skin color, but darker colors will receive a higher dosage with each treatment and lighter skin types will require more treatments, therefore, dosage and treatment schedules will have to be adjusted accordingly by each type of group of Fitzpatrick skin types.

Dispelling Myth #14: Dead Follicles Cannot Come Back with LPT

Hair follicles are remarkable structures within the skin that play an essential role in the growth and regeneration of hair. Unlike certain other cells in the human body, hair follicles do not permanently die due to their unique biological features and regenerative abilities. Remember from Chapter 2 that the average human scalp has about 200 hair follicles per square centimeter. These hair follicles will always be there on the scalp. This density can differ based on factors like genetics, ethnicity, and individual variations.

The fact is that the scalp is under the constant attack of Malassezia furfur (MF). For individuals who are allergic to MF, it can cause inflammation on the scalp due to factors such as seborrheic dermatitis and dandruff, discussed in Chapter 2 as part of the Five Whys.

The final and long-term effect of fungal inflammation is an increase in the production of skin on the scalp due to an increase of epidermal growth factor (EGF). Epidermal growth factor, or EGF, is a special protein that helps skin cells grow and repair themselves. Sometimes, there can be more EGF on the scalp than normal. As the new skin thickens over the old skin, the hair follicles are still under the old skin but devoid of hair follicles and contain only sweat and oil glands. In hair, this results in a narrowing of the pore through which the hair is growing. The final result is the elimination of the thicker hairs with replacement by fine thin hairs. The key structure in the hair follicle (dermal papilla) is now forced to assume a resting phase. DHT is responsible for the formation of EGF. All of the average 200 hair follicles per square centimeter are still there and have not died, per se, but they are now much deeper in the scalp. The combination of hairs getting thinner and the pores getting smaller results in a shinier and slicker-looking scalp in more advanced hair loss individuals.

The good news is that we have seen many hair specialists (Chapter 16) regrow areas of scalps that were barren of hair follicles. The key to regaining one's hair is to reduce or eliminate the inflammation and strengthen the hairs to push through the thicker skin as they have been reduced down by many cycles of DHT and thus, hair will come back.

LPT will not be the only solution for very advanced hair loss, and with today's LPT power and dosage, I believe this will need further research. However, it will necessitate a multi-prong approach. When a hair transplant is performed the new donor hair is positioned in the right depth and this is why it can survive. Patients who do not take care of their scalps will most likely experience loss of these new hair transplants due to the constant inflammation from the MF on their scalp especially as their hairs get longer. This can be remedied with the use of the right medicated shampoo, LPT, and supplements.

A significantly thicker scalp may affect hair follicles and hair growth patterns. It is important to monitor the overall health of the scalp and hair when increasing EGF production to ensure a proper balance is maintained for optimal hair growth and scalp health. Testing to see if the scalp is getting thicker is not possible at the moment but we have seen over and over again that men and women with thicker skins take a much longer time to regrow hair, and the longer they wait, the less chance of regaining their hair back.

Some ridiculous ideas that are circulating on the internet are that men's or women's scalps are somehow tightening and this causes excess tension on the hair follicles causing the skin to become tauter and smoother resulting in a shinier appearance due to the reflection of light on the smooth surface. Another myth is that grooming habits, especially for men who have lost their hair, choose to shave their remaining hair, or maintain a closely cropped hairstyle, further contribute to a smooth, shiny scalp. The use of moisturizers, oils, or other grooming products can also enhance the shine of the scalp. These are absolutely illogical reasons and they do not make sense and should never be accepted by anyone. Unfortunately, the internet is full of these ridiculous claims.

So, this myth is a bit difficult to explain, as it relies on the false premise that hair follicles die (they do not). LPT can, however, bring back hairs that have not been fully covered up by the new skin that covers up the scalp in more advanced hair loss patients. The earlier one starts LPT the more likely their hairs will be recovered.

Dispelling Myth #15: Anyone Can Produce LPT Devices

It's important that a quality medical device designed specifically for the head, our most valuable asset, such as an LPT device helmet, be manufactured in the USA rather than outside of it as the US has strict regulatory guidelines for medical devices. These include quality control, regulatory compliance, and proper implementation of engineering principles throughout the manufacturing process as well as providing customer service throughout the life of the product. In addition, the concept of recalls and other mechanisms that ensure patient safety and clinical reporting is essential for any consumer to consider.

It is important to weigh price versus value when comparing the cost of LPT devices to keep and regrow your hair. Many devices from outside of the US are expensive to manufacture because they use a great deal of manual labor. Having workers solder lasers by hand means that it takes hours to assemble each device. Shipping back to the United States is also costly. Consequently, manufacturers outside of the US are driving up the prices of LPT devices, which is somewhat contrary to conventional thinking of imported devices. Designing the product to be fully automated and built in the US eliminates shipping and manual labor costs, thereby reducing the selling price.

Unfortunately, higher prices are frequently associated with higher quality. A product isn't always better because it has a higher price tag. Getting materials from quality producers and avoiding enormous overseas shipping costs substantially lower manufacturing costs. Many factors affect the end price, so a laser device should be evaluated based on its effects, not its cost.

While there may be cost advantages to producing medical devices in low-cost geographies, the benefits of manufacturing them in the USA can outweigh these considerations, particularly in the case of head-related medical devices, where safety, quality, and compliance are of utmost importance.

Actual Customer Success Stories

A Less-Shining Example

For Richard, hair loss appeared to be a family curse. Every man in his African-American family had thinning hair by their thirties. At family gatherings, it looked like all the men had shiny bald heads and polished their scalps for the special occasion. Richard wanted a different future. When his hair began to thin, he considered laser treatment. His cousins laughed, saying lasers wouldn't work, especially not for people of color. But Richard had done his homework. Ten years later, thanks to laser treatment, he's the only man in the family with a full head of hair at holiday dinners.

CHAPTER 15

Is LPT Right for Me?

"Trust starts with truth and ends with truth."
— Santosh Kalwar, Poet, 2011

LPT Side Effects

There are no significant long-term side effects to LPT treatments. A few people have reported brief tension headaches, sensitive skin, or acne, which cleared up in a couple of weeks or less, though some of the same side effects were experienced by control groups during the research phase using sham devices that didn't work. Other studies reported no LPT side effects. The implication is that short-term side effects, such as tension headaches, could result from wearing a helmet rather than from laser treatment. That is a far cry from the long lists of damaging and potentially fatal side effects from other drugs or surgical treatments being offered today.

A review of hundreds of studies on red light therapies such as LPT found no adverse reactions mainly because the amount of energy exposure during treatments is so low that tissue temperatures don't increase more than a few hundredths of a degree. Because LPT devices can have remarkably potent effects, the nearly non-thermal treatments make them particularly attractive for use on recent hair loss or thinning. As a result of rigorous testing, LPT—already an FDA-cleared treatment for hair growth—is regarded as a Non-Significant Risk device, meaning that the potential for harm is so low that it would be virtually impossible to cause any damage to human tissue.

Anyone who experiences hair loss is a suitable candidate for laser phototherapy. However, not everyone benefits from laser phototherapy in the same way. Patients get the best results when matched with the most appropriate therapy. Laser phototherapy works best for patients who have not reached the regression phase when changes to the scalp are almost irreversible. On the Hamilton-Norwood Scale of male pattern hair loss, people suffering from such severe progression may not see much improvement with laser phototherapy.

Contraindications

A contraindication is a reason not to undergo a certain medical treatment because the treatment may cause harm. Fortunately, there are no absolute contraindications for LPT, only relative ones and warnings.

Although there are no conclusive tests determining any harm, the FDA notes warnings for people with scalp cancer and pregnant women. Yet we can't say for sure that there are no issues with these groups even though no tests have shown problems. And since we don't know whether they're at risk of severe harm, we don't want them to take unnecessary risks. Besides, we consider it unethical to conduct testing on pregnant women, potentially putting the fetus at risk. The fact is that over a billion LPT treatments have been performed over the past forty years and no bona fide medical device complaints have been submitted to date.

Cancer and LPT

Many people don't know too much about lasers. Some believe that a laser emits some kind of mystical "radiation." Yes, radiation (e.g., X-ray or gamma) can be dangerous and can even cause cancer. But can the light from therapeutic laser phototherapy cause cancer? No, *definitely* not. *No* mutational effects have been observed from light with wavelengths above 600 nm at the doses that are used in laser phototherapy. New LPT products are being cleared by the FDA to *treat* cancers, masses, lesions, tumors, and cysts. Individuals with metal plates, cochlear implants, pacemakers, implantable cardiac defibrillators (ICDs), photosensitive medication, and other afflictions and devices are also being cleared for LPT treatment. Therefore, it seems likely that there are few if any additional conditions or populations in which laser phototherapy should be avoided (and only if a doctor recommends avoiding it). The FDA has already cleared the use of laser devices for unsupervised individual use because lasers are safe and effective. That's why it is safe for you to use the LPT helmet to stop your hair loss and regrow hair at home while you're doing your own thing—like reading this book on your tablet.

Shiny Scalps and LPT

In cases of advanced hair loss where the scalp becomes completely devoid of hair or has mostly shiny spots and is unable to regrow hair, those areas of the scalp primarily have a presence of oil and sweat glands. This condition mostly affects men but in rare cases some women have shiny scalps especially after years of hair loss. These are Hamilton-Norwood VI to VII for men and Ludwig-Savin I-5 for women. We do not recommend LPT for these types of patients and only after they have decided to perform a hair transplant as this is the only way to put hair back on their scalp. Once an HT has been performed then we highly recommend using an LPT device to ensure that the HT survives for longer than five years.

Three Ways LPT Affects Hair

LPT will affect your scalp. As I have shown you, both from the scientific and clinical perspective, it has been confirmed and millions of people around the world are enjoying the benefits of LPT.

1. LPT slows down hair loss by converting most hairs from the resting phase to the growth phase, which lasts two to eight years. Less hair loss indicates that the scalp will appear fuller over time due to about 3,000 hairs not shedding over thirty days.

2. LPT reverses the miniaturization phase. In the miniaturizing phase, it appears as if new hairs are growing, but that's not the case. The reality is that hairs are just thicker because they are changing from vellus to terminal hairs.

3. LPT triggers more hairs per square centimeter than we would expect to see in the dormant phase. Patients can go from ten to fifty hairs per square centimeter to fifty-plus hairs in a single square centimeter. This differs from person to person, but everyone has a positive result from LPT. The only exception is someone with a hairless, shiny scalp. This smooth, shiny scalp is a new type of skin that buries hair follicles and contains only sweat and oil glands.

Actual Customer Success Stories

A Bright Future

When Aisha's doctor told her that her cancer treatment had been successful, she was just happy to be alive—to put her year of hell behind her. However, her exposed scalp was a constant reminder of what she'd been through. It didn't seem fair to be left with this visible sign of her ordeal. A friend she'd met at a support group during her treatment had a beautiful head of hair again. In contrast, Aisha's hair was brittle; its color faded from its original deep, rich shade. When Aisha mentioned her sadness about her hair to her friend, that friend told her about laser therapy. Aisha tried her helmet and was amazed at its ease of use. She bought one of her own, and within a couple of months, her hair and confidence were on the road to recovery.

CHAPTER 16:

Meet the Team: Hair Loss Professionals and their Specialties

"The only incurable diseases are those the doctors don't know how to cure." — Charles F. Kettering, Inventor, 1957

Hair Specialists in Today's World

When you have a heart problem, you see a cardiologist. When you have a tooth problem, you know it is time to visit the dentist. It's that simple, and everyone knows which specialist to visit. But can we say the same about hair? Definitely not. The questions many people ask when they are faced with hair loss is, "Where do I get help?" "Who do I turn to?"

Hair loss can be devastating. Especially when we realize that it can happen to young people as well as to older people. It simply doesn't discriminate. In desperation, people turn to Doctor Google: "Where do I go for hair loss help?" Google will give them millions of suggestions, none of which sound right, and they may end up more confused than ever. Remember that companies bid millions of dollars to be at the top of your Google searches! After giving up on Google, they eventually go to the doctor, hoping for help.

Unfortunately, general practitioners know little, and you won't find a hair department at the hospital. The burn unit, plastic surgery unit, and dermatology are about as close as you'll get. The burn unit treats cases of heat, chemical, or electrical burns (so if you use those baseball cap units with hundreds of diodes as we discussed, you just might end up there!). Not a good match for hair loss issues. Plastic surgery may involve the skin, and dermatology treats skin conditions. Hair is included in their scope of treatment but their practice is not the full answer

Dermatologists and Physicians

Hair is one of the three main subjects in dermatology (skin and nails are the other two). Since the structure and function of hair are integral parts of their studies, dermatologists may be able to help you understand the backstory of hair loss. They may be able to diagnose the type of hair loss you have by listening to your history and putting you through different tests. Dermatologists may even provide consultation on hair loss or prescribe oral medications, topicals, or supplements.

Hair loss, however, is only one of the many things that the dermatologists do. Dermatologists are actually more involved with skin than hair loss. Since the skin is the largest organ in the body, it has to battle hundreds of diseases. So, hair loss is not a primary concern for dermatologists. The fact is that over 40% of patients that come visit dermatologists have hair issues, but since the majority of dermatologists don't really market hair services, these patients go unnoticed.

Some dermatologists are trained and certified to give specialized hair loss treatments, which may include steroid injections and platelet-rich plasma (PRP) injections. They can also prescribe medications such as Minoxidil (Rogaine), Finasteride, and certain supplements for the treatment of hair loss. All things considered; we can safely say a dermatologist is qualified to provide treatments that can regrow hair.

Hair Transplant Surgeons

The vast majority of hair transplant surgeons are not dermatologists nor are they trichologists; they restrict themselves to HTs and PRP injections. While some dermatologists are starting to get into HTs, this requires a lot of effort since an HT takes many hours of training and special equipment as well as dedicated resources and staff. There are many services that dermatologists "bolt" onto their clinics, including HTs, but these dermatologists might perform a fraction of the surgeries of a dedicated HT surgeon, who is often booked for months in advance (especially if they are good). In general, the more experienced an HT surgeon, the better the results. So, it's important to know whether they are dedicated to HT surgery or HTs are merely another income stream.

Another consideration is where they stand on LPT, which is still a new concept for most HT surgeons. So, we have a few HT surgeons who aren't familiar with LPT and don't understand its benefits. And we have some HT surgeons who already have LPT devices in their procedure rooms, and while removing the donor graft, they will subject the scalp to red laser light. This helps ensure that new blood vessels form around the hair follicles. These surgeons also apply LPT right after a transplant procedure to reduce swelling and to ensure the formation of new blood vessels (angiogenesis). They are very pro-LPT and claim that their HTs last much longer, which cuts back on the chances of needing another HT in the future. Therefore, it is very important to consider these attributes when considering an HT surgeon.

Despite all the things dermatologists and hair transplant surgeons can do, there's another field where hair has a more central role than it does in dermatology or other specialties. Let me introduce you to trichology, the branch of medical science dedicated to the hair and scalp.

What Is a Trichologist?

In 1860, there was a surge in scientific interest in hair loss and hair care. It began in a barbershop in London and led to an intense study by the self-taught "Professor" Wheeler. By 1902, this interest yielded the field of trichology, which deals with hair disorders and their treatment (the word trichology is taken from *trichos*, meaning *hair* in Greek). In the same year, the first Institute of Trichologists was founded. The International Association of Trichologists was formed in California in 1974. The IAT now offers courses to students around the world who wish to study hair and become certified in its treatments.

Trichologists vs. Physicians

After passing courses in hair and scalp disorders, trichologists are certified, which makes them competent to advise people with hair-related problems. Their recommendations are based on their assessments of patients and their patients' provided histories.

Since trichologists are not doctors, they're not certified to prescribe drugs or perform surgeries. Nor can they request laboratory tests, although they can get test results through a physician who has ordered tests for a patient. For example, a serum vitamin D–level test may be requested to see whether a patient has a vitamin D deficiency.

Recently, there's been greater interest in board-certified physicians to treat hair-related conditions. This has led to the emergence of new fields in medicine and dermatology. In 2010, the term dermatotrichologist was coined to describe board-certified dermatologists who specialize in the scientific study of the hair and scalp. These "hair doctors" may learn about and research treatments such as laser phototherapy. Furthermore, a newer term is being proposed for such dermatologists: *trichiatrist*. This term will be reserved for medical professionals who are expressly involved in managing the health of hair and scalp.

Right now, however, there aren't enough dermatologists to handle the demand.

The practice consensus released by the International Society of Hair Restoration Surgery (ISHRS) in 2021 had quite a few astounding findings:

- It estimated that approximately 703,183 hair restoration procedures were performed worldwide in 2021, a whopping 77% surge as compared to 2014 (397,048 procedures performed). Demand for HTs increased substantially during the COVID-19 era.
- Dermatologists are busy with dermatology, treating disorders affecting the skin such as skin cancer, psoriasis, eczema, leprosy, etc.
- Dermatologists, even if they treat hair, do not have the time needed to handle hair cases.
- Hair patients often have special requirements—they need detailed counseling, including psychological counseling, which is difficult to perform in a busy skin clinic.
- Medical management options for hair disorders are limited with very few drugs and, therefore, are not challenging enough.
- Surgical treatment is time-consuming and has a steep learning curve.
- This has led to the situation where non-dermatologists have assumed the role of trichologists.

At the moment, trichologists are the only specialists focused solely on hair and scalp concerns. Their field of study is narrow to allow specialized knowledge instead of memorizing dozens or hundreds of other fields. And because every patient they treat has hair and scalp issues, their depth of experience cannot be matched.

Physicians and Photonics

Photonics and optics are both branches of physics that study the behavior of light and its properties, and lasers fall in the category of photonics.

Earlier chapters of this book discussed the importance of light in the treatment of hair loss. Therefore, we can assume doctors are taught photonics in medical school, right? Unfortunately, no. Far more emphasis is put on the study of anatomy, physiology, biochemistry, pathology, and pharmacology. Medical training focuses on different systems and areas of the body as well as their diseases. Learning a little bit about everything scatters the physician's knowledge base. Most of the treatments they are taught involve drugs or surgery. X-rays sometimes come into play, but a routine treatment in the hospital probably won't involve light.

Since doctors aren't thoroughly trained in the field of photonics, they're limited in the ways they can use light to treat patients. Although some physicians may have experience with photonics from other fields they studied before going to medical school, that learning is not standard. For example, a doctor who took a physics course may understand the basics of optics and photonics, and a doctor who had some training in bioengineering may be familiar with the uses of light in treatment, but rarely is a doctor who is an expert in physics or optics or photonics. For example, medical devices like PETs (Positron Emission Tomography), MRIs (Magnetic Resonance Imaging, CTs (Computer Tomography), HIFUs (High Intensity Focused Ultrasound), and many others were discovered by physicists (non-physicians) and took several decades until they were fully adopted by hospitals due to the complexity of these devices.

Physicians and Lasers

Laser phototherapy applies the principles of light to the treatment of hair conditions. Since doctors as a rule don't have a strong background in photonics, their understanding of the use of lasers in phototherapy is fairly weak. Not surprisingly, it's difficult for many doctors to appreciate the benefits of laser phototherapy.

Physicians don't necessarily have extensive knowledge of the physics behind the manufacturing, design, and functioning of LPT devices. The fact is that it takes pharmaceutical drugs between seven and fourteen years to gain acceptance amongst physicians; medical devices take about three times as long due to their complex scientific nature. There are currently 141 medical institutions in the U.S. that grant MD degrees and thirty-one accredited DO-granting institutions. Despite these high numbers, LPT is not included as part of any typical medical curriculum. As a result, medical insurance does not usually cover the cost of LPT. However, this is beginning to change in the field of physical therapy and sports medicine. Since the core mechanism of LPT does not vary between medical conditions, the fact that hair loss is viewed differently is contradictory.

A consultation with a dermatologist when hair loss is the problem will usually end with a prescription and some advice on supplements. Although some dermatologists are becoming more aware of the benefits of LPT, it is still not the norm.

Dermatologists who are informed about LPT improve their treatment outcomes by including sessions of LPT in their prescribed therapy. Patients get the combined benefits of a medication that stops, perhaps, their unregulated hormone action and a laser treatment that promotes hair growth and reduces shedding by targeting the hair follicle. LPT is also being encouraged after hair transplants. This usage by dermatologists and hair transplant surgeons shows how doctors are trying to catch up to what trichologists already know: LPT works for hair loss.

Trichology and the Abundant Causes of Hair Loss

There are many hair conditions and diseases, but some are more likely to strike than others. One of the most common is hereditary hair loss as seen in male or female pattern hair loss. This is the condition dermatologists see most frequently.

However, as we know from Chapter 2, hair loss is a complex problem. It might be the simple stoppage of the hair growth cycle, or it can follow from illnesses, surgeries, and other traumatic occurrences. Changes in hormone levels such as those that often come with pregnancy, childbirth, use of birth control pills, or menopause may also lead to hair loss. Underlying medical conditions, including thyroid disease, autoimmune diseases (such as alopecia areata, which attacks hair follicles), or infections of the scalp (such as ringworm) cause hair loss. Scarring from certain types of lupus or a condition known as lichen planus are other potential causes of hair loss. Certain medications can also result in hair loss, including treatments for cancer, high blood pressure, arthritis, depression, and heart disease. Even simple aspirin has been tied to hair loss. High fever, extreme weight loss, or the kind of emotional shock that might result from a death in the family can all lead to hair loss. And then there's trichotillomania, a psychological disorder in which patients compulsively pluck hairs from the head, eyelashes, or eyebrows. Hairstyles that pull on the hair follicles are yet another cause. Finally, a diet lacking essential nutrients, such as protein or iron, may also cause a person to lose their hair.

So you see, we need trichologists. Trichologists specialize in carefully assessing the many potential causes of hair loss in their patients and treating the root cause instead of recommending a one-size-fits-all medication that may not work.

Blood Tests, Trichology, and How Doctors Treat Hair Loss

A visit to the trichologist will typically include an overall assessment. The trichologist will ask questions related to your medical history, eating habits, lifestyle, and haircare routine. The answers will help the trichologist understand the history of your hair loss and the nature of your problem. The goal is to find the right treatment for the specific problem.

They may also request tests that show a complete blood count and the levels of iron, thyroid-stimulating hormones, and vitamin D. These are all associated with hair loss. There are additional tests for women, which include measuring the levels of various sex hormones.

A complete blood workup can help identify some of the causes of damage to hair follicles. These include androgen hormones, thyroid hormones, certain microorganisms, vitamin D levels, iron levels, and certain minerals.

High levels of androgen hormones lead to hair loss because they shrink hair follicles and reduce hair growth.

A deficiency of iron or certain other minerals slows the hair growth cycle. An iron deficiency from 13.5 to 17.5 grams per deciliter (g/dl) directly affects the hair follicles. At such low iron levels, follicles may not be able to grow new cells the way they used to.

Both high and low levels of thyroid hormones cause hair loss by slowing the maturation of hair follicle cells. Normal levels of thyroid hormones in the blood are 0.40–4.50 milli-international units per liter of blood (mIU/mL). Any fluctuation from this normal range can cause numerous complications, including hair loss.

Vitamin D, which we already know is linked to hair loss, is deficient at less than 12 nanograms per milliliter (ng/mL).

Bloodwork can determine these levels, and thorough bloodwork can hint at the outcome of pattern hair loss.

The table below is a summary of the bloodwork done for the underlying causes that may be responsible for hair loss.

Blood Work	Possible Underlying Cause of Hair Loss	Possible Reference ranges
Complete blood count (CBC)	Routine medical test that detects overall abnormalities in the body	If results are inside the reference range, they're considered normal. If your results are higher or lower than the reference range, they're abnormal
Ferritin	Iron deficiency anemia	Female 10-150 ng/ml Male 30-400 ng/ml
Thyroid-stimulating hormone (and thyroid-function tests)	Thyroid diseases	0.45–4.5 mIU/L
Vitamin D 25(OH)	Vitamin D deficiency	30-100 ng/ml
Total testosterone	Androgen excess	Female 8–48 ng/dL Male 264–919 ng/dL
Dehydroepi-androsterone sulfate		Female 84.8–378.0 ug/dL Male 138.5–475.2 ug/dL
Prolactin	Hyperprolactinemia (high levels of prolactin) leading to androgen excess	Male: 4.0-15.2 ng/mL Female: 4.8-23.3 ng/mL
Vitamin B12	Pernicious Anemia (Auto-immune)	160-950 pg/ml
Anti-Nuclear Antibody (ANA)	Check to see if you have an autoimmune disorder	• Negative: <1:80 • Borderline: 1:80 • Positive: >1:80
C-Reactive Protein (CRP)	Help diagnose a chronic inflammatory disease, such as rheumatoid arthritis or lupus	0-10 mg/L

Estradiol (E2) (Women only)	Imbalance raises the telogen/anagen ratio	• Follicular: 12.5-166.0 pg/mL • Ovulation: 85.8-498.0 pg/mL • Luteal: 43.8-211.0 pg/mL • Postmenopausal: <6.0-54.7 pg/mL
Progesterone (Women only)	Inadequate level aids in the conversion of testosterone to DHT	• Follicular: 0.1-0.9/ng/mL • Ovulation: 0.1-12.0ng/mL • Luteal: 1.8-23.9 ng/mL • Postmenopausal: 0.0-0.1 ng/mL
Cortisol, AM	Detects malfunction of the adrenal gland, the pituitary, and the hypothalamus	6.2-19.4 ug/dL

Figure 16.1. Causes and Reference Range. Trichologists use these blood results to determine the root cause of hair loss issues.

The trichologist may provide helpful recommendations for reversing hair loss. In other cases, they may refer the patient to a dermatologist or another specialist for testing.

Trichologists often see hair pattern hair loss in men and women, telogen effluvium, alopecia areata, traumatic hair loss or breakage, and scarring alopecia. The scalp conditions they encounter include different types of eczemas, dandruff, psoriasis, folliculitis, and itching acne. They really see it all, especially when other professionals have given up on a patient.

The uniqueness of trichology lies in its targeted focus on conditions of the hair and scalp. As certified practitioners, they're able to devote their time and effort to assessing patients and providing suitable treatment for hair loss. And trichologists are still improving in their practice through the formation of vibrant international societies. These collaborations allow a global transfer of knowledge among trichologists. Luckily for us, the field is still growing!

LPT for Hair Loss and Scalp Disorders

The main weapon in the trichologist's fight against hair loss is LPT. Trichologists have a sound understanding of LPT because it's a treatment that relates directly to hair. The *International Journal of Trichology*, which reviews scientific studies related to hair loss and other scalp conditions, has published numerous studies that evaluate the effectiveness of LPT.

Common Types of Alopecia

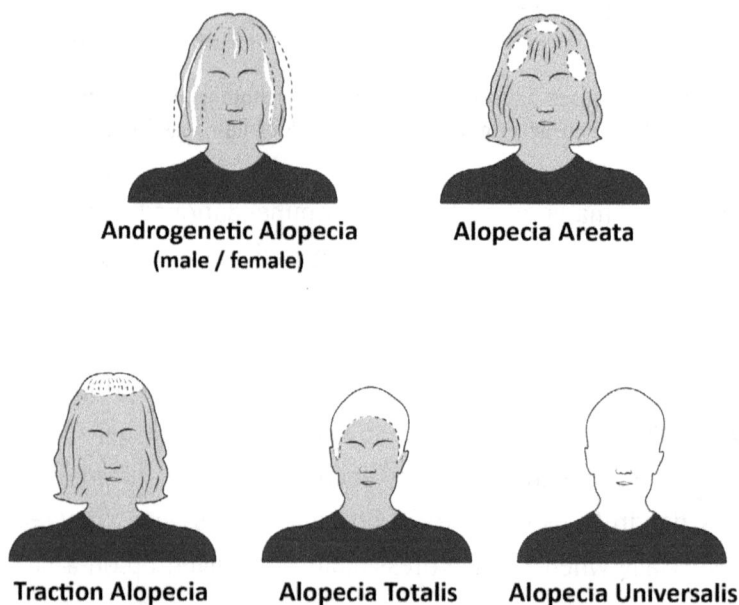

Androgenetic Alopecia
(male / female)

Alopecia Areata

Traction Alopecia   **Alopecia Totalis**   **Alopecia Universalis**

Figure 16.2. Common Types of Alopecia. Androgenetic Alopecia is by far the most popular type of hair loss condition.

Trichologists sometimes use only LPT for treatment, but it can be used in combination with other treatments. Some of the laser devices trichologists recommend for treating hair conditions include laser combs, laser bands, and laser helmets. As you know, laser helmets have proven especially effective and have generated a good deal of excitement in trichology circles over the last decade. Because they work. It's as simple as that. And you have already read why laser combs and laser bands *do not*.

Hair Disease	Condition	Can LPT Treat?
Androgenetic Alopecia	Genetic hair loss/93% of all hair loss	Yes (FDA-cleared)
Telogen Effluvium (TE)	Episodes of severe hair loss	Yes
Alopecia Areata (AA)	Sudden hair loss in patches	Yes
Alopecia Totalis	Complete loss of hair on the scalp	No
Alopecia Universalis	Complete hair loss, autoimmune disorder	No
Cicatricial Alopecia	Scarring hair loss	Yes
Traction Alopecia	Hair loss caused by mechanical stress	Yes
Frontal Fibrosing Alopecia	Scarring hair loss, frontal hairline recession	Yes
Central Centrifugal Cicatricial Alopecia	Scarring hair loss, central region	Yes
Chemo Induced Alopecia	Hair loss due to chemotherapy	Yes
Postpartum Alopecia	Hair loss following pregnancy period	Yes
Diffuse Alopecia	Widespread, thinning hair loss pattern	Yes
Lichen Planopilari	Inflammatory scarring hair loss	Yes
Folliculitis Decalvans	Inflammatory, scarring follicular hair loss	No
Polycystic Ovary Syndrome (PCOS)	Hormonal imbalance, cysts, ovaries, hair loss	Yes
Loose Anagen Syndrome	Easily detached hair, premature shedding	Yes
Trichotillomania (regrowing only)	Compulsive hair pulling disorder	Yes
Dissecting Cellulitis of the Scalp	Inflammatory scalp condition, abscesses	No
Discoid Lupus Erythematosus	Scarring, inflammatory skin lesions	No

Figure 16.3. Hair Diseases and the Probability of Using LPT to Treat These Conditions. There are many trichologists now experimenting with many of these diseases to determine if LPT could help.

The majority of these hair diseases affect fewer than twenty million people in the US. That figure will come down as more trichologists experiment with laser phototherapy as a potential solution for some of these hair diseases. We are fortunate to live in a modern era where medical techniques and innovations such as LPT devices are available with no further harm to patients in terms of potential side effects.

Actual Customer Success Stories

Lasers Are a Girl's Best Friend

Rebecca had always had long hair, and she felt it was essential to her femininity. When she noticed her hair was thinning at the top of her head, she determined she'd do everything to fix it. Her hair was too important to her sense of herself as a woman for her to let it go. Her stylist told her about seeing a trichologist, which she had never heard about. She scheduled an appointment, and the trichologist did a complete set of tests on her, including her blood work, hair sample testing, and about another half a dozen tests. The trichologist determined that she was suffering from a condition called Lichen Planopilari, an inflammatory scalp condition and that wearing a laser phototherapy device would halt the hair loss and promote regrowth. A few months later, she visited her stylist, and they both were impressed with the results.

CHAPTER 17

Frequently Asked Questions

"The important thing is not to stop questioning." — Albert Einstein, Physicist, 1955

How Do I Use a Laser Phototherapy Helmet?

If you've invested your time and money in understanding LPT devices (the fact that you're reading this book says that you have), you've probably come to the conclusion that an LPT helmet is your best option. Now, you most certainly want to know how to use your LPT helmet. We've summarized the information for using a laser-only phototherapy helmet-type of device by addressing the most frequently asked questions about them.

How Long Before I See Results?

Often, the results of laser phototherapy are seen as early as the fourth week of use. The first noticeable change is usually a slow-down in the rate of hair loss. By the eighteenth week, existing hair thickens, reducing miniaturization. By the end of six months, there is actual regrowing and renewing of the hair. So, although it might seem like a bit of a wait before you see results, the good news is that the effects continue beyond a year. It is important to note that LPT treatments are long-term ones that require commitment and consistency. In general, the more you use an LPT device, the sooner you will start to see results.

You may not notice any changes during the first few weeks after starting treatment. That is because LPT devices work below the surface, invisible to the naked eye. Before new hair grows, you will first see a reduction in hair loss, and then hair becomes thicker. That is how you will know the LPT device is working. Remember that slowing down hair loss is the first crucial step in regaining your hair back!

As I did with Melba, it is important that you take consistent pictures to keep track of your hair growth progress.

What Are the Best Treatment Intervals?

Every individual is unique, so there may be slight variations in the intervals that produce the best treatment for laser devices. Generally speaking, the best treatment intervals are two sessions of laser phototherapy per week. As a rule, it's best to space out LPT treatments by at least twelve hours. This is because overstimulating the mitochondria on hair follicles may inhibit new hair growth.

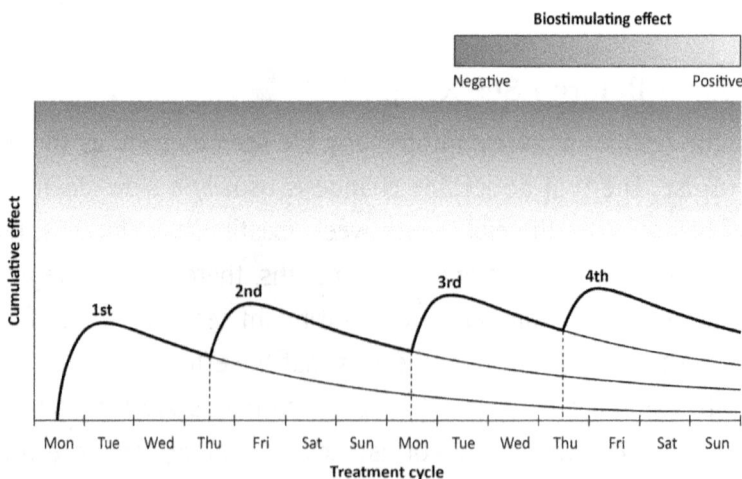

Figure 17.1. The LPT Treatment Cycle. This chart shows the cumulative effect of LPT on the scalp and recommended number of treatments one can do within a one-week period.

How Many Times Per Week Can I Use My LPT Device?

Depending on the power and fluence of the LPT device, the recommended treatment cycle is in the figure above. Since hair follicles are the most active structure, it is advisable to get a daily routine so this will be part of your daily life. This graphic shows that one should do treatments every couple of days, but the fact is that we have found from thousands of our customers that the more they use it the faster and better the outcome. So, power users do a treatment almost every day with absolutely no side effects and with excellent results. If you decide to go beyond the recommended usage, it's advisable to allow a few hours of rest between each treatment. The goal is not to overstimulate the mitochondria in the hair follicles. It will stagnate progress. We do not recommend doing back-to-back LPT treatments; we advise you to give it at least a few hours of rest between treatments.

How Much Is Enough? How Much Is Too Much?

Once you start to see results, keep going! Only taper off once you've achieved the *desired* results. At that point, you can go with a maintenance dosage of LPT. A maintenance treatment schedule of two twenty-minute sessions per week is recommended using an LPT wearable device or four twenty-minute sessions per week for LPT devices with fewer lasers. Laser hair therapy is similar to exercise—you have to integrate it into your lifestyle to continue enjoying the benefits.

How Do I Achieve the Fastest Results Possible?

Look after your hair. Remember, your body is constantly trying to get rid of your hair. Make it easier on your body to keep by avoiding harmful products. When brushing, styling, or grooming your hair, be kind—no excessive pulling, heat such as curling irons, or hair dryers (only use cool rather than heat mode), no tight elastics, or brushing excessively. Do not use pomades, or styling gels, especially alcohol-based products as they dry out the scalp and affect sebum production and cause an imbalanced scalp.

Use the right shampoo and conditioner, choose the right supplements, and use the LPT device as routinely as possible. You cannot force results, and you must be patient. Always take pictures, this is the only way to show yourself that LPT is working for you!

What Are the Best Times to Do an LPT Treatment?

Anytime! The best time for wearing the LPT helmet is whenever is most convenient for you. Since the LPT helmet is a hands-free device, you can use it while you're working at home or relaxing, working at your desk, playing a board game with your kids, watching TV, or even playing video games. We recommend placing the LPT device where you spend the most time privately. If you work from home and have a home or private office, then place your LPT device right on your desk and build up a routine. If you have a long drive or commute, use the LPT device while on your drive. If you tend to watch TV daily, place the LPT device next to your chair or couch. If you take time getting dressed and preparing to go out, then place the LPT device in your closet or bedroom. If you read each night, watch the news, or grade papers, these are perfect times. The goal is to make the LPT accessible and make it a part of your daily routine. Many customers have multiple LPT devices, one in their workplace and one in their bedroom or home office or one in each place. It really depends on where you spend the most time on any day or week.

What Is a Power Treatment?

A power treatment is simply when, after taking a shower, you towel dry your hair leaving it damp-dry and, before using a hair dryer, comb the damp hair to expose the areas that are thinning the most. Then place the LPT device on your head and do a treatment. Exposing those areas of the scalp that have the most thinning will give them better exposure to light. But your hair doesn't need to be damp each time you wear the helmet—only for occasional "power treatments."

We call this a power treatment because you are applying the most amount of laser light to the problem areas of your scalp before putting any creams, mousse, gels, hair products, or hair fibers that might cover the areas. You only need to do this after a shower, and then you can shave and put on your clothes to make this part of your routine.

What Happens When My Hair Starts Growing Back? Then What?

Once the desired results have been achieved, lasers can still penetrate the scalp, and you should continue LPT to maintain your hair. Incorporating LPT into your weekly schedules is a good idea. Remember, LPT is like exercise, you want it to be part of your lifestyle routine. LPT should be seen as something that has both curative and promotional qualities for your hair.

Do I Have to Use LPT for the Rest of My Life?

Yes. The hair is the least required structure in the human body so whether it is stress, an underlying medical condition, or aging-related issues, the body is always trying to get rid of it. Hair loss gets worse with aging, especially if it's compounded by androgenetic alopecia. Therefore, it will be a continuing effort to maintain a great head of hair. Consistency is vital for the effectiveness of LPT.

The quality and reliability of an LPT device are important if you want to continue to have a full head of hair. Your LPT device is a solid-state device (e.g., no moving parts) and should be built to have at least 18,000 treatments which is years of treatments—if so, replace the battery every three to five years. But as long as you take care of an LPT device it should last for a lifetime.

What Can I Expect Based on My Hair Loss Condition?

Everyone's hair and scalp are different which means each person requires an individual assessment of their situation. We recommend taking our short quiz (at the back of this book) or discussing your situation with a trichologist. We can't emphasize enough the need for consistent pictures as this is the only way to objectively measure the progress of LPT.

Remember that LPT is a lifelong commitment and should be used for the rest of your life to keep up the renewed result of your hair regrowth. Hair loss gets worse every year after the age of forty for both men and women. Getting ahead of hair loss should always be the goal and if you use the right LPT device, the right topical products, and the right supplements, all of this will be part of your daily regimen and you will have a regular hair loss prevention system.

Can I Use the LPT by Itself or Should I Use Other Products?

Most LPT devices can work perfectly on their own, but many users either have been using a hair loss regimen that they feel has been successful or have built some history using the treatments. The truth is that LPT should not be the only tool for hair loss issues. As stated in Chapter 4, using LPT, topicals, and supplements maintains hair in a four-pronged approach. There are no other solutions that provide as many benefits for scalp health as LPT. It's not worth wasting time or money or scalp health on other products that are not clinically proven.

Does My Scalp Have to Be Clean Prior to Using an LPT Device?

Light from lasers prefer no interference before entering the scalp so shiny scalps are not a good choice since they will reflect a portion of the light and prevent full dosage. You can use an LPT at any time but the fewer products on the hair and scalp that are present, the better the ability for laser light to be absorbed by the scalp.

Is There Anything I Should Avoid If I'm Considering Using LPT?

Before considering any hair growth treatment, you should visit a physician or trichologist to properly diagnose the cause of your hair loss. You may have an underlying medical condition, such as thyroid disease or anemia. Visiting the doctor before starting LPT is also helpful if you're taking medication. In the case of scalp conditions, such as psoriasis, it's important to visit a doctor. Unresolved medical issues can slow the hair growth rate typical of laser phototherapy.

Will the LPT Device Reach through Extensions, Wigs, and Other Products?

Using an LPT device in combination with wigs and weaves can be a useful approach to promoting hair growth while maintaining a desired hairstyle. It is very important to have some hair on your scalp when using wigs, as having no hair on the scalp makes it difficult for it to stay in place properly. Hair provides the necessary friction.

To make the most of your LPT treatment while wearing wigs or weaves, follow these steps:

1. Come up with a regular LPT schedule, using the device ideally at least three to four times a week, depending on the recommendations of

the LPT device manufacturer or your hair loss professional. Consistency is key for the effectiveness of LPT helmets.

2. Remove your wig or weave. Before starting your LPT session, gently remove your wig or weave to expose your natural hair and scalp. This ensures the laser light can reach your scalp and hair follicles without any obstruction.

3. Clean your scalp. This is not necessary every time for every LPT session, but a clean scalp will allow the laser light to penetrate more effectively, increasing the effectiveness of the treatment. Wash your hair and scalp using a gentle shampoo, ensuring that any product residue, dirt, or oil is removed.

4. Dry your hair. Make sure your hair and scalp are completely dry before starting the LPT session. Damp or wet hair can reduce the laser light's effectiveness.

5. Use the LPT device. Follow the instructions for proper usage by the LPT manufacturer. Place the device on your head through your hair, ensuring even coverage and exposure to the laser light. Treatment duration may vary, but most sessions last about twenty minutes.

6. Reapply your wig or weave. Once your LPT treatment is complete, you can reapply your wig or weave as desired.

Remember that LPT is not a quick fix, and consistent use over several months is necessary to see optimal results. LPT will help wig and weave users.

Can I Use the LPT Device Outdoors?

In general, it depends on the ambient weather outside. If it is above 68° Fahrenheit or 20° Celsius, we would strongly discourage using it. Same goes if the skies are sunny, as the sun could heat the device and cause internal temperatures to increase thus affecting the sensitive electronics, especially the lasers, which are extremely sensitive to high temperatures.

We highly suggest storing and using LPT devices indoors at all times. Remember, LPT devices are medical devices and should be treated with the utmost care and should really be used indoors.

Will I Feel the LPT Device Working?

Well-designed LPT devices will not generate any heat, so one would not feel any heat. In terms of other sensations, it's a painless treatment. There is also no tingling during treatment, though sometimes users have experienced a slight tingling sensation after using LPT devices, because of increased blood flow because every muscle and tissue in the scalp is being affected. This means the LPT device is working which is a great sign. Some users experience tightening of the scalp, which is usually another sign the LPT is working. A very small percentage (less 1%) experience a tension headache that usually goes away after about one week. Again, this is a great sign that the LPT device is working as intended.

The weight of the LPT sometimes might cause some issues if the user is not used to wearing hats or headgear, even though a well-designed LPT device should weigh less than 16 oz and not cause any issues.

How Will the LPT Device Grow Hair Where There Is No Coverage?

This is a very common question, especially with users that have thin areas in places like above the ears, around the back of the head by the hairline, or at the sides. The good news is that lasers do penetrate the scalp and spread the light around as explained in Chapter 1. We even have many of our users state that their eyebrows have started filling in after using our LPT helmet to regrow their hair.

Once I Grow Back My Hair, Will My Thicker Hair Block the Lasers?

When your hair starts to fill, many people ask if their new hair will block some or all of the lasers from penetrating the scalp. Even if some of the hairs might be "blocking" the laser light, there are many beams of light that will still pass through as the scalp just needs at least one good laser beam to stimulate it. For example, if the LPT device has eighty lasers, we estimate that for someone with very thick hair, about 30% to 50% of the laser light will penetrate the scalp. This is more than enough to see great results. However, we recommend that a "power treatment" should be done weekly to ensure maximum efficacy.

Can I Take a Vacation and Not Use the LPT Device While I Am Away?

The quick answer is, it depends on how long you'll be gone. The main goal of LPT is to continually apply trillions of photons on the scalp as the body is continuously trying to get rid of hair. If you'll only be away for two to three weeks then, yes, it will be ok to take a break from using your device. But if you're going through a difficult hair-shedding period, then we suggest taking the LPT device on your vacation. It is ok to place it in a carry-on and travel with the LPT device. It will pass airport security and most well-designed LPT devices will operate in any country's power grid which is important to note.

Can I Color My Hair and Use LPT?

The short answer is yes. In fact, many users are reporting back to us that using the LPT device right after hair coloring substantially improves the outcome. Hair coloring is achieved by using chemicals to open up the hair's cuticle (outer layer) and attempting to insert the color inside the hair follicle. Chemicals cannot seal the cuticles back up resulting in frizzy hair, inconsistent hair coloring, or rapid return of the original coloring.

LPT comes to the rescue by closing the cuticle with light providing smooth hair and avoiding any leakage or premature color evaporation. Hair coloring plus LPT will theoretically provide a much better experience. We have been getting great feedback.

We have not done any clinical trials or studies on this, but it is interesting to see feedback from hundreds of LPT users with the same results. We encourage you to test this if you do hair coloring and let us know the results, we would love to know more!

Why Do I Have Less Gray Hair Using LPT?

Another misconception is that LPT reduces graying. LPT enhances hair growth but doesn't prevent hair from going gray although it may *look* that way. This is an illusion. What happens is that, as LPT stimulates hair growth, new strands with color start to outnumber the grays. As the new hairs become thicker, gray hairs are hidden between them. In other words, LPT works wonders for increasing hair growth and volume but does not affect gray hair.

Lots going on in that scalp of yours. And that's why it's so hard to manage your hair growth. Most products offering instant hair-repair remedies don't even consider—much less explain—all the moving parts. They get you to slather some nutrients on your hair or swallow some supplements and then tell you that's good enough. Since they're not paying attention to all the factors that go into hair health, it's little wonder the results aren't what you want.

The way to attain a great head of hair is to maximize the growth cycle of each hair on your scalp. I'll explain as we go along how this can be accomplished and how to reduce hair loss. The combination of these two strategies is the ultimate goal.

What Are the Minimum and Maximum Age Users of an LPT Device?

Since hair loss affects nearly the whole human population, we receive a lot of inquiries from very young customers to older patients as old as ninety-seven! The youngest LPT which their parents asked us if our LPT device could treat was six months old! During our FDA submissions, we only tested patients from eighteen to sixty-five years old. The fact is that androgenetic alopecia technically starts right at puberty and gets progressively worse as one ages, and by the time someone is eighty years old, up to 70% of their hairs can be lost. When the scalp stops hair loss, it is technically unable to regrow any new hairs. We believe that LPT can keep the scalp active until the end of someone's life—we have many customers in their late nineties with a great head of hair.

Younger patients (ages eight to eighteen) who are suffering from che-mo-induced alopecia (CIA) often use our product to recover their lost hairs, which has been successfully accomplished. We do not market or foresee attaining FDA clearance for CIA, as this is a very tiny market and the clinical trials would cost millions to conduct. Therefore, we do not market this feature but, interestingly, many research academic institutions such as the University of Miami and others are looking at LPT as a solution for CIA.

What If the Lasers Shine onto My Eyes?

We covered this in Chapter 1, and a good LPT device will have a proximity sensor that will only turn on the lasers if it detects the scalp or head. This will avoid any potential issues with lasers shining in the eyes. But again, no one in the world has ever been hurt by red lasers shining on their eyes, so this is a non-issue and not a potential hazard.

Will the LPT Device Help with My Dermatitis or Other Scalp Disorder?

There hasn't been a study on this as it relates to the scalp but there are red light devices that are FDA-cleared for dermatitis or even eczema. But in terms of LPT devices for hair loss, these claims cannot be made at this time. We do get feedback from many of our customers that their dermatitis has either disappeared or minimized. But again, this is just ad hoc data received from our customers. This has never been clinically confirmed by anyone. If someone has dermatitis, they should take pictures and document their progression and show their physicians, and maybe this might be a good application for LPT devices in the near future!

Can I Use LPT If I Take Photosensitizing Medications?

LPT hair devices that operate at a wavelength that will not affect them should you use LPT while under these medications.

The fact is that the sun emits many types of wavelengths and photo-sensitive medications are primarily sensitive to UV (ultraviolet) wavelengths. To be more specific, wavelengths within the UVA spectrum (320–400 nm) and UVB (290–320nm) cause drug-induced photosensitivity reactions.

Since LPT devices emit at around 680 nm which is closer to the near-infrared spectrum, there is absolutely no effect when customers are on drugs that have photosensitivity warnings or labels.

What about If I'm Undergoing Cancer Treatment?

During ongoing cancer treatment, you should contact your physician for medical advice. LPT is not advised for people with scalp cancer. This is because it *hasn't* been clinically tested for use with cancer patients. That said, many recovering cancer patients who have used laser helmets for hair restoration have experienced an improvement in the quality of their hair. There are new LPT devices in the near-infrared spectrum that are used to treat lesions, masses, tumors, polyps, and other "cancerous" growths with great success. This new technology is demonstrating that light energy will destroy these cancerous cells. We will be watching this closely over the next few years and maybe a new helmet with anti-cancer (scalp) and hair loss/growth capabilities will be an interesting solution!

There's also been great feedback from many people who've reactivated hair follicles that became dormant due to chemo treatments. Since no formal treatment protocol has been developed specifically for chemo-therapy-induced alopecia (CIA), this potential new application of LPT should help many patients. Other technologies use a cooling device during the chemo process, but these devices are very expensive and the treatments are limited during the chemo treatment periods. What's good about LPT is that one can utilize it before, during, and long after the chemo treatments have been administered and in the comfort of your home instead of in a clinical setting.

What If I Have Implants in My Skull or Scars on My Scalp?

This question comes up if someone has a cochlear implant or some type of plate (e.g., metal or other material) in their skull, and the answer is that this will not affect them as it will not affect the implant or any metal plates. Some users have had surgical procedures on their scalp/skull. Hair does not normally grow on scars, especially fibroid scarring, which is almost completely void of any hair follicles. Hair does grow along the sides of these scars and those will grow and prosper using LPT. These longer hairs can be used to cover the scars as long as the hairs are left a bit longer than normal.

What Happens If You Stop Using LPT?

Hair loss, unfortunately, gets worse with age, especially combined with androgenetic alopecia which is about 93% of all hair loss. Just like brushing one's teeth to avoid periodontal diseases, it requires the regular and continuous use of LPT devices to prevent a return of hair loss. Therefore, maintenance use of the device at least once a week, preferably daily, is required to keep a healthy head of hair.

If you stop using an LPT device, it will take about three months or less to start seeing hair loss again. You must have a daily routine or some weekly routine for the LPT device to prevent hair loss from resuming.

Note that the LPT device will become part of your daily routine just like brushing your teeth or exercising. So, a great LPT device is designed to be easy to use and completely wireless so you can use it anytime like in bed, at your computer, while watching TV, and more.

We strongly encourage using an LPT device as much as possible to combat hair loss and never stop using it for more than eight weeks.

What About If I'm Pregnant or Breastfeeding?

Pregnancies may also cause hair to become brittle and thin. The use of laser phototherapy is not recommended during pregnancy or breastfeeding. However, LPT can be started for hair regrowth and thickening after your child is no longer breastfeeding.

How Do I Know the LPT Is Working?

To tell whether LPT is growing hair, photographs are absolutely necessary. Just as you don't notice hair loss overnight, hair growth is also a very gradual process that you won't notice right away. Follow the steps below to help you document your hair growth journey.

- **Use a Reliable and High-Quality Camera:** The latest iPhone may be perfect for taking selfies, but it's not good for taking pictures of progress with LPT! It doesn't matter whether you have the latest iPhone or what its zooming capabilities are. You need a much better camera if you want clear results of hair growth. Of course, the iPhone is great for social media testimonies when your hair is fully grown. But in the early stages, a high-resolution camera will allow you to zoom in on the scalp and fully capture burgeoning hair follicles.

- **Get the Lighting Right:** Lighting is one of those variables where more is not necessarily better. Artificial light from a camera flash is the main culprit when it comes to poor before and after photos. It creates glare, which can make it hard to compare photos as you progress on your journey. Natural lighting makes for the best clinical photos, so it's best to pick a spot in the house that's well-lit but where the light is diffuse and there's no direct sunlight. Also, it's helpful to keep in mind where the camera is in relation to the light. It is best if the light is coming from behind the camera, shining towards the hair.

- **Style Your Hair Normally:** You should style your hair how you normally style your hair then take a hair growth photo. Whatever style you choose, use the same one every time so the way your hair lies doesn't affect the photo. Also, tight hairdos should be avoided for the pictures, and I discourage accessories, such as hats or hair bands. You want to be as precise and clinical as possible.

- **Ask for Help:** Sometimes it may be necessary to bring in another person to help you take pictures. This often permits different angles of the hair to be captured with precision. The use of a timed camera to take pictures is good, but it can sometimes be a daunting task. An extra hand can be a real help. I also recommend you find a "hair buddy" who has a similar hair restoration goal. This will keep you motivated on your hair growth journey. Moreover, you can help each other with taking hair photos.

- **Take Hair Growth Pictures Monthly:** As with weight loss, there's no need to step on the scale daily, but progress must be monitored. Your scalp and hair follicles are unique, so the results of LPT will differ from person to person. It's a good idea to take monthly pictures, especially because this may enable you to make the right modifications, if called for, to your treatment.

- **Capture All Areas of the Scalp:** It's important that all parts of the scalp are captured when you take your laser phototherapy photographs. This will allow you to view an objective measure of growth. If you just do one section of your hair you will miss seeing the growth in relation to the rest of your hair, and this can skew your interpretation of your new hair growth.

How to Take a Before & After Picture

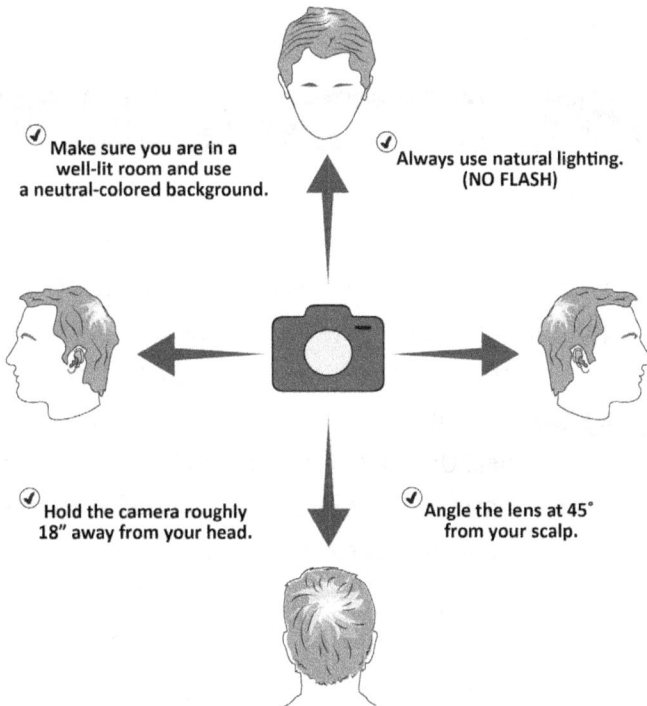

Make sure you are in a well-lit room and use a neutral-colored background.

Always use natural lighting. (NO FLASH)

Hold the camera roughly 18" away from your head.

Angle the lens at 45° from your scalp.

Figure 17.2. How to Take Before and After Pictures During Your Hair Growth Journey. Taking pictures should be one of the most important tasks for any LPT user. Seeing is believing and pictures help one understand the progress of LPT.

Success with LPT – Before and After Pictures

The only remaining step in this presentation is to show you the photographic evidence. We mentioned how you can take your own pictures to monitor your hair regrowth journey, yet we'd like to show you some results from people who have already used LPT. We know the best proof of regrowing hair is showing you how hair has grown on actual human beings using genuine pictures taken under identical conditions. These pictures are all over the Internet, on the review pages of various LPT companies, the personal pages of people who have used laser phototherapy, and the websites of dermatologists and trichologists. I have taken the liberty of posting results from LPT users in Appendix A.

After answering all your questions about LPT helmets, there's only one thing left to talk about . . .

Actual Customer Success Stories

The Success You Deserve

Angela lost her parents in the pandemic. 2020 was a challenging year, and when she tried to put it behind her, she noticed tufts of hair falling out in the shower. She lost her parents, and now losing her hair too was too much to bear. She tried to hide it, but the thinning was too fast. She considered wearing a wig but was uncomfortable with the idea. One day, scrolling social media, she stumbled upon a post about laser therapy. The before-and-after pictures were impressive. It was a small investment compared to everything she had been through. After a few months, her hair was thicker than it had been in years. She was able to optimize the LPT device as she joined public forums about this new technology. After a few months of continued success, she cried in relief in the shower.

CHAPTER 18

The Future of Laser Phototherapy

"We can easily forgive a child who is afraid of the dark; the real tragedy of life is when men are afraid of the light." — Seneca, Philosopher, first century CE

The Future of Laser Phototherapy

Laser phototherapy has been proven to be the most effective hair loss treatment of all time, yet it's still in its infancy in terms of its visibility. The estimated marketplace awareness of LPT for hair growth is only about 5%. This isn't because it hasn't been sufficiently proven; it's just a stage every useful device goes through to make sure it's safe to use and worth the cost. Also, its adoption in different clinical and home settings is still very low.

While this may look discouraging on the surface, it's a rather good statistic. The current level of awareness suggests that there will come a day when that 5% awareness has grown to 10%. A short time later, 10% will become 50%. Then global awareness will follow. If the device shows measurable results, the word will spread, and awareness will grow.

We are in the early stages of LPT being introduced into the marketplace. By 2030, we believe that almost every home will have some form of an

LPT device. It is my opinion that LPT devices will be as common as hair dryers one day, and for all types of ailments—not just hair loss!

Just look at cell phones. A couple of decades ago, people on the go were forced to find payphones to make a call. Very few people owned cell phones. Now they're so common you might be reading this book on one. What drove this explosive growth over such a short time? The cell phone proved useful. Everyone needed it.

When it comes to hair loss, LPT is equally useful. And since about 50% of the world's population suffers from hair loss, it's only a matter of time before LPT devices become part of the average household.

One reason to anticipate this kind of growth for LPT is the increased recognition it's enjoying in medical schools and the medical community. Scientific journals are showing a growing interest in LPT, and an increasing number of high-quality studies are being published by experts in photomedicine, biomedical scientists, and by companies involved in the production of laser devices. Actions such as these always contribute to the growth of fields of specialization.

When we compare the degree of understanding of laser phototherapy today to the days of Dr. Mester and his mouse experiments in the 1960s, a vast difference is apparent. Dr. Mester observed growth in the hair of his lab animals and wondered, "Why?" Now we know the phases of hair growth with precision and understand how light energy from lasers results in biostimulation. This understanding has brought a great deal of scientific interest to the field of laser phototherapy.

Emerging international bodies are actively involved in LPT application. Greater numbers of associations, organizations, and international groups—both new and more established—are beginning to throw their weight behind LPT for hair growth. Examples of such groups include the World

Association of Laser Therapy (WALT) and the North American Association for Photobiomodulation Therapy (NAALT). A strong international community such as this is key to driving stronger public awareness.

Photobiomodulation as a Drug?

A drug is an agent that can produce changes in the body. Going by this definition, we can see that LPT, which achieves results through biomodulation, falls into this category. When laser light is applied to the tissues of the body, it produces the desired effects in the cells (biomodulation). The fact remains that all forms of light affect living organisms, and we still have so many unknowns about light even though it is essential to the survival of our world. An important consideration with any drug is its dosage, which is the amount of the drug needed to get the results you want. In photobiomodulation, we see a therapeutic window—the minimum and maximum effective dosage—which is similar to the therapeutic window of a drug. With LPT, the therapeutic window is defined by the wavelength of the light. More specifically, it's the wavelength of light capable of producing biostimulation. For hair growth, we know this wavelength to be around 680 nm.

LPT shares other qualities with drugs, such as the interval between doses, the concentration of the dose, and more. We are still not sure of the exact dosage to stimulate hair follicles with LPT, nor the minimum and maximum length for treatments. We do not know the exact rest needed between each LPT hair session, as there is no research on this yet. We assume that hair follicles treated with LPT need some type of rest between treatments. We also know that the optimal energy dosage must be delivered to the tissue, but this still needs more studies and a dosage chart must be constructed. Conventional drugs like acetaminophen have pretty clear dosage limits for minimum and maximum consumption and dosages for what ailments are most optimal. These similarities, between medicinal drugs and photobiostimulation convince me that phototherapy is indeed equivalent to a drug.

As evidence continues to emerge from the ever-expanding research into LPT, we can expect to see a greater degree of standardization. This will make it easier to use LPT more precisely. With the emergence of sub-specialties in dermatology, I think we can expect doctors to prescribe LPT much more frequently.

If you are still with me after all these discussions, I want to highlight the fact that while laser phototherapy has shown promising results in promoting hair growth, the optimal dosage for this treatment is still unknown. The effectiveness of laser phototherapy can be influenced by factors such as wavelength, energy output, duration of treatment, and the individual's hair and scalp characteristics. Therefore, it can be challenging to determine the ideal dose for each individual. While there is ongoing research in this area, healthcare professionals must use their clinical experience and judgment to tailor the treatment to the individual's needs.

LPT is NOT a One-Stop-Shop

People throughout the world desperately need safe and effective ways to resolve their hair loss issues. People want therapies that work and don't have dangerous side effects. Healing and restoration are the goals.

Laser Phototherapy (LPT) has the potential to work on many ailments that are based on inflammatory issues and reduces the need for expensive, damaging drugs that have side effects or that might not resolve the issues. Light as a medicine and the sweet spot for optimal dosages for each application is yet to be exploited. Even though there are many LPT devices for all kinds of ailments, one has to be knowledgeable about the new devices and their applications.

As people become more informed and fearless about choosing devices that are safe and effective for at-home treatments that deliver so many benefits, we will see a quick and easy shift to LPT right before our eyes.

Laser phototherapy isn't a cure for all diseases, but it does optimize cellular function, support the immune system, and accelerate the healing process.

The Many Other Uses of LPT

Although my main goal with this book has been to dive deep into LPT, hair loss, and hair regrowth, I also want to share the many benefits of Laser phototherapy. We are on the cusp of a revolution in medical light therapy!

The fact is that there is a new revolution of light and there are now hundreds of new products that are hitting the marketplace such as light beds that douse the body with all types of light, from UV to IR and beyond. Unfortunately, these are usually not FDA-cleared and so they are marketed as health or cosmetic gadgets, which means there have not been any clinical trials or the manufacturers' claims have not been legitimatized.

In the next few sections, I will be discussing light technologies that are going through the right processes to get FDA clearance and be properly introduced into the marketplace.

The Ultimate Anti-Aging Hack

The currently aging population refuses to grow old. The quest to slow down the aging process is a daunting one with a plethora of options that seem to be ever-changing. The term "anti-aging hack" has become a popular buzzword in recent years as more people are looking for ways to stay youthful and healthy for as long as possible and to promote longevity while preventing the signs of aging.

Laser hair loss phototherapy is not only the ultimate anti-aging hack by promoting hair growth and improving skin health, but it can also be a powerful confidence booster. Fuller, healthier-looking hair can make a person feel more vibrant, youthful, and confident in their appearance.

LPT (red light) therapy also helps stimulate cellular metabolism and repair. As we've learned, spectrums of light in the 680-800 nm range activate light-sensitive receptors in the energy-making processes of our cells (the mitochondria). This process enhances molecular exchange in the skin that allows for the removal of accumulated toxins while promoting the infusion of molecules specific to cellular repair.

Since the publication of NASA research in the 1990s, many research studies on red light and infrared therapy have demonstrated their benefits on wound healing, metabolism enhancement, and the reduction of fine lines, wrinkles, and acne.

How exactly does it work for other aging-related conditions? LPT therapy causes an increase in fibroblast creation and activation, which can enhance the cellular functions of deep skin layers. Simply put, LPT therapy stimulates the production of collagen and fibroblasts which until now, relied on injecting fake implants or foreign materials (e.g., fillers) into the skin. These implants and fillers can cause potential damage and only offer short-term solutions.

Collagen is what is responsible for the elasticity, firmness, and fullness of your skin. The increased production of collagen and fibroblasts is what will smooth out your fine lines and wrinkles, smooth the texture of the skin, and reduce pore size over time. Collagen cells grow slowly, so be patient, and expect to see "before and after" results at about three months of consistent treatment.

Below is a list of some of the anti-aging results of LPT therapy for the skin:

- It prevents hair loss and stimulates regrowth
- It repairs sun damage
- It reduces wrinkles including crow's feet, under-eye wrinkles, forehead wrinkles, and laugh lines
- It creates a healthy glow about your face
- It speeds the healing of blemishes, acne, and rosacea
- It brings more moisture to your skin
- It fades scars and stretchmarks

Many LED-based masks are flooding the market but unfortunately, LEDs cannot penetrate more than one or two layers of the skin; they need to be twenty-five times stronger to reach and stimulate collagen production. Only be hundred times stronger a laser can do this.

Improving Cognitive Function

LPT has been clinically proven to improve cognitive function. Specifically, it has been studied in a wide variety of conditions including stroke, Alzheimer's, Traumatic Brain Injury (TBI), Parkinson's disease, depression, and cognitive enhancement in healthy subjects.

In a recent study by the Harvard School of Medicine, when a helmet device with multiple LPT lasers was used on dementia patients, it showed that memory, attention, and executive function improved. The caretakers of almost all these patients noticed improvements in their patients' abilities to tie their shoes or remember recent events or names. These were people who hadn't been able to speak in connected sentences for weeks or months, yet who suddenly started having a conversation, speaking in full sentences, understanding, and replying. In addition, LPT is an effective treatment for psychiatric disorders including major depression, bipolar disorder, anxiety, and post-traumatic stress disorder.

Scientists believe that LPT works by stimulating the mitochondria within cells to produce more ATP, the energy that powers cellular activity. However, getting to the brain requires a high dosage since it must penetrate through the cranium (bone) which takes a lot of energy density and the wavelength should be between 804 nm to 904 nm. For LPT to work on the brain, it must be able to reach it. Measurements of light penetrating through the cranium and into the brain are about 3% of the total applied light meaning that it does not take much to stimulate the brain. Dosage is the key here and as we continue to discover more about how much light energy is required, we further advance humankind so we can advance as a society.

This type of new modality for brain reparation will be the future, as LPT also stimulates the formation of new brain cells and the formation of new connections between existing ones. Therefore, even people with normal brain functions will be able to improve their intelligence and use more of their brain functions than ever before.

We believe that all our customers are now the smartest people in the world!

Autoimmune Conditions

Autoimmune diseases are among the most frustrating conditions to treat, usually caused by organs and tissues in the body that are just not functioning correctly. Unfortunately, there are no medications that succeed in treating autoimmune diseases, and they often worsen the condition.

Inflammation usually accompanies these conditions. Since LPT is used for reducing inflammation, there has been success in treating the inflammation. A recent study of patients with thyroid issues due to autoimmune conditions showed that an 810 nm laser successfully treated this condition with only ten laser treatments.

Usually, these conditions are treated with some type of steroid which can only be used a few times before it stops working. LPT will greatly benefit women since they tend to suffer from autoimmune conditions more than men. And yes, these autoimmune conditions also cause hair loss!

LPT for Pain Management

In recent years, professional sports teams have been increasingly incorporating laser phototherapy into their injury management protocols, recognizing its potential to expedite the recovery process and optimize player performance. Almost every US professional football, soccer, hockey, basketball, and baseball team has multiple LPT devices for all of their players and training staff. Even tennis players like the famous USTA sisters each have two devices (one for home and one for travel) since these are used for their ankles. Recovery time for joint injuries is substantially reduced by using LPT. This type of product can get a highly paid player back into the game due to the fast-healing process and save the team millions of dollars. What is interesting is that they regard this type of tool as a trade secret, and do not disclose this to any of their competitors or the public since it is a competitive advantage.

In addition, veterinarians are using this for horses and dogs for their injuries instead of putting down the animal. Now soft injuries and broken bones can be healed at the speed of light, using LPT devices.

For a cutting-edge, non-invasive treatment, low-level laser light is employed to effectively combat knee and back pain. By penetrating the affected tissues, the therapy promotes cellular regeneration, expediting the body's innate healing capabilities. The process not only enhances blood circulation in the targeted area, supplying vital nutrients and oxygen, but also facilitates the release of endorphins and serotonin, natural analgesic, and mood-enhancing chemicals.

LPT also assists with repairing nerve function, diminishing the transmission of pain signals from the knee and back to the brain, thereby alleviating pain perception. Through the activation of cartilage, collagen, and elastin fiber production, the therapy fosters the repair of damaged ligaments, joints, and tendons, leading to long-lasting pain relief and improved joint functionality. Consequently, laser phototherapy presents a comprehensive approach to addressing both the symptoms and the underlying causes of knee, joint, and back pain. I believe that every home will have an LPT device specifically tuned for these types of injuries. Especially as one ages, these types of devices will be a lifesaver.

Ophthalmology

Today there are thousands of laser-assisted procedures like LASIK and PRK which reshapes the cornea to improve the eye's ability to focus light onto the retina. But these are hot lasers that use high heat to alter tissue. This results in clearer vision and reduced dependency on corrective lenses for individuals with nearsightedness, so lasers are used in ophthalmology applications.

The development of new devices using LPT and standardized dosage could lead to an increase in its use in ophthalmology which is painless and has no side effects. One potential application for LPT is age-related macular degeneration (an eye disease that blurs central vision) as the main cause is mitochondria weakness. LPT, as we have learned in this book, will stimulate the mitochondria. Therefore, light phototherapy could repair the targeted cells with weak mitochondrial activity and reduce inflammation without monthly injections directly into the cornea, as they are doing today. The present method for age-related macular degeneration is costly and painful for the patient.

Many early reports of LPT applications have helped regenerate damaged retinal tissue. Work still needs to be done to apply LPT safely and to maximize the benefits within ophthalmology, but we are moving in that direction.

Gastrointestinal Tract (GI Tract) and LPT

Previously in my career, I was a young engineer working on gastrointestinal video endoscopy for Pentax, a very famous Japanese company known for its cameras. One of the projects I worked on was a swallowable camera pill that took pictures as it traversed the almost 30-foot journey of the large and small intestines.

A potential LPT application could be to outfit similar pills with laser light to treat inflammation along the GI tract. As we've learned LPT is highly effective in treating inflammation. Since many inflammatory diseases start within the GI tract, swallowing a pill with LPT capabilities every month for routine treatment of bowel diseases, ulcers, masses, lesions, polyps, and tumors would be ideal.

Laser Phototherapy: Light up the World

In the beginning, there was light. I started this book with that line because light started it all. Light is the energy that supports all life on earth, either directly or indirectly.

Humans need light and we will always benefit from the energy that light produces. The fact that our planet Earth is the third rock from the sun, which means that the intensity of the sun is near perfect, our oceans can remain liquid without getting too hot or cold and life thrives because of this perfect alignment.

We already know that light gives plants the energy they need for photosynthesis. We also know that humans need light to stay healthy and happy. Seasonal Affective Disorder is a good example of how the absence of light can impact our mental health, leading to emotional changes and often depression.

But beyond that, I hope I have shown you that LPT therapy offers tremendous health and quality-of-life benefits. We've already seen its use in the treatment of hair conditions and hair loss. Each one of us will get to a stage when we experience hair loss if we live long enough. At that point, LPT becomes a potential treatment for all of us.

The prospects for photobiostimulation, especially through red-light therapy, are virtually unlimited. The future is lasers, baby! And the best news is that we're seeing increased interest in the field today along with greater awareness and more frequent use of LPT. Soon, everyone will be enjoying the benefits LPT brings to their hair health, physical, and mental needs.

You're a decade ahead of everyone else—enjoy it! Make the best of laser phototherapy. Keep and grow your hair back with lasers and live the rest of your life with a healthy scalp full of thick hair. When someone asks how you did it, you can smile and say, "In the beginning, there was light."

Actual Customer Success Stories

The Ultimate Matriarch

Elsie had a thick head of hair for nine decades, but on her ninety-second birthday, she noticed that her silver full head of hair wasn't as thick as the years before. And that was not good enough. Determined to address it, she recalled a recent TV segment about an FDA-cleared hair rejuvenation device. She placed an order. After about six months, she was delighted by the results, but when the company refused her second order, Elsie was outraged and called them up. "Madam, you seem to have ordered nine helmets—this must be a mistake." "I ordered nine helmets because that is the exact number I require," Elsie retorted. "I have nine grandchildren, and this could give some of them hope to look as good as I do come my age...it might even shine some light into their minds, too."

LPT in the Age of COVID

Since COVID-19 was a very recent event as of writing this, I wanted to make sure I addressed the fact that COVID-19 affected everyone and especially with hair loss. We had never seen so many customers complain about hair loss as we did during these very trying times. Therefore, I wanted to share my thoughts on CCOVID-19 and hair loss.

COVID-19 and Hair Loss

Can COVID Cause Hair Loss?

Some common questions asked by people having post-COVID hair loss include: "Does

COVID cause hair loss?"; "Is hair loss a side effect of COVID?"

The answer to these questions is that the COVID-19 virus *is* involved in causing hair loss by weakening the body and its immune system.

The spike proteins of COVID-19 facilitate the entry of the virus into the healthy cells of the body. After its entry, the COVID virus reduces the body's immune system, leading to the infection. Due to this infection, the body weakens, and the immune system can't produce a proper response to combat the virus.

In such a critical situation, the body goes into lockdown mode and only focuses on essential functions to retain itself. *Since hair growth is not as essential* as other body functions, it receives the least amount of nutrients and energy, and the patient ends up having hair loss.

Possible Side Effect

The hair loss that's been observed post-COVID-19 infection is consistent with telogen effluvium (TE).

Telogen effluvium (TE) is temporary hair loss due to high fever or during recovery from an illness (such as a COVID-19 infection). In TE, people may lose up to 300 hair strands a day instead of only fifty to one hundred hairs per day (regular hair loss count during the resting stage of hair). The cases of telogen effluvium have grown by over 400% since the beginning of the COVID-19 pandemic because of infection and the stress of being quarantined.

How Long Does COVID Hair Loss Last?

People who develop TE have noticeable hair loss roughly two to three months after recovering from COVID-19 infection, and hair loss can last for six to nine months. After this period, most patients observe hair regrowth.

Other Reasons for Post-COVID Hair Loss:

There are many reasons why you may have hair loss after a COVID-19 infection.

Stress is a common cause and potential trigger for post-COVID hair loss. Experiencing a COVID-19 infection can cause both emotional and physical stress.

Being diagnosed with such a deadly virus can lead to mental anxiety and emotional stress. This emotional stress shifts more of a person's hair to the resting phase of the hair growth cycle, ultimately leading to hair loss. In fact, hair loss from COVID has also been observed in some people due to the stress of being quarantined. The sheer fact that billions of people around the world were sequestered in their homes, not able to see family, and friends, go to work, or enjoy normal activities raised stress levels around the world.

COVID-19 puts the body under great physical stress by interfering with its essential systems and functions. Such physical stress on the body weakens which can cause hair loss.

Another reason for hair loss is vitamin D deficiency. Since vitamin D is mostly obtained from direct sunlight, lockdowns during the COVID-19 pandemic limited people's access to direct sunlight. Many people became deficient in vitamin D and started losing their hair.

Besides viral infection, stressful events, and vitamin D deficiency, it is suspected that hair loss after COVID-19 may be a side effect of medications and treatments. However, there is no conclusive research and evidence available that indicate the occurrence of hair loss due to COVID-19 treatments and medications. We are still in the early stages of understanding them.

Hair Loss After COVID Vaccines
COVID vaccines are used worldwide to control the spread of the COVID-19 virus.

These vaccines have proved very efficient in the fight against the COVID-19 pandemic. Besides their valuable benefits in combating the COVID-19 virus, COVID-19 vaccines also show some side effects such as headache, fever, chills, fatigue, hair loss, pain in joints and muscles, etc.

Among these side effects, as noted, hair loss is mostly observed after mRNA—Pfizer or Moderna vaccines. The reason for hair loss after mRNA vaccines is actually because of their mechanism of action.

How Do COVID mRNA Vaccines Work?

The mRNA vaccines work by inoculating the body with the piece of mRNA that codes for the spike proteins of the COVID-19 virus. These mRNAs are used by the body's cells to synthesize the spike proteins. The spike proteins are responsible for the pathogenicity of the actual COVID-19 virus leading to the weakening of the body and immune system.

These spike proteins, produced from the mRNA vaccine, are detected by the body's immune system as foreign particles. In response, the activated immune system starts producing antibodies and other immune cells to combat what looks like a real COVID-19 infection. This triggers the antibodies remaining in the body to act as a defense system against the actual COVID-19 virus. Then, if the body encounters these spike proteins again in the future (for example, from an actual COVID-19 virus), the immune system can quickly respond to it and protect the body from a severe form of COVID-19 infection.

Why Does Hair Loss Occur after mRNA Vaccines for COVID?

The mRNA vaccines are very helpful in preparing the body against future COVID infection. But recently, these vaccines are known to cause hair loss as their side effect. Many people from different parts of the world have complained of hair loss after the COVID-19 vaccination.

These complaints and concerns from people drew the attention of scientists, doctors, and researchers to this issue. Many studies and research have been done to determine the mechanism behind this issue.

Despite conducting different studies, scientists have not yet been able to determine the exact mechanism behind the hair loss. So, the COVID-19 vaccines have not been medically proven to cause it. However, some experts explain that it may be caused by a weakened immune system due to vaccination. The mechanism of this reaction is very similar to the infection of the actual COVID-19 virus.

The spike proteins produced by the body cells using mRNA vaccines work as pathogens just like the actual COVID-19 virus. These spike proteins, although later killed by antibodies, remain in the body for some time. During this time, these spike proteins act as infectious agents and start infecting the body. As a result of this infection, the body and its overall immune system are weakened. The weakened body starts showing different symptoms and side effects.

In this critical situation, the body tries to retain itself by focusing on the essential functions and systems. Since hair growth is not an essential function for survival and hair is the last thing the body may need, the body limits the delivery of nutrients and energy to the hair growth process. Eventually, the hair strands become weak due to a lack of nutrition, and the patient starts losing hair.

The good news is that, for most people, hair loss after COVID-19 is not permanent and hair regrowth starts within a few months. Once people get back out into their daily lives and routines, this unique type of hair loss should subside quickly as the global pandemic gets resolved and stress levels are reduced.

How Can an LPT Helmet Help in Controlling Post-COVID Hair Loss?

Having hair loss after a COVID-19 infection or after getting a shot of the COVID mRNA vaccine can be distressing for some people. A laser photo-therapy helmet can be very helpful in controlling this type of hair loss.

Post-COVID-19 hair loss is due to a lack of energy provided to the hair follicles by the body. In this condition, using an LPT helmet will provide photonic energy to the hair follicles to stimulate their mitochondria. This will improve the health of the hair follicles which leads to the strengthening of existing hair and the growth of new hair strands. In this way, an LPT device can help in controlling post-COVID-19 hair loss. And it can be done in the privacy and comfort of your own home.

EPILOGUE

Born at the Perfect Time

I was born in Afghanistan in the early 1960s and at that time, Afghanistan did not have a TV station—only radio stations—so the words "technology" and "Afghanistan" rarely went hand in hand. To say I was born in a place with very little technology is not an exaggeration. The mountains of Afghanistan made a lot of the population very remote and difficult to relay information. Afghanistan in the 60s was so primitive that the best way to communicate announcements and news to the population, about 93% of which was illiterate, was to use helicopters to drop papers and leaflets with simple messages (with pictures) from the sky.

My father and mother finally moved us out of Afghanistan after he finished medical school to Toulouse, France where he specialized in ENT (Ears/Nose/Throat) medicine. It was at this time that I finally got to see my first TV—but it had only two channels, and was black and white at that! One summer evening in 1969, my neighbors in our apartment building in Toulouse yelled out that the Americans had landed on the moon! We rushed over to their apartment to watch this amazing sight—it was a day I would never forget. I couldn't stop thinking about the moon landing. I knew then that I definitely wanted to be involved in the world of space somehow. It was around this time that my family started watching the new TV show *I Dream of Jeannie* ("Jinny de mes rêves"), starring the magnificent Barbara Eden as Jeannie, on French television. I was a huge fan of Ms. Eden's work, and quickly fell in love with the show. Watching *I Dream of Jeannie*, an American fantasy sitcom featuring an astronaut, convinced me that I wanted to be in the space industry and live in Cocoa Beach Florida!

Several years later, my family and I moved to the United States and ended up in Kansas City, Missouri, where my grandfather had moved prior as a physician at the Baptist Memorial Hospital. My first impression was that Kansas City was huge and plentiful—and it was also the city where my grandfather introduced me to my first-ever color TV, complete with thirteen channels! It was amazing! The only issue was that I was my father's new remote control, always sitting next to the TV for my dad to tell me which channel he wanted me to navigate to. This experience convinced me I wasn't going to go into medicine like all of my other family members, but rather that I should go into technology and come up with a better way to turn TV channels!

Therefore, at the University of Missouri, I went into Electrical Engineering and tried to come up with technologies to improve the overall lives of everyday people. Then the Challenger space shuttle incident happened on January 1986. Fortunately, despite the tragedy, this incident gave me the opportunity to finally go into my ultimate dream job and work at NASA: one step closer to my dream of living out *I Dream of Jeannie!*

NASA ended up hiring about brand new engineers to specifically come in to automate and improve the Kennedy Space Shuttle (KSC) program after the report from Rogers Commission was presented to Congress, and I was one of those lucky engineers selected to do just that. My first project was working on voice recognition and speech synthesis, as well as developing new lasers to measure the thermal protection system, and nine other high-tech projects over my ten-year career at KSC. I was finally able to get my top-secret clearance (DoD), even though Afghanistan was still considered to be part of the USSR after being invaded in the 1980s. Getting my clearance took a little bit over two years due to the fact I was born in Afghanistan—they really wanted to make sure I wasn't some Russian spy! I remember celebrating with my friends the day I finally received this top-secret clearance, as all my other KSC friends had received their DoD clearances in six months or fewer!

After getting my DoD top-secret clearance, I genuinely thought the government was going to tell me what really happened with the assassination of JFK, or what was really in Area 51 or in Roswell, New Mexico; but unfortunately, I was simply instructed to never talk about my work during those space flight missions. The good news is that getting my clearance boosted my confidence quite a bit, to the point that I was beginning to think about becoming an astronaut. Why not? I had made it this far! Part of my projects required meeting with astronauts to improve space flight operations, and I had already met several astronauts at Kennedy Space Center. One of my favorite astronauts was named John Young. John had an amazing character and had a formidable career as the only astronaut to be in at least the Apollo/Gemini and Space Shuttle Program. After I shared with him my new dream of becoming an astronaut during a project we worked on together, he suggested that I should apply and try to become a mission specialist. He suggested that I first learn how to fly and get more heavily involved in aviation. He said, "Look, if you're the only person left on the space shuttle while in space, you will need to learn to become a pilot really fast!" So, I went and received my pilot's license and my glider rating, as well as did about fifty skydiving jumps and helped my friends put airplanes together in their plane hangars. One such friend was astronaut Fernando Caldeiro, may he rest in peace, with whom I built a DIY micro-jet aircraft. When I got my master's and then was working on my Ph.D., I decided that I was going to submit an application to be an astronaut and become Major Anthony Nelson, the protagonist in *I Dream of Jeannie*. Given that I was already living in Cocoa Beach, Florida and working at Kennedy Space Center, my dream was coming true!

My first application was rejected, basically explaining that I was too young. At twenty-seven years, I needed more experience; I was devastated, but I vowed to try harder. At the age of twenty-eight, one full year later, I decided to try again, but again, I was rejected. They finally told me that they said the average age for becoming an astronaut was thirty-eight years old, and I was much too young and inexperienced!

This is where my impatience got the best of me, and I decided that I couldn't wait another ten years to try again. I decided then to follow in my father's and grandfather's footsteps and go towards medicine by going into biomedical engineering, helping people with new technology and designing medical devices to further advance humankind.

Starting my company to help sufferers of androgenetic alopecia has been an amazing experience, as prior to doing so there was really nothing that could stop hair loss or regrow hair. But now, with over 80,000,000 laser phototherapy treatments from our device to date, I am receiving daily "thank you" messages from our customers showing their gratitude for inventing this device. This is what motivated me to write this book and to show that there is a great solution for hair issues using lasers.

One of the reasons I decided to ensure that our LPT device was made in the USA, right here in heart of Silicon Valley, California, was because obtaining my American Naturalized Citizenship is one of my proudest accomplishments. My citizenship certificate is the only thing that I hang on my wall—not my degrees, not awards nor pictures with famous people—but just this certificate with a small American flag on the frame. Only in the US can someone like me come from a distant land and make something like the Theradome with only a dream and hard work. Yes, other countries have very educated citizens and people much smarter than me, but unfortunately, they are not often given the opportunity to start a company like this and prosper. Therefore, the only thing is that I have of value is my US citizenship plaque, which I proudly hang on my wall.

For this reason, even though making our device in the States is much more expensive than outsourcing the job to somewhere in Asia, for example, I would rather invest in the United States. Given that this device is worn on the head, there is even more reason to make sure we at Theradome incorporate all the safety and regulatory measures to achieve a very safe medical device—measures that are guaranteed when constructing products in a country with robust regulatory procedures.

All in all, in my almost sixty years of living on this earth, I went from being born in one of the most rugged, underdeveloped countries in the world with near zero technology, to now having the privilege of having saved more hairs and growing more hairs than any human being on earth with one single piece of technology. To have had the privilege to experience such accomplishments is humbling, and I wouldn't trade it for anything. Becoming an astronaut like Major Anthony Nelson would have been great, but if I had gone down this path, I would have missed out on inventing and sharing the most effective hair loss and hair growth tool our society has seen. And, as I found out later on when living in Cocoa Beach, Florida, there's more than one way to connect with your heroes...

Remember when I mentioned what a big Barbara Eden fan I had become after watching her star in *I Dream of Jeannie*? As it turns out, Ms. Eden liked to frequent the yearly Cocoa Beach parade, which is where I was able to first see her from a distance—although we had never met.

Despite only ever seeing Ms. Eden from afar, my dream of one day meeting my favorite actress was not dead yet. And, as fate would have it, that dream finally came true one day, years after first seeing Barbara at the parades, when out of the blue, I received a phone call from an unknown person asking about hair loss and the Theradome helmet. It somehow came up on the call that the client in question had worked on the *I Dream of Jeannie* set making replica props for the show and knew Barbara Eden and fellow actor Bill Daily personally! I knew this was my chance to thank the actors and their show for inspiring me to go work with NASA and set out on a journey that would eventually lead me to invent the Theradome. I sent both of them a helmet, along with my thanks for the role they played in my life.

But the story doesn't end there. If getting the chance to share my product with Ms. Eden weren't enough, most recently, in 2018, I had the immense privilege of being presented with the Hollywood Beauty Awards' Best Aesthetic Product of the Year Award by Ms. Barbara Eden herself! With this latest meeting, my dream was complete—I knew for certain that I had taken the right path in setting out on my own to become a businessman and inventor. The fact is that Ms. Eden has played a pivotal role in my life, and I will forever be grateful.

Although my life didn't turn out exactly as I had dreamed it would when I was younger, when I reflect on all of the experiences and feats I have been a part of, I can't help but feel that I was born at the perfect time in history.

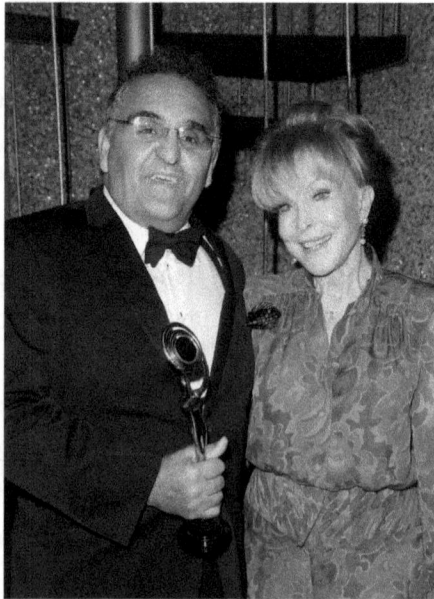

Barbara Eden and Tamim Hamid at the Hollywood Beauty Awards in 2018.

APPENDIX A

"A picture is worth a thousand words." — *Fred R. Barnard*

GALLERY OF SUCCESS STORIES

When done correctly, laser phototherapy (LPT) to stop hair loss and promote new hair is the safest and fastest way to grow back your own, natural hair. The people in photos below are real users of the Theradome LPT helmets, which deploys the ideal wavelength, dosage, and beam divergence. Each user has had fewer than 120 days of treatments and, with continued use, their results will get even better. No other technology or medication can produce such results.

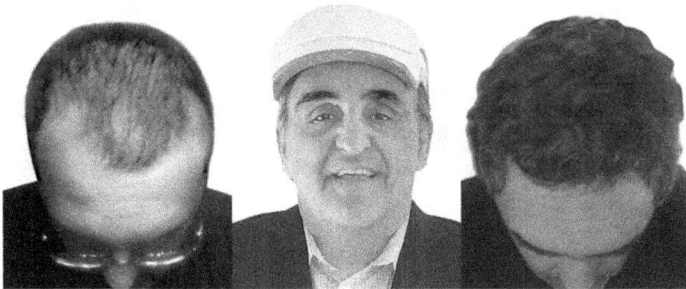

Tamim Hamid, the Author, Before, During, and After.

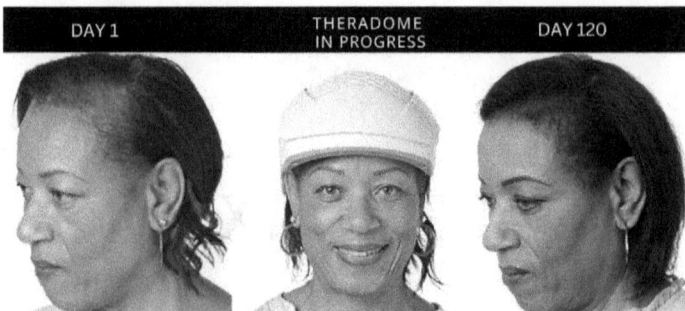

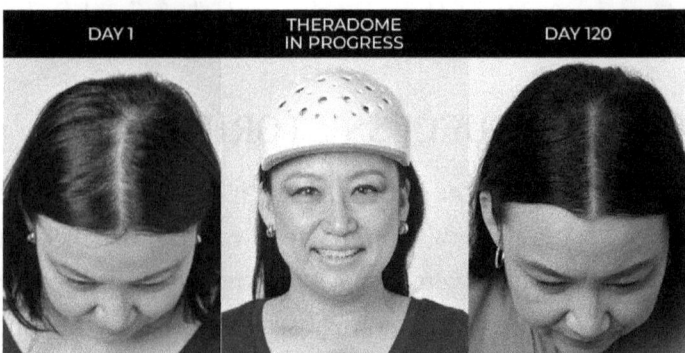

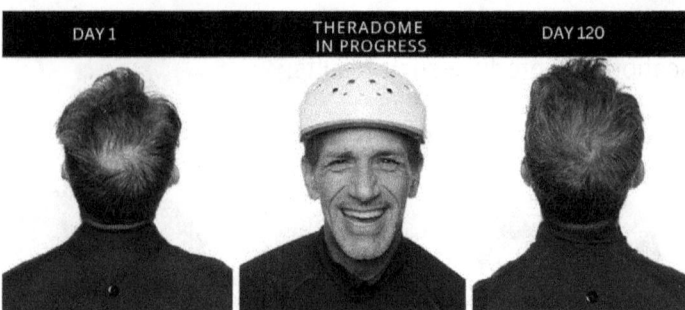

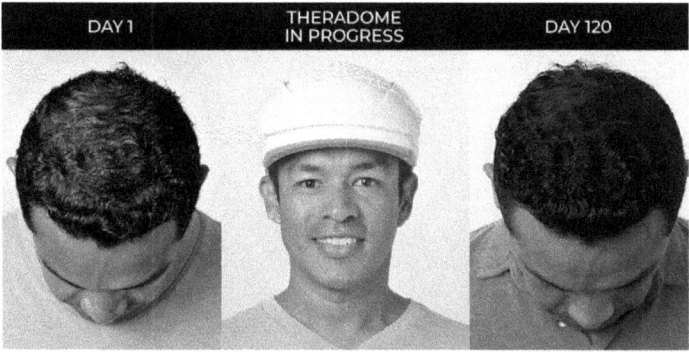

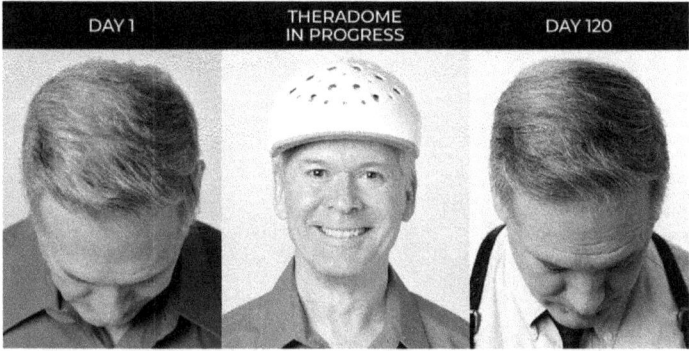

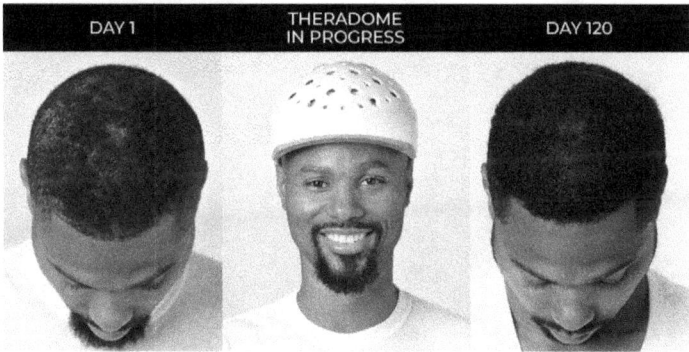

APPENDIX B

100 MOST INTERESTING HAIR FACTS

1. Hair grows faster in summer than in winter for everyone.
2. Hairs have a natural inclination to grow in the direction of the sun.
3. The only thing that can't be identified by hair is gender.
4. On average, a person can lose up to 150 strands of hair during a shampoo.
5. Hair above the scalp is composed of 90% dead cells, while the remaining 10% is made up of water and proteins.
6. Hair is electrically conductive, which is why it can stand on end in certain weather conditions.
7. Hair grows faster during the day than at night.
8. Female hair grows faster than male hair
9. Hair contains small amounts of gold, as traces of the element can be found in the bloodstream.
10. Regular trimming does not make hair grow faster, but it can help prevent split ends and improve overall hair health.
11. The common thought that hair continues to grow after death is a MYTH!
12. Combing or brushing wet hair can cause more damage than doing it when dry.
13. Hair follicles are the second fastest-growing tissue in the body after bone marrow.
14. A single hair can support the weight of 100,000 times its own mass.
15. Hair can stretch up to 30% of its length when wet.

16. Hair loss can be as devastating as a death in the family to some.
17. Castrated men have near little or no hair loss as well as no dan-druff—this indicates that hair production is heavily dependent on hormones (e.g., Testosterone/DHT).
18. The length of the growing phase of hair follicles shortens as you age.
19. A new hair begins to grow as soon as it is plucked from its follicle.
20. Hair can respond to sound waves, causing it to vibrate slightly in response to certain frequencies.
21. The protein structure of hair is similar to that of wool and feathers.
22. All of human hair follicles were formed when we were five months in the womb.
23. On average, women's hair is half the diameter of men's hair.
24. Hair and nails share similar characteristics in terms of growth and durability.
25. Hair can act as a protective barrier against UV radiation.
26. Hair has a tensile strength of about 14 MPa (megapascals).
27. Hair has a natural pH level of around 4.5 to 5.5.
28. African hair grows slower and is more fragile than European hair.
29. Asian hair grows the fastest and has the best elasticity.
30. A strand of hair is stronger than a copper wire with the same diameter.
31. When we are cold or scared, goosebumps happen when the muscle for each hair strand contracts.
32. In some cultures, hair is considered a symbol of fertility and vitality.
33. Hair is an excellent insulator, helping to regulate body temperature.
34. Hair is incredibly strong and can withstand temperatures of up to 451°F (232°C).
35. The scientific study of hair is called trichology.
36. At different times, 90% of hair is growing, while the other 10% is resting.
37. Hair contains carbon, hydrogen, oxygen, nitrogen, and sulfur.
38. A single hair has an average lifespan of about five years and some cases up to eight years.

39. The phrase "bad hair day" was first coined in the 1970s.
40. Hair can change texture over time due to hormonal changes or aging.
41. The word "hair" comes from the Old English word "hǣr."
42. The word "wig" is short for "periwig," which was a popular hairstyle in the 17th century.
43. Bald eagles are not bald; they have white feathers on their heads, giving the appearance of baldness.
44. The term "frizz" describes the uneven texture of hair caused by a lack of moisture.
45. The term "blond" comes from the Old French word "blund," which originally meant "a color midway between golden and light chestnut."
46. Frequent exposure to chlorinated water, like in swimming pools, can damage hair and lead to dryness and brittleness.
47. When you add up how much each hair on your head grows over a year's time, you get ten miles worth of hair!
48. Ancient Romans used hair color as a way to indicate their social status.
49. Hair color can change naturally due to age, hormonal fluctuations, and other factors.
50. Hair color is influenced by the amount and type of melanin pigment present in the hair shaft, with eumelanin causing black and brown colors, and pheomelanin leading to red and blond colors.
51. Beards were often considered a symbol of power and wisdom in ancient civilizations.
52. The ancient Greeks believed that lightning bolts were the cause of gray hair.
53. The word "shampoo" comes from the Hindi word "champu," which means massage.
54. Leonardo da Vinci was one of the first people to study human hair under a microscope.
55. The growth rate of hair can be affected by factors such as stress, illness, and certain medications.

56. Human hair can be used to clean oil spills due to its ability to absorb oil.
57. Hair mats and booms made from human or animal hair are effective in containing and absorbing oil spills in water.
58. Human hair has been used in art and fashion to create intricate sculptures and unique designs.
59. Human hair has been used in various ways throughout history, including creating brushes for painting and calligraphy, as well as being woven into jewelry and artwork.
60. Hair contains a history of the body's exposure to toxins and heavy metals.
61. Hair contains information about drug use, as drug metabolites can be detected in hair follicles for several months.
62. Hair has been used as a symbol of beauty, identity, and social status in various works of art and literature.
63. Stress and traumatic events can cause hair loss, a condition known as telogen effluvium.
64. The average person will spend around six months of their life styling their hair.
65. The world's first-ever patented hairbrush was created in 1854 by Hugh Rock.
66. Hair and skin color are both influenced by the same pigment, melanin.
67. Hair follicles go through growth phases called anagen, catagen, and telogen.
68. The iconic hairstyle of Marie Antoinette was created to hide a bald spot on her head.
69. The world's first electric hair dryer was invented in 1890 by Alexandre Godefroy.
70. Hair color can be influenced by the level of copper, iron, and zinc in the body.
71. Believe it or not, humans have the same amount of hair follicles per square inch as a chimpanzee!

72. Hair density and texture can vary significantly among different ethnic groups.
73. Hair has a unique structure, with three layers: the medulla, cortex, and cuticle.
74. The average person has around 100,000 to 150,000 hair follicles on their scalp.
75. Pubic hair serves as a cushion and helps reduce friction during sexual activity.
76. Blond hair is more common in children but tends to darken as they age.
77. Hair can become more porous with age, making it more susceptible to damage.
78. Hair grows at an average rate of about 0.5 inches (1.25 cm) per month.
79. The diameter of a hair strand can range from 0.017 to 0.18 millimeters.
80. The act of twirling one's hair absentmindedly is known as "trichotemnomania."
81. Ancient Egyptians used combs made from bone and ivory to groom their hair.
82. The cross-section shape of hair can be round, oval, or flattened, influencing the texture and appearance of the hair.
83. Hair can hold on to scents for a long time, which is why certain smells trigger memories.
84. Hormonal changes during pregnancy can cause an increase in hair thickness and fullness.
85. Hair contains small amounts of metallic elements, including aluminum, copper, and nickel.
86. The most common hair color worldwide is black, found in approximately 75–80% of people.
87. Hair is electrically conductive, which is why it can stand on end in certain weather conditions.
88. The hair on your head contains different types of hairs, including vellus hair and terminal hair.

89. Different ethnicities have varying hair characteristics, such as density, thickness, and curl pattern.
90. The chemical structure of hair is similar to that of a fingerprint, making each person's hair unique.
91. Hair is not only found on the head but covers almost the entire human body, with the exception of the palms of the hands, soles of the feet, lips, and certain parts of the genitals.
92. The total length of all the hair on your scalp can reach up to 100,000 miles in a lifetime—that's more than four times around the Earth.
93. The longest recorded hair belongs to Xie Qiuping from China and measured 18 feet 5.54 inches (5.62 meters) when measured on May 8, 2004.
94. In rare cases, a person can be born with congenital hypertrichosis, also known as "werewolf syndrome," where excessive hair growth covers their face and body.
95. Hair can be used in forensic investigations to determine a person's DNA, providing valuable evidence in criminal cases.
96. Some people have a condition called "trichotillomania," which compels them to pull out their hair, leading to bald patches.
97. On average, people with naturally red hair have fewer hair strands (about 90,000) than people with other hair colors.
98. The world's oldest-known hairbrush is over 2,000 years old and was made from boar bristles and a gold handle.
99. If a man never shaved with, his beard would grow to over thirty feet in his lifetime.
100. The longest beard on record belonged to Shamsher Singh from India and measured over 8.2 feet (2.49 meters).

APPENDIX C

100 MOST INTERESTING LASER FACTS

1. Lasers can produce light that is billions of times more intense than sunlight.
2. Lasers do not occur in nature and are a 100% man-made invention.
3. Lasers have been used to measure the thickness of a single human hair with incredible accuracy.
4. Fiber optic technology, which uses lasers to send data as light pulses through thin glass fibers, powers over 99% of the internet, making it a critical backbone for high-speed data transmission.
5. Laser phototherapy can be used to treat both acute and chronic pain conditions, such as arthritis, back pain, and sports injuries. Even professional athletic teams have LPT devices for their injured players.
6. The *Star Wars* franchise popularized the concept of laser weapons with the term "blasters."
7. Lasers are essentially really bright, colored torches.
8. In 1917, Albert Einstein proposed the concept of (Light Amplification by Stimulated Emission of Radiation (LASER) theory.
9. Lasers have been used in art conservation to remove dirt and debris from delicate historical artifacts.
10. Laser measuring is accurate to more than a nanometer—which is a billionth of a meter!
11. Lasers are used to cut and shape gemstones.
12. Laser phototherapy may help reduce the duration and severity of cold sores and canker sores.

13. Lasers cannot be seen in space because they have no matter. The matter causes the scattering effect which would actually give the appearance of a light bulb.
14. Studies suggest that broken bones heal much faster using highly focused laser beams.
15. Laser phototherapy may help reduce the formation of scar tissue and improve the appearance of scars.
16. In 1974, lasers were utilized in supermarket barcode scanners to read, identify, and provide a price on products sold.
17. High-powered lasers have been proposed as a means of diverting asteroids on a collision course with Earth.
18. In 1971, researchers used lasers to transmit digital data for the first time, laying the foundation for modern optical communication systems.
19. Lasers have been used in dentistry for procedures like teeth whitening and gum reshaping.
20. Lasers are used in art and entertainment, creating stunning visual effects in concerts and shows.
21. In the medical field, lasers have been used to treat skin conditions like tattoos, birthmarks, and scars.
22. Laser phototherapy works by stimulating the mitochondria in cells, promoting the production of adenosine triphosphate (ATP), the energy currency of cells.
23. Lasers have been employed in nuclear fusion research to create and sustain high-temperature plasmas.
24. Lasers are used in non-destructive testing (NDT) to inspect materials and structures for flaws or defects.
25. Lasers help in creating intricate patterns in fabrics and determine how fabrics behave when worn on a human body.
26. Laser eye surgery, also known as LASIK (Laser-Assisted In Situ Keratomileusis), is a common procedure to correct vision problems such as nearsightedness and farsightedness.

27. X-ray lasers produce coherent X-ray beams and have applications in imaging and probing atomic and molecular structures.
28. Laser light can travel in a vacuum, making it an essential tool for space exploration and communication.
29. Lasers have been used in particle accelerators to manipulate and control charged particles.
30. Class 1 lasers are safe under normal operating conditions, while Class 4 lasers are high-power lasers that can cause serious injuries.
31. Lasers have been proposed as a means of harvesting energy from space-based solar power systems, providing clean and abundant energy to Earth.
32. Some animals, like certain species of sharks, have specialized cells in their eyes that can detect faint laser light in the ocean.
33. Lasers have been tested as a means of transmitting power wirelessly over long distances.
34. Lasers can be used in studying art by analyzing paint strokes and other fine details.
35. Lasers were first introduced in 1960, with the ruby laser being the first type to be developed.
36. The term "laser" stands for "Light Amplification by Stimulated Emission of Radiation."
37. The first laser was demonstrated on May 16, 1960, by Theodore Maiman, who used a synthetic ruby crystal to produce red laser light.
38. Lasers produce a concentrated, coherent beam of light that can be precisely controlled and focused.
39. Lasers have been used in military applications, such as laser rangefinders and target designators.
40. The first practical and widely used application of lasers was in barcode scanners, which revolutionized retail and inventory management.
41. Some lasers can emit terahertz radiation, which lies between microwaves and infrared light.
42. Lasers are used in laser pointers, which emit a narrow, bright beam of light used for presentations and educational purposes.

43. Laser light is monochromatic, meaning it has a single color or wavelength.
44. Laser phototherapy may help reduce muscle soreness and fatigue after intense physical activity.
45. Blue lasers were historically challenging to develop, but the invention of the blue laser diode in the 1990s enabled the creation of blue laser pointers and Blu-ray technology.
46. Lasers are now used to remove rust and paint from various surfaces without damaging the surface.
47. Green lasers are often used by astronomers to point out celestial objects and stars during public stargazing events and educational programs.
48. Laser weapons capable of directly damaging or destroying a target in combat are still in the experimental stage.
49. Laser light has been found to be effective in treating various skin conditions, such as acne and psoriasis.
50. Lasers are utilized in the manufacturing industry for cutting, welding, and engraving metals and other materials.
51. Lasers are used in cutting-edge scientific research, such as studying subatomic particles or creating controlled nuclear fusion reactions.
52. Laser beams can be invisible, visible, or ultraviolet, depending on the wavelength of the light.
53. Laser additive manufacturing uses lasers to selectively melt or solidify materials, layer by layer, to create complex 3D objects.
54. The first laser light show was displayed in 1968 during the Olympics in Mexico City.
55. Lasers are utilized in fiber-optic communication, enabling high-speed data transmission over long distances.
56. Lasers have been used in experimental propulsion systems for spacecraft, potentially enabling faster interstellar travel.
57. Rangefinders employ laser technology to precisely calculate the distance to a target.

58. Laser-induced fluorescence is used in forensic investigations to detect trace evidence like blood and fingerprints.
59. In 2008, scientists transmitted a laser beam from Earth to the Moon and detected its reflection, demonstrating the precision of laser technology.
60. The process of "quantum squeezing" has been utilized to detect gravitational waves using lasers.
61. The most powerful lasers in the world are found in research facilities and can generate pet watts (quadrillions of watts) of power.
62. A laser creates light by special actions involving a material called an "optical gain medium."
63. Lasers are commonly used in laser printers and photocopiers to create high-quality prints.
64. The most common type of laser used in everyday life is the semi-conductor laser, also known as a diode laser.
65. Gas lasers use gases as the gain medium, and common types include helium-neon (HeNe) lasers and carbon dioxide (CO_2) lasers.
66. Gas lasers are widely used in research, industry, and medical applications.
67. Lasers can be used to stimulate plant growth and improve crop yields in agriculture.
68. Laser phototherapy has a wide range of medical applications, including wound healing, pain management, and inflammation reduction.
69. The term "laser" was first coined by Gordon Gould in 1959, who independently developed the laser concept.
70. Lasers emit coherent light, meaning the light waves are aligned and in phase with each other.
71. The world's largest laser is the National Ignition Facility (NIF) in the USA, which aims to achieve nuclear fusion ignition. This facility is only two miles away from our company's headquarters.
72. Some animals, like cats, have a reflective layer in their eyes that causes them to glow when exposed to laser light.

73. The laser is considered one of the most significant man-made inventions of the 20th century.
74. Laser ablation is a process where high-power lasers are used to remove material from a surface, often used in manufacturing and artistic applications.
75. Photobiomodulation, also known as low-level light therapy, uses low-power lasers to stimulate cell function and promote tissue repair.
76. Laser hair removal works by targeting the pigment in hair follicles, damaging them and inhibiting future hair growth.
77. Laser phototherapy may help reduce the risk of infection in wounds and surgical incisions.
78. Ultraviolet (UV) light is used for phototherapy to treat conditions like psoriasis, vitiligo, and eczema.
79. Light-emitting diodes (LEDs) are used in photodynamic therapy for mostly topical skincare, wound healing, and acne treatments.
80. LIDAR (Light Detection and Ranging) uses lasers to measure distances and create detailed 3D maps of the environment and is in nearly every new car now.
81. Light therapy is used to treat Seasonal Affective Disorder (SAD), a type of depression associated with changes in seasons and reduced sunlight exposure.
82. Ultraviolet germicidal irradiation (UVGI) is a technique that uses UV light to disinfect air, water, and surfaces by inactivating microorganisms.
83. The US Food and Drug Administration (FDA) has cleared LLLT for specific medical indications, including carpal tunnel syndrome and chronic pain.
84. Laser phototherapy has been investigated for its potential in treating conditions related to the eyes, such as macular degeneration and retinitis pigmentosa.
85. The therapy has been studied as a potential treatment for temporomandibular joint disorder (TMJ) and associated pain.
86. In 1961, the first laser diode was invented by Robert N. Hall.

87. Lasers have been used in "optical storage devices" like CDs and DVDs to read and write data.
88. Lasers have been used to detect explosives and hazardous chemicals from a safe distance.
89. Laser tag or Laser Quest type games were developed as a non-lethal training program for the US Army in the 1970s.
90. With the aid of lasers, scientists can manipulate and examine biological cells and tiny particles using the optical trapping technique.
91. Scientists have long been working on a laser that draws lightning strikes away from airports and power plants.
92. Lasers can be hazardous if not used properly.
93. Military forces have explored the development of laser weapons for various applications, including defense against missiles, drones, and other threats.
94. Laser weapons have the potential for high precision and reduced collateral damage.
95. A method for measuring minute changes in distance is called laser interferometry.
96. Precision measurements, gravitational wave detection, and other areas of science can all benefit from laser technology.
97. Laser Doppler velocimetry is a method for measuring the speed of moving particles or fluids.
98. Lasers are commonly used for engraving intricate designs or markings on various materials, including wood, glass, metal, and plastics.
99. The world's most powerful laser has the power of a hydrogen bomb.
100. Though it sounds ancient, the strength of early lasers was measured in "gillettes," which are the number of razor blades a beam is capable of breaking through.

APPENDIX D

LPT STUDIES WITH SUMMARIES:

The Science of Low-Level Light Therapy (LLLT) and Laser Phototherapy (LPT)

This appendix outlines and summarizes various clinical trials behind low-level light therapy (LLLT) for hair loss and hair growth. We have referenced several peer-reviewed journals in support of the information contained in this book.

Note: The new term laser phototherapy (LPT) is used since LLLT devices may use weaker light sources, such as LEDs. Theradome uses the acronym LPT as it uses only lasers.

The following is a list of studies conducted and the summarized results.

Clinical and Scientific Studies that Demonstrate LLLT Treatment Efficacy

1. LLLT Accelerates Hair Growth in Chemotherapy-Induced Alopecia

Wikramanayake, TC; Villasante, AC; Mauro, LM; Nouri, K; Schachner, LA; Perez, CI; Jimenez, JJ. Low-level laser treatment accelerated hair regrowth in a rat model of chemotherapy-induced alopecia (CIA). *Lasers Med Sci.* 2013 May; 28(3):701–6. doi: 10.1007/s10103-012-1139-7.

Summary: This study tested the effects of low-level laser treatment for alopecia areata in a mouse module. In the current study, young rats were given chemotherapy and they developed full-body alopecia. After chemotherapy, a few of them were treated with LLLT, and others with sham devices. The results showed that rats receiving laser treatment regrew hair five days earlier than rats receiving chemotherapy alone or sham laser treatment. Moreover, LLLT treatment didn't compromise the chemotherapy or its effects. Keeping the results in mind, it was suggested that LLLT should be explored for the treatment of chemotherapy-induced alopecia (CIA) in clinical trials for humans.

Conclusion: The results demonstrated that LLLT significantly accelerated hair regrowth after CIA without compromising the efficacy of chemotherapy in the rat model. Based on the positive results in rats, testing of LLLT for CIA is also suggested in humans.

2. LLLT Promotes Hair Growth in Women with Alopecia

Lanzafame, RJ, et al. The growth of human scalp hair in females using visible red-light laser and LED sources. *Lasers Surg Med.* 2014 Oct; 46(8):601–7. doi: 10.1002/lsm.22277.

Summary: Twenty-four females with androgenic alopecia used a bicycle-helmet-like LLLT apparatus for twenty-five minutes, every other day for sixteen weeks. Eighteen females with androgenetic alopecia used similar helmets with incandescent red lights (sham treatment). A 37% increase in hair growth was observed in the LLLT group as compared to the placebo group. No adverse events or side effects were reported. Overall, LLLT of the scalp significantly improved hair counts in women with androgenetic alopecia. Similar results were observed one year prior in males using the same parameters.

Conclusion: Results indicate that LLLT for CIA would produce similar outcomes.

3. LLLT Promotes Hair Growth in Men with Alopecia

Lanzafame, RJ et. al. The growth of human scalp hair mediated by visible red-light laser and LED sources in males. *Lasers Surg Med.* 2013 Oct; 45(8):487–95. doi: 10.1002/lsm.22173.

Summary: Twenty-two males with androgenetic alopecia used a bicycle-helmet-like LLLT apparatus for twenty-five minutes, every other day for sixteen weeks. Nineteen males with androgenetic alopecia used similar helmets with incandescent red lights (sham treatment). A 39% increase in hair growth was observed in the LLT group as compared to the placebo group. No adverse events or side effects were reported. Overall, LLLT of the scalp at significantly improved hair counts in men with androgenetic alopecia.

Conclusion: Similar outcomes are expected from LLLT treatment for CIA.

4. LLLT Promotes Hair Growth and Increased Hair Diameter

Kim, H, et al. Low-level light therapy for androgenetic alopecia: a 24-week, randomized, double-blind, sham-device-controlled multicenter trial. *Dermatol Surg.* 2013 Aug; 39(8):1177–83. doi: 10.1111/dsu.12200.

Summary: Forty subjects (male and female) were randomized into different LLLT groups in which they wore a helmet-like device for eighteen minutes daily. After twenty-four weeks, the LLLT group showed significantly greater hair density in comparison to the sham-treatment group. Larger improvements in hair diameter were also observed for the LLLT group in comparison to the sham treatment group. No serious adverse reactions were detected.

Conclusion: The results of this study not only show that LLLT not only promotes hair regrowth, but also has the ability to increase hair diameter as well.

5. LLLT Increases Hair Count and Shaft Diameter

Avram, MR, Rogers, NE. The use of low-level light for hair growth: part I. Journal of Cosmetic and Laser Ther. 2009 Jun; 11(2):110-7. doi: 10.1080/14764170902842531.

Summary: Five patients were exposed to LLLT twice weekly for twenty minutes for three months; two received the same treatment for six months. The results indicate that several of the patients had a decrease in the number of vellus hairs, an increase in the number of terminal hairs, and an increase in shaft diameter.

Conclusion: Although the sample size was small, the results provided early supportive evidence of the efficacy of LLLT to promote hair regrowth and increase shaft diameter.

6. LLLT for the Prevention, Reduction, and Reversal of Hair Loss

Avci, P; Gupta, GK; Clark, J; Wikonkal, N; Hamblin, MR. Low-level laser (light) therapy (LLLT) for treatment of hair loss. *Lasers Surg Med.* 2014 Feb; 46(2):144–51. doi: 10.1002/lsm.22170.

Summary: This review describes the results of several animal and human studies regarding LLLT, some of which have previously been discussed. The general consensus is that LLLT safely and effectively stimulates hair growth in men and women who have various forms of hair loss, such as alopecia areata and androgenetic alopecia. Proposed mechanisms include the stimulation of epidermal stem cells in the hair follicle bulge and the shifting of follicles into the growth (anagen) phase.

Conclusion: It is hypothesized that chemotherapy-induced hair loss may be prevented, reduced, and reversed by LLLT through the same mechanisms.

7. LLLT for Androgenetic Alopecia: Systematic Review

Afifi, L, et al. Low-level laser therapy as a treatment for androgenetic alopecia. *Lasers Surg Med.* 2017 Jan; 49(1):27–39.

Summary: Investigation of 680 patients who underwent phototherapy with LaserComb or TOPHAT: 444 males and 236 females. The assessment involved hair count as well as hair density. Depending on the device, the sessions ranged from five to twenty minutes. The treatment period ranged from twelve to forty-eight weeks. The treatment frequency ranged from daily, every other day, or three times a week. Significant improvements in hair thickness as well as tensile strength were observed.

Conclusion: LLLT is described as a promising therapy for androgenetic alopecia, particularly for individuals who want to avoid medicinal approaches or surgery.

8. A New Helmet-Type LLLT Device for Androgenetic Alopecia

Yoon, JS, et al. *Medicine* (Baltimore). 2020; 99(29): e21181. Low-level light therapy using a helmet-type device for the treatment of androgenetic alopecia. A 16-week, multicenter, randomized, double-blind, sham-device-controlled trial.

Summary: To evaluate the safety and efficacy of a new helmet-type device for androgenetic alopecia treatment, sixty subjects (forty men and twenty women) were randomized into two groups: LLLT helmet-type device or a sham device (red light 0 output) with recommended treatment at home for twenty-five minutes, every other day for sixteen weeks. Results demonstrated an increase in hair density (41.90 hairs/cm^2) and hair thickness (7.50 μm) in the treatment group as compared to increased hair density of 0.72 hairs/cm² and a decrease in hair thickness of 15.03 μm for the control group. Prior to the intervention, tattooing with blue dye was performed at the central point of the vertex (scalp) for subsequent measurements.

Conclusion: The new helmet-type LLLT device produces a significant increase in hair density for people with androgenetic alopecia.

9. Theradome PRO LH80 Clinical Trial (Unpublished)

Gold, et al. Clinical Laser Phototherapy Study: NCT02528552.

Efficacy and safety of low-level laser phototherapy with Theradome PRO LH80 for promoting hair growth in males with androgenetic alopecia: a multicenter, randomized, sham-device-controlled, double-blind study.

Summary: Evaluated the efficacy of LLLT Theradome PRO LH80 red-laser device (680 nm) to boost hair growth and hair follicle number in comparison to a sham device (red-light placebo 680 nm). Forty-nine males with androgenic alopecia were randomized to use Theradome (n = 27) or a sham device (n = 22) at home for ≤20 minutes, twice weekly for twenty-six weeks. The Theradome group experienced hair growth at twenty-six weeks while the placebo (sham device) group experienced a decrease in hair growth.

Conclusion: Results demonstrated that all participants who had active hair loss experienced positive benefits from the Theradome PRO LH80 therapy since hair count increased for the treatment group. The most significant hair growth and the greatest benefits were observed in men ≤40 years of age who had androgenetic alopecia and Hamilton-Norwood scale scores of II–IV.

10. Theradome PRO LH80 Versus Other Forms of LLLT for Hair Growth

Theradome is the only device in the world that emits laser energy at 680 nm (other LLLT devices emit laser energy at wavelengths of 630 nm–655 nm. The absorption into the scalp at 680 nm is 2.5x greater than at wavelengths of 630 nm–655 nm. (T Karu. IEEE J. *Quantum Electronics.* 20:2. Mar/Apr 2014).

Theradome PRO LH80 therapy helps reduce the frequency of necessary treatments: The Theradome group demonstrated benefits after twice weekly sessions of ≤20 minutes (Gold, et al., publication year).

Conversely, individuals typically must use other devices daily, every other day, or three times a week before benefits are experienced (Afifi, et al., 2017; Yoon, et al., 2020).

Research shows that other devices typically deliver LLLT in the range of 630–655 nm (± 20 nm) (Afifi, et al., 2017; Yoon, et al., 2020), which is lower than that of Theradome PRO LH80 (Gold, et al., publication year).

Theradome treatment in women and men demonstrates an increase in hair count in the absence of adverse effects and, unlike other LLLT devices, reduces hair shedding.

A systematic review indicates that certain LLLT devices (e.g., HairMax LaserComb or TOPHAT 655) may cause headaches, dry skin, pruritus, scalp tenderness, and scalp irritation, among other side effects for some patients (Afifi, et al., 2017).

11. LLLT for Pattern Hair Loss: RCTs Analysis

Gentile, P; Garcovich, S. "The Effectiveness of Low-Level Light/Laser Therapy on Hair Loss." *Facial Plast Surg Aesthet Med.* 2021 Sep 20. doi: 10.1089/fpsam.2021.0151. Epub ahead of print. PMID: 34546105.

Summary: A systematic review of low-level light/laser therapy (LLLT) in male pattern hair loss (MPHL) and female pattern hair loss (FPHL) was performed. Of the 298 articles initially identified, 136 articles focusing on MPHL and FPHL were selected, of which only thirty-six articles focused exclusively on LLLT. Of this number, twenty-three articles were clinical trials while thirteen were systematic reviews. Systematic reviews were excluded, and only seven articles were analyzed as RCTs.

Conclusions: All the articles selected and analyzed reported positive effects of LLLT for MPHL and/or FPHL treatment without side effects.

12. Critical Assessment of LLLT Trials and Evidence

Gupta, AK; Foley, KA. "A Critical Assessment of the Evidence for Low-Level Laser Therapy in the Treatment of Hair Loss." *Dermatol Surg.* 2017 Feb; 43(2):188–197. doi: 10.1097/DSS.0000000000000904. PMID: 27618394.

Summary: Nine trials were identified for comb and helmet/cap devices, five of which were randomized, controlled trials. Data comparison across LLLT trials along with traditional hair loss therapy (Minoxidil, Finasteride) was not straightforward because there was a lack of visual evidence, sample sizes were low, and there were large variations in study duration and efficacy measurements.

Conclusion: There are several unanswered questions about the optimum treatment regimen, including maintenance treatment and the long-term consequences of LLLT use. Moving forward, protocols should be standardized across trials. Moreover, it is recommended that future trials include visual evidence and that trial duration be expanded to twelve months.

13. Effectiveness of LLLT for Pattern Hair Loss Treatment

Egger A, Resnik SR, Aickara D, Maranda E, Kaiser M, Wikramanayake TC, Jimenez JJ. "Examining the Safety and Efficacy of Low-Level Laser Therapy for Male and Female Pattern Hair Loss: A Review of the Literature." *Skin Appendage Disord.* 2020 Sep; 6(5): 259–267. doi: 10.1159/000509001. Epub 2020 Jul 7. PMID: 33088809; PMCID: PMC7548873.

Summary: Ten randomized, controlled trials were included, of which eight compared LLLT to a sham device and one to no treatment. The study populations varied, with three studies evaluating only women. All sham-device-controlled studies demonstrated statistically significant increase in hair diameter or density (p < 0.01) following LLLT. LLLT appears to be effective for treating pattern hair loss in both men and women. The laser devices have good safety profiles, with only minor adverse effects reported. However, physicians should be cautious when drawing conclusions since some studies included have a relationship with industry.

Conclusion: All the trials included demonstrated that LLLT is effective for pattern hair loss treatment since an increase in hair diameter or density was observed. Laser devices also appeared to safe and had minor adverse effects, but they must be used very carefully.

14. LLLT Increases Hair Density During PHL Treatment

Lueangarun S, Visutjindaporn P, Parcharoen Y, Jamparuang P, Tempark T. "A Systematic Review and Meta-analysis of Randomized Controlled Trials of United States Food and Drug Administration-approved, Home-use, Low-level Light/Laser Therapy Devices for Pattern Hair Loss." *Device Design* and *Technology.* J Clin Aesthet Dermatol. 2021 Nov; 14(11) :E64–E75. PMID: 34980962; PMCID: PMC8675345.

Summary: The overall quantitative analysis yielded a significant increase in hair density in those treated by LLLT versus sham groups (SMD: 1.27, 95% confidence interval [CI]: 0.993-1.639). The subgroup analysis demonstrated increased hair growth in male and female subjects with both comb- and helmet-type devices. There were significant LLLT sources in the LDs alone (SMD: 1.52, 95% CI: 1.16-1.88) and the LDs combination (SMD: 0.85, 95% CI: 0.55-1.16) (p=0.043).

Conclusion: LLLT is potentially effective for PHL treatment. Nonetheless, long-term follow-up study in patients with severe PHL with combined standard treatment and comparison between LLLT devices and energy sources is recommended.

15. Effectiveness of LLLT in Combination with Minoxidil

Liu Y, Jiang LL, Liu F, Qu Q, Fan ZX, Guo Z, Miao Y, Hu ZQ. Comparison of low-level light therapy and combination therapy of 5% Minoxidil in the treatment of female pattern hair loss. *Lasers Med Sci.* 2021 Jul; 36(5):1085-1093. doi: 10.1007/s10103-020-03157-1. Epub 2020 Oct 17. PMID: 33068178.

Summary: The effectiveness of reducing oil secretion in the LLLT group and the combination group was higher than the Minoxidil group (P < 0.05). For improving hair diameter and hair density, the combination group was better than the LLLT and Minoxidil groups. No side effects were reported. Our study illustrated that LLLT is a safe and effective treatment for FPHL. Furthermore, LLLT can significantly improve its efficacy when used in combination with 5% Minoxidil.

Conclusion: LLLT proved effective in reducing oil secretion and as a treatment for FPHL. A combination of LLLT and Minoxidil was better for increasing hair diameter and density than either procedure performed individually.

16. Effects of LLLT in FPHL and TE patients

Amer M, Nassar A, Attallah H, Amer A. "Results of Low-level Laser Therapy in the Treatment of Hair Growth: An Egyptian Experience." *Dermatol Ther.* 2021 May; 34(3) :e14940. doi: 10.1111/dth.14940. Epub 2021 Apr 17. PMID: 33713522.

Summary: Low-level laser therapy of the scalp significantly improved hair counts in FPHL, but there was no significant difference in telogen effluvium (TE) patients. There were no serious adverse reactions. Additional studies should be considered to determine the long-term effects of low-level laser therapy treatment on hair growth and maintenance and to optimize laser modality.

Conclusion: LLLT was found to be effective in treatment of female pattern hair loss (FPHL) but not in telogen effluvium (TE).

17. LLLT Devices are Safe and Effective for PHL Treatment

Zarei M, Wikramanayake TC, Falto-Aizpurua L, Schachner LA, Jimenez JJ. "Low-level Laser Therapy and Hair Regrowth: An Evidence-based Review." *Lasers Med Sci.* 2016 Feb; 31(2):363–71. doi: 10.1007/s10103-015-1818-2. Epub 2015 Dec 21. PMID: 26690359.

Summary: Based on all the available evidence about the effectiveness of LLLT with regard to alopecia, we found that the FDA-cleared LLLT devices are both safe and effective in patients with MPHL and FPHL who did not respond or were not tolerant to standard treatments. Future randomized, controlled trials of LLLT are strongly encouraged. They should be conducted and reported according to the Consolidated Standards of Reporting Trials (CONSORT) statement in order to facilitate analysis and comparison.

Conclusion: This review demonstrates that LLLT devices are safe and effective for PHL treatment. However, more trials and studies are encouraged for further analysis and information.

18. Uses of LLLT in Many Hair Conditions

Afifi L, Maranda EL, Zarei M, Delcanto GM, Falto-Aizpurua L, Kluijfhout WP, Jimenez JJ. "Low-level Laser Therapy as a Treatment for Androgenetic Alopecia." *Lasers Surg Med.* 2017 Jan; 49(1):27–39. doi: 10.1002/lsm.22512. Epub 2016 Apr 25. PMID: 27114071.

Summary: The majority of studies covered in this review found an overall improvement in hair regrowth, thickness, and patient satisfaction following LLLT therapy. Although we should be cautious when interpreting these findings, LLLT seems to be a promising monotherapy for androgenetic alopecia (AA) and may serve as an effective alternative for individuals unwilling to use medical therapy or undergo surgical options.

Conclusion: This review emphasized the uses of LLLT in different hair conditions, including AA and as an alternative for many other medical and surgical procedures.

19. LLLT as a Treatment for Androgenic Alopecia

Darwin E, Heyes A, Hirt PA, Wikramanayake TC, Jimenez JJ. "Low-level Laser Therapy for the Treatment of Androgenic Alopecia: A Review." *Lasers Med Sci.* 2018 Feb; 33(2):425–434. doi: 10.1007/s10103-017-2385-5. Epub 2017 Dec 21. PMID: 29270707.

Summary: LLLT appears to be a safe, alternative treatment for patients with androgenic alopecia. Clinical trials have indicated efficacy for androgenic alopecia in both men and women. LLLT may be used independently or as an adjuvant of Minoxidil or Finasteride. More research needs to be undertaken to determine the optimal power and wavelength to use in LLLT as well as LLLT's mechanism of action.

Conclusion: Final words about the review are that LLLT can be used as treatment for androgenic alopecia, independently or with Minoxidil or Finasteride. But more research is still needed to ensure optimum results.

20. Combined use of Micro-needling, LLLT and PRP

Gentile P, Dionisi L, Pizzicannella J, de Angelis B, de Fazio D, Garcovich S. A randomized, blinded, retrospective study: the combined use of micro-needling technique, low-level laser therapy and autologous non-activated platelet-rich plasma improves hair regrowth in patients with androgenic alopecia. *Expert Opin Biol Ther.* 2020 Sep; 20(9):1099–1109. doi: 10.1080/14712598.2020.1797676. Epub 2020 Jul 27. PMID: 32678725.

Summary: The combined use of biotechnologies, such as the association of PRP with micro-needling and low-level laser therapy, may improve the results in terms of hair count and hair density compared with those obtained with PRP alone. All the procedures must be performed with full respect to international and local rules.

Conclusion: The study concludes that the combined use of PRP, micro-needling, and LLLT shows better results than PRP alone.

21. Effectiveness of LLLT in Treatment of AA

Faghihi G, Mozafarpoor S, Asilian A, Mokhtari F, Esfahani AA, Bafandeh B, Nouraei S, Nilforoushzadeh MA, Hosseini SM. "The Effectiveness of

Adding Low-level Light Therapy to Minoxidil 5% Solution in the Treatment of Patients with Androgenetic Alopecia." *Indian J Dermatol Venereol Leprol.* 2018 Sep-Oct; 84(5):547–553. doi: 10.4103/ijdvl.IJDVL_1156_16. PMID: 30027912.

Summary: The percentage of recovery from androgenetic alopecia and the patients' satisfaction with their treatment were significantly higher in the case group compared to the control group. The patients' mean hair density and diameter were found to be higher in the case group after the intervention compared to the control group. As a new method of treatment, low-level light therapy can help improve the percentage of recovery from androgenetic alopecia and increase patients' satisfaction with their treatment.

Conclusion: LLLT proved very effective in AA treatment in terms of recovery and patient satisfaction. Mean hair density and diameter were improved, and recovery percentage from AA was found to be higher with the use of LLLT.

22. LLLT is Effective in Drug-intolerant Patients

Paquet P, Orduz M, Franchimont C, Nikkels AF. "Quel est l'intérêt des lasers de basse énergie dans le traitement de l'alopécie androgéno-génétique?" [What is the value of low-energy lasers in the treatment of androgenetic alopecia?]. *Rev Med Liege.* 2017 Dec;72(12):540–546. French. PMID: 29271134.

Summary: Used as monotherapy, LLLT offers a safe and potentially effective therapeutic option in the short and medium term for AA, both in men and women, in patients who do not respond or are intolerant to drug treatments. In combination with topical Minoxidil and oral Finasteride, the LLLT may also act synergistically with these treatments to stimulate hair growth.

Conclusion: The review concludes that LLLT is effective in drug-intolerant or non-responsive patients. LLLT increases hair growth in combination with Minoxidil and Finasteride.

23. Combination Therapies: Analysis and Results

Zhou Y, Chen C, Qu Q, Zhang C, Wang J, Fan Z, Miao Y, Hu Z. "The Effectiveness of Combination Therapies for Androgenetic Alopecia: A Systematic Review and Meta-analysis." *Dermatol Ther.* 2020 Jul; 33(4) :e13741. doi: 10.1111/dth.13741. Epub 2020 Jul 2. PMID: 32478968.

Summary: The study evaluated the effectiveness of three common combination therapies of Minoxidil with Finasteride, low-level laser light therapy (LLLT) or micro-needling versus Minoxidil monotherapy. We conducted meta-analysis for three groups of combined treatment separately, and all were superior to monotherapy in terms of global photographic assessment (P < .05). Combination of LLLT or micro-needling with Minoxidil also showed significant increase in hair count (P < .05) compared to monotherapy.

Conclusion: The present study suggests that combination therapy of three therapies with Minoxidil could be an effective, safe, and promising option for the treatment of AA as opposed to monotherapy.

24. Earlier Treatment Methods for Alopecia

Najem I, Chen H. Use of low-level laser therapy in treatment of the androgenic alopecia, the first systematic review. *J Cosmet Laser Ther.* 2018 Aug; 20(4):252–257. doi: 10.1080/14764172.2017.1400174. Epub 2017 Dec 11. PMID: 29227728.

Summary: Some earlier studies had shown that the use of low-level laser therapy stimulated hair growth when mice were treated with chemotherapy, which induced alopecia, as well as another type of alopecia (alopecia areata). The researchers hypothesized that the primary mechanism of treating androgenic alopecia was the stimulation of the epidermal stem cells, which are in the hair follicle, making them bulge and shift the follicles into the anagen (growth) phase.

Conclusion: The review shows that LLLT was proved experimentally in mice as treatment for chemotherapy-induced alopecia. It was also hypothesized that the stimulation of the epidermal stem cells in hair follicles could be used to treat androgenetic alopecia.

25. LLLT devices: Comparison and Effectiveness

Torres AE, Lim HW. "Photobiomodulation for the Management of Hair Loss." *Photodermatol Photoimmunol Photomed.* 2021 Mar; 37(2):91–98. doi: 10.1111/phpp.12649. Epub 2021 Jan 13. PMID: 33377535.

Summary: Photobiomodulation (PBM) or LLLT is a safe and potentially effective modality for the management of hair loss. It can be conveniently administered from home, and certain models offer hands-free, discreet use. Available data (tested on different types of hair loss). However, further large-scale studies on the different LLLT devices are needed to corroborate efficacy data, establish an optimal treatment protocol, and determine the ideal patient candidate. Based on currently available data, PBM may be recommended as an alternative for failed standard therapy or as an adjunct to prevailing treatments. The cost of PBM devices is a limitation although combined laser-LED devices are less expensive options. Lastly, management of patient expectations is an essential part of patient education.

Conclusion: Different models and forms of LLLT devices are available. PBM is also a recommended option, but it is quite costly.

26. Helmet-type LLLT Device for Androgenetic Alopecia

Suchonwanit P, Chalermroj N, Khunkhet S. Low-level laser therapy for the treatment of androgenetic alopecia in Thai men and women: a 24-week, randomized, double-blind, sham device-controlled trial. *Lasers Med Sci.* 2019 Aug; 34(6):1107–1114. doi: 10.1007/s10103-018-02699-9. Epub 2018 Dec 19. PMID: 30569416.

Summary: At week twenty-four, the laser helmet was significantly superior to the sham device for increasing hair density and hair diameter (p = 0.002 and p = 0.009, respectively) and showed a significantly greater improvement in global photographic assessment by investigators and subjects. Reported side effects included temporary hair shedding and scalp pruritus. The novel helmet-type LLLT device appears to be an effective treatment option for AA in both male and female patients with minimal adverse effects. However, the limitations of this study are the small sample size, no long-term follow-up data, and use of inappropriate sham devices, which do not reflect a true negative control.

Conclusion: In the clinical trial, the laser helmet was proved to be better than the sham device and to be an effective treatment for AA with some temporary side effects. Nonetheless, the study was questionable due to its different limitations.

27. Analysis of Photobiomodulation for the Treatment of AA

Gupta AK, Carviel JL. "Meta-analysis of Photobiomodulation for the Treatment of Androgenetic Alopecia." *J Dermatolog Treat.* 2021 Sep; 32(6):643–647. doi: 10.1080/09546634.2019.1688755. Epub 2019 Nov 20. PMID: 31746251.

Summary: Using hair density (hairs/cm^2) as a measure of efficacy, the standardized mean difference (SMD) was 1.02 (95% CI: 0.68, 1.36) in

favor of treatment over control (fifteen studies, pooled N = 795, p <
.00001). A subgroup analysis comparing comb-style devices versus hel-
met/hat-style devices did not reveal a significant difference (p = .08). A
second subgroup analysis suggested that laser treatment was significantly
more effective (p = .009) than a combination of laser/LED treatment
although the combination treatment was still significantly better than
the control treatment.

Conclusion: The photobiomodulation group showed better results than
the control group in the above study. Also, laser treatment alone was
more effective than the combination of laser/LED treatment.

28. Effectiveness of LLLT for AA: a Systematic Review

Liu KH, Liu D, Chen YT, Chin SY. Comparative effectiveness of low-level
laser therapy for adult androgenic alopecia: a systematic review and
meta-analysis of randomized controlled trials. *Lasers Med Sci.* 2019
Aug;34(6):1063–1069. doi: 10.1007/s10103-019-02723-6. Epub 2019 Jan
31. PMID: 30706177.

Summary: The quantitative analysis showed a significant increase in
hair density for those treated by LLLT versus the sham group (SMD
1.316, 95% confidence interval, CI 0.993 to 1.639). The subgroup analysis
demonstrated that LLLT increases hair growth in both genders, for both
comb- and helmet-type devices, and in short- and long-term treatment
courses. The subgroup analysis also showed a more significant increase
in hair growth for the LLLT. LLLT significantly increased hair density in
AA. The meta-analysis suggests that low treatment frequency with LLLT
produces a better hair growth effect than a high treatment frequency.
LLLT represents a potentially effective treatment for AA in both males
and females. The types of LLLT devices and the duration of the course
of LLLT treatment did not alter the effectiveness in hair growth.

Conclusion: LLLT treatment showed better results in terms of increasing hair density and hair growth in AGA. Also, LLLT treatment results are not affected by gender, type of device, or treatment course.

29. The Effectiveness of Treatments for AA

Adil A, Godwin M. "The Effectiveness of Treatments for Androgenetic Alopecia: A Systematic Review and Meta-analysis." *J Am Acad Dermatol.* 2017 Jul; 77(1):136–141.e5. doi: 10.1016/j.jaad.2017.02.054. Epub 2017 Apr 7. PMID: 28396101.

Summary: This meta-analysis strongly suggests that Minoxidil, Finasteride, and low-level laser light therapy are effective for promoting hair growth in men with androgenetic alopecia and that Minoxidil is effective in women with androgenetic alopecia. A meta-analysis was conducted separately for five groups of studies that tested the following hair loss treatments: low-level laser light therapy in men, 5% Minoxidil in men, 2% Minoxidil in men, 1 mg Finasteride in men, and 2% Minoxidil in women. All treatments were superior to placebo (P < .00001) in the five meta-analyses. Other treatments were not included because the appropriate data were lacking.

Conclusion: The above clinical trial proved the effectiveness of Minoxidil, Finasteride, and LLLT in men with AA but only of Minoxidil in women with AA.

30. Efficacy of LLLT in AA Treatment

Qiu J, Yi Y, Jiang L, Miao Y, Jia J, Zou J, Hu Z. "Efficacy Assessment for Low-level Laser Therapy in the Treatment of Androgenetic Alopecia: A Real-world Study on 1383 Patients." *Lasers Med Sci.* 2022 Feb 8. doi: 10.1007/s10103-022-03520-4. Epub ahead of print. Erratum in: *Lasers Med Sci.* 2022 Mar 23: PMID: 35133519.

Summary: More than 80% of users were between eighteen and forty years old. The median use times were 133 for mild AA patients and 142 for moderate-to-severe AGA patients, which equated to thirty-eight weeks and forty weeks, respectively. The overall clinical effectiveness was nearly 80%. PSM analysis revealed that gender (P = 0.002), use period (P = 0.068), and scalp conditions, with dandruff, rash, and itchy symptoms, were associated with the grading of efficacy assessment. Male users (ordinal OR: 1.35, CI: [1.01, 1.79]); use of more than 180 times or use period of one year (ordinal OR: 1.40, CI: [1.11, 1.96]); and those with scalp dandruff (ordinal OR: 1.34, CI: [1.01, 1.87]), rash (ordinal OR: 1.47, CI: [1.04, 2.07]), and itchy symptoms (ordinal OR: 1.51, CI: [1.12, 2.03]) had better efficacy assessments. The recommended treatment regime with low-level laser helmet was more than one year or 180 use times. Male patients with dandruff, rash, and scalp itching tended to have a better outcome.

Conclusion: Efficacy of LLLT in AA treatment is dependent on gender, period of use, and scalp conditions. Efficacy of LLLT is greater in males, in longer period use, or with scalp conditions.

31. LLLT Role in AA: RCTs and Analysis

Pillai JK, Mysore V. "Role of Low-Level Light Therapy (LLLT) in Androgenetic Alopecia." J Cutan *Aesthet Surg.* 2021 Oct–Dec; 14(4):385–391. doi: 10.4103/JCAS.JCAS_218_20. PMID: 35283601; PMCID: PMC8906269.

Summary: Studies have shown that LLLT stimulated hair growth in both men and women. Studies with the largest randomized controlled trials demonstrated statistically significant hair regrowth by terminal hair count in both males and females. One study also showed that LLLT and Minoxidil had similar efficacy in hair growth and that combination therapy was even more effective. LLLT represents a non-invasive, safe, and potentially effective treatment option for patients with AA who do not respond to or are not tolerant of standard treatment for AA. Moreover, combining LLLT with topical Minoxidil solution and oral Finasteride may act synergistically to enhance hair regrowth.

Conclusion: RCTs demonstrated that LLLT improves hair growth and acts as an effective treatment for AA patients. A combination of LLLT, Minoxidil, and Finasteride had greater efficacy than monotherapy.

32. Efficacy of Non-surgical treatments for AGA

Gupta AK, Bamimore MA, Foley KA. Efficacy of non-surgical treatments for androgenetic alopecia in men and women: a systematic review with network meta-analyses, and an assessment of evidence quality. J Dermatolog Treat. 2022 Feb;33(1):62–72. doi: 10.1080/09546634.2020.1749547. Epub 2020 Apr 13. PMID: 32250713.J Dermatolog Treat. 2022 Feb;33(1):62–72. doi: 10.1080/09546634.2020.1749547. Epub 2020 Apr 13. PMID: 32250713.

Summary: The networks for male and female AGA included thirty and ten RCTs, respectively. We identified the following treatments for male AGA in decreasing rank of efficacy: platelet-rich plasma (PRP), low-level laser therapy (LLLT), 0.5 mg dutasteride, 1 mg Finasteride, 5% Minoxidil, 2% Minoxidil, and bimatoprost. For female AGA the following were identified in decreasing rank of efficacy: LLLT, 5% Minoxidil, and 2% Minoxidil. The evidence quality of the highest ranked therapies, for male and female AGA, was judged to be low.

Conclusions: While newer treatments like LLLT may be more efficacious than more traditional therapies like 5% Minoxidil, the efficacy of the more recent treatment modalities needs to be further validated by future RCTs.

33. Combination therapy of LLLT and Minoxidil

Esmat SM, Hegazy RA, Gawdat HI, Abdel Hay RM, Allam RS, El Naggar R, Moneib H. "Low-level light–Minoxidil 5% Combination Versus Either Therapeutic Modality Alone in Management of Female pattern Hair Loss: A Randomized Controlled Study." *Lasers Surg Med.* 2017 Nov; 49(9):835–843. doi: 10.1002/lsm.22684. Epub 2017 May 10. PMID: 28489273.

Summary: The efficacy and safety of both topical Minoxidil and LLLT were highlighted with comparable results within all parameters. The combination group (iii) occupied the top position regarding Ludwig classification and patient satisfaction. UBM and dermoscopic findings showed significant increase in the number of regrowing hair follicles at four months in all groups, whereas only UBM showed such significant increase at two months in the combination group (iii). A non-significant increase in the hair diameter was also documented in the three groups.

Conclusion: LLLT is an effective and safe tool with comparable results to Minoxidil 5% in the treatment of FPHL. Owing to the significantly better results of combination therapy, its usage is recommended to hasten hair regrowth.

34. Comparison of LLLT and Sham Devices

Mai-Yi Fan S, Cheng YP, Lee MY, Lin SJ, Chiu HY. "Efficacy and Safety of a Low-Level Light Therapy for Androgenetic Alopecia: A 24-Week, Randomized, Double-Blind, Self-Comparison, Sham Device-Controlled Trial." *Dermatol Surg.* 2018 Nov; 44(11):1411–1420. doi: 10.1097/DSS.0000000000001577. PMID: 29957664.

Summary: This twenty-four-week, randomized, double-blind, self-comparison, sham-device-controlled trial enrolled one hundred patients with AGA. All participants were randomly assigned to receive the investigational LLLT on one side of the head and sham light treatment on the contralateral side three times weekly for thirty minutes each over a twenty-four-week period. After twenty-four weeks of treatment, the LLLT-treated scalp exhibited significantly greater hair coverage than the sham-device-treated side (14.2% vs. 11.8%, $p < .001$). A significantly greater improvement from baseline in hair thickness, hair count, hair coverage, and IGA were also observed in the LLLT-treated side than in the sham-device-treated side at the twelve- and twenty-four-week visits. No serious adverse events were observed.

Conclusion: The trial compared use of LLLT on one side of the head and a sham device on the other. The LLLT treated side of the head showed better results in terms of hair coverage, hair count, and thickness than the other side.

35. LLLT for treatment of AGA: Clinical Trial

Yoon JS, Ku WY, Lee JH, Ahn HC. "Low-level Light Therapy Using a Helmet-type Device for the Treatment of Androgenetic Alopecia: A 16-week, Multicenter, Randomized, Double-blind, Sham-device-controlled Trial." *Medicine* (Baltimore). 2020 Jul 17; 99(29):e21181. doi: 10.1097/MD.0000000000021181. PMID: 32702878; PMCID: PMC7373546.

Summary: A randomized, sham-device-controlled, double-blind clinical trial was conducted at two institutions. Sixty participants diagnosed with androgenic alopecia, aged nineteen to sixty-five years, were recruited. LLLT was performed through a helmet-type device that emitted light with a mean output power of 2.36 mW/cm. Participants were divided into two groups, which used the experimental device and a sham device respectively. After tattooing at the central point of the vertex, phototrichograms at that point were obtained at zero, eight, and sixteen weeks. Comparing the results at baseline and week sixteen, the experimental group showed an increase in hair density of 41.90 hairs/cm and an increase in hair thickness of 7.50 μm, whereas the control group showed an increase of 0.72 hairs/cm and a decrease of 15.03 μm, respectively (P < .001).

Conclusion: Clinical trial of LLLT and sham devices showed that LLLT provides better treatment option for AA. The LLLT group showed a greater increase in hair thickness and hair density than the sham-device group.

36. Studies Supporting LLLT for AGA

Martínez-Pizarro S. "Low-level Laser Therapy for Androgenetic Alopecia." *Actas Dermosifiliogr* (Engl Ed). 2021 Feb; 112(2):99–102. English, Spanish. doi: 10.1016/j.ad.2020.03.010. Epub 2020 Oct 29. PMID: 33130013.

Summary: This review analyzed nine different studies that proposed low-laser therapy as a treatment for androgenetic alopecia. All the studies that were analyzed concluded that LLLT is a potentially effective treatment for AA, and their findings support the benefit of LLLT in the treatment of AA. It was also demonstrated in these studies that the new laser devices achieved promising results without any observable adverse effects. The review found hardly any negative articles on LLLT. However, the studies showing positive outcomes of LLLT in humans are also limited in number. This limitation and the lack of sufficient evidence suggest that further high-quality clinical trials should be conducted to ensure safety and establish the general recommendation of LLLT for AA.

Conclusion: The review concludes that all the studies on LLLT support its benefits in the treatment of AA. No study negating its benefit in treating AA was found. Nonetheless, studies supporting LLLT are limited, and further trials are suggested to properly establish the use of LLLT for AA.

37. Review of Different Treatment Modalities for AA

Galadari H, Shivakumar S, Lotti T, Wollina U, Goren A, Rokni GR, Grabbe S, Goldust M. "Low-level Laser Therapy and Narrative Review of Other Treatment Modalities in Androgenetic Alopecia." *Lasers Med Sci.* 2020 Aug; 35(6):1239–1244. doi: 10.1007/s10103-020-02994-4. Epub 2020 Mar 11. PMID: 32162134.

Summary: This review focused on the various treatment options available in the management of AA. The reviewed options include the use of anti-androgens, Minoxidil, platelet-rich plasma therapy, adipose-derived stem cells, hair transplantation, micro-needling, fractional radio frequency, electrotrichogenesis, and carboxytherapy, with special emphasis on the role of low-level laser therapy (LLLT) in AA treatment. Different studies and trials on these methods of treatment were analyzed to evaluate the efficiency of these treatments for AA. The studies on LLLT demonstrated that a significant improvement in hair thickness, hair density, and hair coverage was observed. Although studies on the effectiveness of LLLT are scarce, this review was focused on bringing to light this new and promising treatment option for AA.

Conclusion: All treatment options for AA analyzed in this review differ in their efficacy for treating AA and in terms of the chances of side effects. LLLT is a relatively new treatment option, but its benefits are highlighted by the RCTs reviewed in this study. However, there is a need for larger RCTs on LLLT to clarify its effectiveness.

Appendix E

DIVING DEEPER INTO PHYSICS OF LPT

In this book, *Grow It Back*, I avoided discussing any equations, formulas, or physics since I wanted this book to be read by anyone experiencing hair loss or looking to grow back their hair.

Laser phototherapy (LPT) is a minimally invasive treatment that uses a range of laser light wavelengths to stimulate cellular activity within hair follicles. The aim for applying laser light is to curb hair loss, enhance hair thickness, and foster hair growth. The device used for laser phototherapy emits low-intensity coherent light, mainly in the red or near-infrared spectrum. This light is absorbed by the mitochondria of the hair follicle cells, boosting cellular metabolism and leading to photobiomodulation, which increases cellular activity, enhances energy production, and reduces inflammation. These factors facilitate the hair follicles' transition back into the anagen (growth) phase, yielding thicker and healthier hair strands.

We will be going over about eight calculations, which will explain LPT for specific wavelengths and other factors covered in this book. This section is for anyone to understand how certain key calculations are derived, especially as it relates to LPT and hair loss and growth.

Following are the sub-appendices topics covered in this appendix:

1. Frequency of light
2. Beam divergence
3. Energy of a photon
4. Total number of photons delivered
5. Power density
6. Energy density
7. Pulsed versus continuous laser beam energy
8. Bioabsorption of light on scalp and dosage

1. Frequency of Light

LPT involves the use of a laser beam with a wavelength λ of 680 nanometers in vacuum. Light travels at a speed of approximately $3 \cdot 10^8$ meters per second (c), still in vacuum. We would want to know at what frequency the laser light will have when it enters the human tissue specifically the scalp.

The frequency of light remains constant regardless of the medium it enters. This is because frequency is an intrinsic property of the light wave (photon). The fact is, when light enters a different medium, such as human tissue, its speed and wavelength change, but its frequency remains the same.

To calculate frequency, the formula of wave equation used is:

$$c = f\lambda$$

From which we obtain

$$f = \frac{c}{\lambda}.$$

Putting the values $c = 3 \cdot 10^8$ m/s and $\lambda = 680$ nm $= 680 \cdot 10^{-9}$ m in the previous equation, we can calculate the frequency

$$f = \frac{3 \cdot 10^8 \text{ m/s}}{680 \cdot 10^{-9} \text{ m}} = 4.41 \cdot 10^{14} \text{ Hz}.$$

Thus, light has a frequency of $4.41 \cdot 10^{14}$ Hz when entering the human tissue.

Vice versa, if we know the frequency at which light enters the human body and we want to calculate the wavelength, we can use the previous formula to extract λ as $\lambda = \frac{c}{f}$.

2. Beam Divergence

Although we can think laser beams to be perfectly collimated (all photons are travelling in parallel), they will always diverge to a certain degree because of diffraction. The beam divergence is a measurement of this spreading.

To calculate the beam divergence, we can use the diffraction-limited beam divergence formula:

$$\vartheta_d = \frac{\beta \lambda}{D},$$

where λ is the wavelength of the laser beam, β is a numerical factor representing the beam quality (in terms of collimation), and D is the output beam diameter. For a perfect diffraction-limited gaussian beam, β is equal to 1. In our calculation, we can use $\beta = 1.22$: It derives from the diffraction of a plane wave through an aperture with the same diameter as our laser. Despite not being the actual value of our laser, it is acceptable.

Given:

$\lambda = 680 \text{ nm} = 680 \cdot 10^{-9} \text{ m}$

$D = 0.64$ mm $= 0.64 \cdot 10^{-3}$m

$\beta = 1.22,$

we obtain that the beam divergence ϑ_d in radians as

$$\vartheta_d = \frac{\beta\lambda}{D} = \frac{1.22 \cdot 680 \cdot 10^{-9}\text{m}}{0.64 \cdot 10^{-3} \text{ m}} = 1.296 \cdot 10^{-3} \text{ rad} .$$

To convert the beam divergence to degrees we use the degree-radians relationship

$$\vartheta_d{}^{(\circ)} = \vartheta_d \cdot \frac{180}{\pi}$$

from which we obtain a value of 0.0743 degrees.

3. Energy of a Photon

The wavelengths for LPT are those that can be absorbed by biological components, in particular by chromophores of hair follicles cells as they enter the scalp and light transmits below the scalp and eventually stimulates the mitochondria. The power with which photons may penetrate tissues determines how well light can produce photo biomodulation or other therapeutic effects.

As said before, LPT uses a laser with a wavelength λ of a 680 nm. We want to calculate how much energy is contained in each photon of this light.

The energy E of a photon can be determined using the equation:

$E=hf$,

where $h = 6.626 \cdot 10^{-34}$J·s is Planck's constant and f is the frequency of the light.

In laser terminology, a Joule (J) measures the total energy the laser emits in a single pulse or over a specific duration.

From Section 1 we know that the frequency is related to the speed of light c and the wavelength λ:

$$f = \frac{c}{\lambda}$$

From which we derive that

$$E = h\frac{c}{\lambda}.$$

Putting the values for $c = 3 \cdot 10^8$ m/s and $\lambda = 680$ nm $= 680 \cdot 10^{-9}$ m, the energy of each photon is approximately:

$$E = \frac{6.626 \cdot 10^{-34} \text{ J·s} \cdot 3 \cdot 10^8 \text{ m/s}}{680 \cdot 10^{-9} \text{ m}} \cong 2.92 \cdot 10^{-19} \text{ J}.$$

4. Total Number of Photons Delivered

We want now to calculate the total number of photons delivered by a laser diode with power $P = 5$ mW during 20 minutes of operation or treatment. Since the power is defined as the amount of energy E_{tot} delivered over a certain time interval t

$$P = \frac{E_{tot}}{t}$$

we derive that the total energy delivered by the laser in 20 minutes is $E_{tot} = P \cdot t.$

Expressing the power in Watts (W) and the time in seconds (s) we have that

$P = 5$ mW $= 5 \cdot 10^{-3}$ W and $t = 20$ minutes $= 20 \cdot 60$ s $= 1200$ s, thus leading to an energy of $E_{tot} = 6$ J.

If each photon has an energy $E = 2.92 \cdot 10\text{-}19$ J, we can obtain the number of photons delivered in 20 minutes as

$$N = \frac{E_{tot}}{E} \sim 2.05 \cdot 10^{19}.$$

5. Power density

Power density, also known as irradiance, is a crucial element in LPT. It refers to the amount of laser energy that is delivered to a certain region of tissue over the course of a specified amount of time. Power density is an essential factor in determining the effectiveness and safety of laser treatment because it regulates the amount of energy received by the target tissues.

We want to calculate the power density of a laser phototherapy device that produces laser light with a power $P = 5$ mW over a surface $A = 0.64$ cm^2.

To determine the power density D for the treatment area, we'll use the formula $D = \frac{P}{A}$, leading to

$$D_{\frac{mW}{cm^2}} = \frac{5 \text{ mW}}{0.64 \text{ cm}^2} = 7.8125 \text{ mW/cm}^2$$

6. Energy density

Energy density, also known as fluence or dose, is a crucial element of LPT. It shows the total amount of energy that the laser delivered over time to a unit area of tissue. Energy density significantly influences how much energy is absorbed by the target tissues, which has an impact on the effectiveness and safety of laser treatment.

Let's assume that the continuous laser beam used for phototherapy delivers a power of 5 mW over a 0.64 cm² area. We want to determine the energy density of the laser beam.

For a continuous laser beam, the energy density J_0 is the product of power density D and time of exposure

$$J_0 = D \cdot t$$

The power density D is:

$$D = \frac{P}{A}.$$

Given $P = 5$ mW $= 5 \cdot 10^{-3}$ W, $A = 0.64$ cm² and a time of exposure $t = 1200$ s, the energy density can be calculated as follows:

$$J_0 = \frac{P}{A} \cdot t = \frac{5 \cdot 10^{-3} \text{W}}{0.64 \cdot \text{cm}^2} \cdot 1200 \text{ s} = 9.375 \text{ J/cm}^2.$$

7. Comparing Pulsed Laser Beam versus Continuous Laser Beam Output

We want to compare the output of a pulsed laser with the one of a continuous laser. The idea is to calculate the energy delivered by two laser beams, a continuous one and a pulsed one, both with a 5 mW power output and a wavelength of 680 nm. An operation time of 20 minutes will be considered.

We can proceed by calculating the energy delivered by each beam separately.

a. Continuous Laser Beam:

Given $P_{continuous}$ = 5 mW = 5 $\cdot 10^{-3}$ W and

t_{total} = 20 minutes = 1200 s,

the total energy delivered by the continuous laser beam in the time t_{total} is:

$$E_{continuous} = P_{continuous} \cdot t_{total} = 6.0 \text{ J.}$$

b. Pulsed Laser Beam:

Let us consider a pulsed laser beam with a pulse duration of 100 ms and an off-time of 900 ms: it emits light for 100 ms while stays off for 900 ms, making a complete cycle of 1 s.

The energy delivered in one pulse is $E_{pulse} = P_{pulse} \cdot t_{pulse}$, where t_{pulse} = 0.1 s, obtaining that

$$E_{pulse} = 5 \cdot 10^{-3} \text{ W} \cdot 0.1 \text{ s} = 5 \cdot 10^{-4} \text{ J.}$$

In 20 minutes, the laser completes a number of cycles (each with duration of t_{cycle} = 1 s) given by

'

which means that the laser emits light 1200 times in 20 minutes. Therefore, we can multiply the energy of the single pulse by the number of pulses N_pulses to obtain the total energy

$$N_{pulses} = \frac{t_{total}}{t_{cycle}} = \frac{1200 \text{ s}}{1 \text{ s}} = 1200 ,$$

The continuous laser beam delivers 10 times more energy than the pulsed laser beam over the 20-minute duration. This is because the pulsed laser is only emitting for 10% of the time (100 ms out of every 1 second), while the continuous laser is emitting for the entire time duration. By pulsing lasers, we modulate the energy output, minimizing thermal buildup and keeping delicate human tissue from potential heat damage. Therefore, the lasers pulse rate depends on the desired dosage vs. heat output and proper design must be considered for pulsed laser applications.

8. Bioabsorption of Light into Scalp Tissue

In this section, we will discuss and calculate how laser light penetrates the scalp at the most critical depth, which is 0.5 cm, the location of the papilla and bulge. We will show that the longer wavelengths (680 nm) and higher dosage will be superior to lower wavelengths (635 nm) and lower dosages. We will show via calculations the difference as a function of energy density.

The Beer-Lambert Law describes the relationship between light absorption and the properties of the material through which the light flows. According to the Beer-Lambert Law, the luminous intensity of light penetrating a material decreases exponentially with the depth from the material surface

$$I(x) = I_0 e^{-\alpha x} ,$$

where

$I(x)$ is the intensity of light at depth x,

I_0 is the initial intensity of light at the surface (in this case, the energy density at the surface),

α is the absorption coefficient of the material (the unit of measurement is the inverse of a length),

x is the depth of penetration (in cm).

Once the angle of emission and the distance are fixed, the light intensity has a linear relationship with the energy density.

To calculate the energy density in the human scalp at a depth of 5 mm with an initial energy density $J_0 = 9.375$ J/cm^2 (obtained in Section 6), we just need α.

The absorption coefficient α for the human scalp at the wavelength of 680 nm is not a fixed value and can vary based on several factors, including individual variations, hair density, and hydration levels. However, for the sake of providing an illustrative example, let's assume a hypothetical absorption coefficient: A common range for near-infrared light (like 680 nm) is between 0.1 cm^{-1} and 1 cm^{-1}.

Let's use an average value of $\alpha = 0.5$ cm^{-1} for this calculation.

Putting these values in $J(x) = J_0 e^{-\alpha x}$, we have that the energy density at a depth of 5 mm in the human scalp is approximately 7.301 J/cm^2.

Please note that this value is based on an estimated absorption coefficient, and the actual energy density can vary based on the specific properties of the individual's scalp and the exact absorption coefficient at the given wavelength.

For comparison, let's do the same thing but for a different laser source, like an Edge Emitting Laser (EEL) diode, so we can show you the difference between high dosage and low dosage (lower energy density) using inferior laser diodes such as EEL's. The laser has a wavelength of 635 nm.

We are once more using the Beer-Lambert Law, now with an energy density of $J_{(0)} = 1.1$ J/cm^2 while the depth remains the same x = 5 mm = 0.5 cm.

Again, we are considering an average value of $\alpha = 0.5$ cm for this calculation. We can repeat the previous calculation using this value to obtain 0.8567 J/cm^2.

In conclusion, the energy density at 680 nm and applying 9.375 J/cm^2 will deliver at least 11 times more energy to a hair follicle than a 635 nm laser diode source and with 1.1 J/cm^2. Therefore, a laser diode with longer wavelengths (680 nm) accompanied with a higher energy density will result in better results hair growth (635 nm) and a lower energy.

BIBLIOGRAPHY

Chapter 1: Light Is the Foundation of Growing It Back

Alberts, B; Johnson, A; Lewis, J.; et al. (2002). Molecular Biology of the Cell, Fourth Edition (4th ed.). Garland Science.

AlGhamdi MAI. Comparative Effectiveness Research in Photodynamic Therapy for Oral Lichen Planus. University of California, Los Angeles; 2016.

Ascherio, A; Munger, KL; Simon, KC; Vitamin D and Multiple Sclerosis. The Lancet Neurology. 2010 Jun 1;9(6):599–612.

Bowers, B. Historical Review of Artificial Light Sources. IEE Proceedings A (Physical Science, Measurement and Instrumentation, Management and Education, Reviews). 1980 Apr 1;127(3):127–33.

Bernstein EF. Hair Growth Induced by Diode Laser Treatment. Dermatologic Surgery (2005): 31(5): 584–586.

Bozzetto, S; Carraro, S; Giordano, G; et al. Asthma, Allergy and Respiratory Infections: The Vitamin D Hypothesis. Allergy. 2012 Jan;67(1):10–7.

Dainty JC. Laser Speckle and Related Phenomena. Springer Science & Business Media; 2013.

De Freitas, LF; Hamblin, MR. Proposed Mechanisms of Photobiomodulation or Low-Level Light Therapy. IEEE Journal of Selected Topics in Quantum Electronics. 2016 Jun 9;22(3):348–64.

Haddad JG, Matsuoka LY, Hollis B, Hu YZ, and Wortsman J. Human Plasma Transport of Vitamin D after its Endogenous Synthesis. The Journal of Clinical Investigation. 1993;91(6):2552-5.

Early History of Laser. Laserfest. Available from: https://laserfest.org/lasers/history/early.cfm.

Farivar S, Malekshahabi T, and Shiari R. Biological Effects of Low Level Laser Therapy. Journal of Lasers in Medical Sciences. 2014;5(2):58.

Gáspár, L. Professor Endre Mester, the Father of Photobiomodulation. Journal of Dental Lasers. 2009;17(3):146–8.

Geldenhuys. S; Hart, PH; Endersby, R; et al. Ultraviolet Radiation Suppresses Obesity and Symptoms of Metabolic Syndrome Independently of Vitamin D in Mice Fed a High-Fat Diet. Diabetes. 2014 Nov 1;63(11):3759–69.

Ghali L, and Dyson M. Angiogenesis: Key Principles—Science—Technology—Medicine. Springer; 1992:411-4.

Glickman, G; Byrne, B; Pineda, C; et al. Light Therapy for Seasonal Affective Disorder with Blue Narrow-Band Light-Emitting Diodes (Leds). Biological Psychiatry. 2006 Mar 15;59(6):502–7.

Goldman, L; Blaney, DJ; Freemond, A. The Biomedical Aspects of Lasers. JAMA. 1964 Apr 20;188(3):302–6.

Grossweiner, LI; Grossweiner, JB; Rogers, BG (2005, Jan 27). The Science of Phototherapy: An Introduction. Dordrecht, The Netherlands: Springer.

Hamblin, MR. Photobiomodulation or Low-Level Laser Therapy. Journal of Biophotonics. 2016 Dec;9(11–12):1122.

Hönigsmann, H. History of Phototherapy in Dermatology. Photochemical & Photobiological Sciences. 2012 Jan;12(1):16–21.

Kim MM, and Darafsheh A. Light Sources and Dosimetry Techniques for Photodynamic Therapy. Photochemistry and Photobiology. 2020;96(2):280-94.

King PR. Low Level Laser Therapy: A review. Lasers in Medical Science. 1989;4:141-50.

Klotter, J. Colored Light Therapy. Townsend Letter. 2011 Feb 1(331–332):2--30. Laser Theory. Available from: https://minerva.union.edu/newmanj/Physics100/Laser%20Theory/laser_theory.htm.

Kubota J. Effects of Diode Laser Therapy on Blood Flow in Axial Pattern Flaps in the Rat Model. Lasers in Medical Science. 2002;17:146-53.

Lightforce. The Science behind How Laser Therapy Works. Available from: https://lightforcemedical.com/photobiomodulation-therapy-pbm/.

Lim, HW (1993, Mar 19). Clinical Photomedicine. CRC Press.

Maisels, MJ; McDonagh, AF. Phototherapy for Neonatal Jaundice. New England Journal of Medicine. 2008 Feb 28;358(9):920–8.

Mathieu, C; Badenhoop, K. Vitamin D and Type 1 Diabetes Mellitus: State of The Art. Trends in Endocrinology & Metabolism. 2005 Aug 1;16(6):261–6.

Mccarthy, D. Laser Control Photosynthesis. Photonics. Available from: https://www.photonics.com/Articles/Laser_Controls_Photosynthesis/a13314.

Møller, KL; et al. How Finsen's Light Cure Lupus Vulgaris. Photodermatology, Photoimmunology & Photomedicine (2005): 21(3): 118–24.

Moriarty, C. Vitamin D Myths "D"-Bunked. Yale Medicine. Available from: https://www.yalemedicine.org/stories/vitamin-d-myths-debunked/.

Morimoto Y, Arai T, Kikuchi M, Nakajima S, and Nakamura H. Effect of Low-Intensity Argon Laser Irradiation on Mitochondrial Respiration. Lasers in Surgery and Medicine. 1994;15(2):191-9.

Oregon University. Laser Safety and Hazards. Oregon University. Available from: https://safety.uoregon.edu/laser-safety.

Paschotta R. Optical Power. RP-Photonics. Available from: https://www.rp-photonics.com/optical_power.html.

Pathak, MA; Fitzpatrick, TB. The Evolution of Photochemotherapy with Psoralens and UVA (PUVA): 2000 BC to 1992 AD. Journal of Photochemistry and Photobiology B: Biology. 1992 Jun 30;14(1-2):3–22.

Population Inversion. Physics and Radio Electronics. Available from: https://www.physics-and-radio-electronics.com/physics/laser/laser-populationinversion.html.

Powell, K; Low, P; McDonnell, PA; et al. The Effect of Laser Irradiation on Proliferation of Human Breast Carcinoma, Melanoma, and Immortalized Mammary Epithelial Cells. Photomedicine and Laser Surgery. 2010 Feb 1;28(1):115–23.

Roelandts R. The History of Phototherapy: Something New Under the Sun? Journal of the American Academy of Dermatology. 2002;46(6):926–30.

Silfvast WT. Laser Fundamentals. Cambridge University Press; 2004.

Suchkov S, and Herrera AS. The Role of Human Photosynthesis in Predictive, Preventive and Personalized Medicine. EPMA Journal. 2014;5(Suppl 1):A146.

Tunér, Jan & Lars Hode. The New Laser Therapy Handbook. Gragensberg, Sweden: Prima Books AB, 2010.

Unique Hair Concepts. Are Premature Graying and Hair Loss Related? (2018, February 15). https://www.uniquehairconcepts.com/blog/are-premature-graying-and-hair-loss-related.

Weller RB. The Health Benefits of UV Radiation Exposure through Vitamin D Production or Non-Vitamin D Pathways. Blood Pressure and Cardiovascular Disease. Photochemical & Photobiological Sciences. 2017;16:374–80.

Xu, C; Zhang, J; Mihai, DM; et al. (2014). Light-Harvesting Chlorophyll Pigments Enable Mammalian Mitochondria to Capture Photonic Energy and Produce ATP. Journal of Cell Science, 127(Pt 2), 388–399. https://doi.org/10.1242/jcs.134262.

Yamazaki M, Miura Y, Tsuboi R, and Ogawa H. Linear Polarized Infrared Irradiation Using Super Lizer™ is an Effective Treatment for Multiple-Type Alopecia Areata. International Journal of Dermatology. 2003;42(9):738–40.

Chapter 2: Human Hair 101

Abate M, Festa A, Falco M, Lombardi A, Luce A, Grimaldi A, et al. Seminars in Cell & Developmental Biology. Elsevier; 2020:139–53.

Alonso, L; Fuchs E. The Hair Cycle. Journal of Cell Science. 2006 Feb 1;119(3):391–3.

Barth, JH. Measurement of Hair Growth. Clinical and Experimental Dermatology. 1986 Mar;11(2):127–38.

Buffoli B, Rinaldi F, Labanca M, Sorbellini E, Trink A, Guanziroli E, et al. The Human Hair: from Anatomy to Physiology. International Journal of Dermatology. 2014;53(3):331–41.

Chang YC, and Goldberg LJ. Alopecias and Disorders of the Hair Follicle. Dermatoanthropology of Ethnic Skin and Hair. 2017:331–57.

Commo S, Gaillard O, and Bernard BA. Human Hair Greying is Linked to a Specific Depletion of Hair Follicle Melanocytes Affecting Both the Bulb and the Outer Root Sheath. British Journal of Dermatology. 2004;150(3):435–43.

Fuchs, E. (2007). Scratching the Surface of Skin Development. Nature, 445(7130), 834–842.

Higgins, CA; Westgate, GE; Jahoda, CA. From Telogen to Exogen: Mechanisms Underlying Formation and Subsequent Loss of the Hair Club Fiber. Journal of Investigative Dermatology. 2009 Sep 1;129(9):2100–8.

InformedHealth.org [Internet]. Cologne, Germany: Institute for Quality and Efficiency in Health Care (IQWiG); 2006. What is the Structure of Hair and How Does it Grow? 2019 Aug 29. Available from: https://www. ncbi.nlm.nih.gov/books/NBK546248/.

Jordan, A. How Much Money Is Your Hair Worth? Life Hacker. 2022, April 8. Available from: https://lifehacker.com/how-much-money-is-your-hair-worth-1846638883.

Joulai Veijouye S, Yari A, Heidari F, Sajedi N, Ghoroghi Moghani F, Nobakht M. Bulge Region as a Putative Hair Follicle Stem Cells Niche: A Brief Review. Iran J Public Health. 2017 Sep;46(9):1167-1175. PMID: 29026781; PMCID: PMC5632317.

Linch CA, Whiting DA, Holland MM. Human Hair Histogenesis for the Mitochondrial DNA Forensic Scientist. J Forensic Sci 2001;46(4):844–853.

Matsumura H, Mohri Y, Binh NT, Morinaga H, Fukuda M, Ito M, et al. Hair Follicle Aging is Driven by Transepidermal Elimination of Stem Cells via COL17A1 Proteolysis. Science. 2016;351(6273):aad4395.

Murphrey MB, Agarwal S, Zito PM. Anatomy, Hair. [Updated 2022 Aug 8]. In: StatPearls [Internet]. Treasure Island (FL): StatPearls Publishing; 2023 Jan-. Available from: https://www.ncbi.nlm.nih.gov/books/NBK513312/.

Paus R, and Cotsarelis G. The biology of hair follicles. New England Journal of Medicine. 1999;341(7):491–7.

Rompolas, P; & Greco, V. Stem Cell Dynamics in the Hair Follicle Niche. Seminars in Cell & Developmental Biology, 25–26, 34–42.

Sharquie KE, and Jabbar RI. COVID-19 Infection is a Major Cause of Acute Telogen Effluvium. Irish Journal of Medical Science (1971-). 2022;191(4):1677≠81.

Sperling LC. Hair Anatomy for the Clinician. Journal of the American Academy of Dermatology. 1991;25(1):1–17.

Chapter 3: Hair Loss: Causes and Consequences

Almohanna, HM; Ahmed, AA; Tsatalis, JP; et al. The Role of Vitamins and Minerals in Hair Loss: A Review. Dermatology and Therapy. 2019 Mar;9(1):51–70.

Alshahrani FM, Almalki MH, Aljohani N, Alzahrani A, Alsaleh Y, and Holick MF. Vitamin D: Light side and best time of sunshine in Riyadh, Saudi Arabia. Dermato-endocrinology. 2013;5(1):177–80.

American Academy of Dermatology. "African American hair: Dermatologists' tips for everyday care, processing and styling." News release issued Aug 24, 2014.

American Academy of Dermatology Association. (n.d.). Do You Have Hair Loss or Hair Shedding? Retrieved from https://www.aad.org/public/diseases/hair-loss/insider/shedding.

Arca E, Açıkgöz G, Yeniay Y, and Çalışkan E. Erkeklerde Androgenetik Alopesi Tedavisinde Topikal Saw Palmetto ve Trichogen Veg Kompleksinin Etkinlik ve Güvenirliğinin Değerlendirilmesi. Turkish Journal of Dermatology/Turk Dermatoloji Dergisis. 2014;8(4).

Asadi S. The Role of Mutations on Gene AR, in Androgenetic Alopecia Syndrome. Int J Mol Biol Open Access. 2020;5(2):46–49.

Avci, P; Gupta, GK; Clark, J; et al. (2014). Low-Level Laser (Light) Therapy (LLLT) for Treatment of Hair Loss. Lasers in Surgery and Medicine, 46(2), 144–151.

Avram, M; et al. The Current Role of Laser/Light Sources in the Treatment of Male and Female Pattern Hair Loss. Journal of Cosmetic and Laser Therapy (2007): 9(1): 27–28.

Bartsiokas A, and Arsuaga J-L. Hibernation in Hominins from Atapuerca, Spain Half a Million Years ago. L'Anthropologie. 2020;124(5):102797.

Binkley N, Novotny R, Krueger D, Kawahara T, Daida YG, Lensmeyer G, et al. Low Vitamin D Status Despite Abundant Sun Exposure. The Journal of Clinical Endocrinology & Metabolism. 2007;92(6):2130–5.

Bories M, Martini M, Et M, and Cotte J. Effects of Heat Treatment on Hair Structure. International Journal of Cosmetic Science. 1984;6(5):201–11.

Casey, A. (2021, Feb 9). Low-Level Light Therapy Shows Promise for Hair Regrowth After Chemotherapy. Oncology Nursing News. Available from: https://www.oncnursingnews.com/view/lowlevel-light-therapy-shows-promise-for-hair-regrowth-after-chemotherapy.

Clarke, C. (2022, Jan 5). Keto Hair Loss: 5 Common Causes & Tips to Prevent Hair Loss. Ruled Me. https://www.ruled.me/keto-hair-loss/.

Finner AM. Nutrition and Hair: Deficiencies and Supplements. Dermatologic Clinics. 2013;31(1):167–72.

Gade VKV, Mony A, Munisamy M, Chandrashekar L, and Rajappa M. An Investigation of Vitamin D Status in Alopecia Areata. Clinical and Experimental Medicine. 2018;18:577–84.

Ghanaat M. Types of Hair Loss and Treatment Options, Including the Novel Low-Level Light Therapy and its Proposed Mechanism. South Med J. 2010;103(9):917–21.

Grant W, Strange R, and Garland C. Sunshine is Good Medicine. The Health Benefits of Ultraviolet-B Induced Vitamin D Production. Journal of cosmetic dermatology. 2003;2(2):86–98.

Grover C, and Khurana A. Telogen Effluvium. Indian Journal of Dermatology, Venereology and Leprology. 2013;79:591.

Grymowicz M, Rudnicka E, Podfigurna A, Napierala P, Smolarczyk R, Smolarczyk K, et al. Hormonal Effects on Hair Follicles. International Journal of Molecular Sciences. 2020;21(15):5342.

Gupta, AK; Batra, R; Bluhm, R; et al. Skin Diseases Associated with Malassezia Species. J Am Acad Dermatol. 2004;51:785–98.

Hewings-Martin, Y, PhD. (2017, Aug 25). Why Does Chemotherapy Cause Hair Loss? Medical News Today. https://www.medicalnewstoday.com/articles/319146.

Higgins, CA; Westgate, GE; Jahoda, CA. From Telogen to Exogen: Mechanisms Underlying Formation and Subsequent Loss of the Hair Club Fiber. Journal of Investigative Dermatology. 2009 Sep 1;129(9):2100–8.

Hillmer AM, Flaquer A, Hanneken S, Eigelshoven S, Kortüm A-K, Brockschmidt FF, et al. Genome-Wide Scan and Fine-Mapping Linkage Study of Androgenetic Alopecia Reveals a Locus on Chromosome 3q26. The American Journal of Human Genetics.

Ho CH, Sood T, Zito PM. Androgenetic Alopecia. [Updated 2022 Oct 16]. In: StatPearls [Internet]. Treasure Island (FL): StatPearls Publishing; 2023 Jan-. Available from: https://www.ncbi.nlm.nih.gov/books/NBK430924/.

Hwang, K (n.d.). Anti-Androgens for Hair Loss: Everything You Need to Know. WebMD. https://www.webmd.com/connect-to-care/hair-loss/what-to-know-about-anti-androgens-for-hair-loss.

Kim, HS. Sunlight, Vitamin D Receptor Polymorphisms, and Colorectal Cancer. University of Washington; 2002.

Kivi, R. (2019, June 11). Male Pattern Baldness. Healthline. Available from: https://www.healthline.com/health/male-pattern-baldness.

Kunz M, Seifert B, and Trüeb RM. Seasonality of hair shedding in healthy women complaining of hair loss. Dermatology. 2009;219(2):105–10.

Lee, Y; Kim, YD; Hyun, HJ; et al. Hair Shaft Damage from Heat and Drying Time of Hair Dryer. Annals of Dermatology. 2011 Nov 1;23(4):455–62.

Mayo Clinic Staff. (2022b, Feb 26). Chemotherapy and Hair Loss: What to Expect during Treatment. Mayo Clinic. https://www.mayoclinic.org/tests-procedures/chemotherapy/in-depth/hair-loss/art-20046920.

McKenzie PL, and Castelo-Soccio L. Localized Hair Loss in Infancy: A Review. Current Opinion in Pediatrics. 2021;33(4):416–22.

Migala, J & Grieger, L. R. (2020, May 26). Why the Keto Diet Is Making Your Hair Fall Out (and How to Stop It). https://www.everydayhealth.com/ketogenic-diet/keto-diet-hair-loss-how-to-stop/.

Mirmirani P. Age-Related Hair Changes in Men: Mechanisms and Management of Alopecia and Graying. Maturitas. 2015;80(1):58–62.

Mutti DO, and Marks AR. Blood Levels of Vitamin D in Teens and Young Adults with Myopia. Optometry and Vision Science: Official Publication of the American Academy of Optometry. 2011;88(3):377.

Nina van, B; Enikő, B; Arno K et al. Thyroid Hormones Directly Alter Human Hair Follicle Functions: Anagen Prolongation and Stimulation of Both Hair Matrix Keratinocyte Proliferation and Hair Pigmentation, The Journal of Clinical Endocrinology & Metabolism, Volume 93, Issue 11, 1 November 2008, Pages 4381–4388, https://doi.org/10.1210/jc.2008-0283.

Osborn, C. O. (2018, September 18). Your Guide to Anti-Androgens. Healthline. https://www.healthline.com/health/anti-androgen#uses.

Park HK, Ha M-H, Park S-G, Kim MN, Kim BJ, et al. (2012) Characterization of the Fungal Microbiota (Mycobiome) in Healthy and Dandruff-Afflicted Human Scalps. PLoS ONE 7(2): e32847. doi:10.1371/journal.pone.0032847.

Pan C-W, Qian D-J, and Saw S-M. Time Outdoors, Blood Vitamin D Status and Myopia: A Review. Photochemical & Photobiological Sciences. 2017;16:426–32.

Phillips TG, Slomiany WP, and Allison R. Hair Loss: Common Causes and Treatment. American Family Physician. 2017;96(6):371–8.

Piérard-Franchimont C, Quatresooz P, and Piérard GE. Aging Hair. Springer; 2010:113–21.

Pillai JK, and Mysore V. Role of Low-Level Light Therapy (LLLT) in Androgenetic Alopecia. Journal of Cutaneous and Aesthetic Surgery. 2021;14(4):385.

Powell, K; Low, P; McDonnell, PA; et al. The Effect of Laser Irradiation on Proliferation of Human Breast Carcinoma, Melanoma, and Immortalized Mammary Epithelial Cells. Photomedicine and Laser Surgery. 2010 Feb 1;28(1):115–23.

RANDALL VA, and Ebling F. Seasonal Changes in Human Hair Growth. British Journal of Dermatology. 1991;124(2):146–51.

Roland, J. (2019, Oct 28). How to Prevent Hair Loss with a Ketogenic Diet. Healthline. https://www.healthline.com/health/hair-loss-ketosis.

Saini K, and Mysore V. Role of vitamin D in Hair Loss: A Short Review. Journal of Cosmetic Dermatology. 2021;20(11):3407–14.

Sanghvi AS. How to Regrow Lost Hair.

Shapiro, J & Kaufman, KD. Use of Finasteride in the Treatment of Men with Androgenetic Alopecia (Male Pattern Hair Loss). In Journal of Investigative Dermatology Symposium Proceedings 2003 Jun 1 (Vol. 8, No. 1, pp. 20–23). Elsevier.

Sharquie KE, and Jabbar RI. COVID-19 Infection Is a Major Cause of Acute Telogen Effluvium. Irish Journal of Medical Science (1971-). 2022;191(4):1677–81.

Slominski AT, Zmijewski MA, Plonka PM, Szaflarski JP, and Paus R. How UV Light Touches the Brain and Endocrine System through Skin, and Why. Endocrinology. 2018;159(5):1992–2007.

Strazzulla LC, Wang EHC, Avila L, Sicco KL, Brinster N, Christiano AM, et al. Alopecia Areata: Disease Characteristics, Clinical Evaluation, and New Perspectives on Pathogenesis. Journal of the American Academy of Dermatology. 2018;78(1):1–12.

Suchonwanit P, Chalermroj N, and Khunkhet S. Low-Level Laser Therapy for the Treatment of Androgenetic Alopecia in Thai Men and Women: A 24-Week, Randomized, Double-Blind, Sham Device-Controlled Trial. Lasers in Medical Science. 2019;34:1107–14.

Tobin D. Human Hair Pigmentation–Biological Aspects. International Journal of Cosmetic Science. 2008;30(4):233–57.

Tobin DJ. The Cell Biology of Human Hair Follicle Pigmentation. Pigment Cell & Melanoma Research. 2011;24(1):75–88.

Tortelly VD, Melo DF, Ghedin BS, Lima CdS, Garcia TU, and Barreto TdM. Pressure-Induced Alopecia: Presence of Thin Hairs as a Trichoscopic Clue for the Diagnosis. Skin Appendage Disorders. 2020;6(1):48–51.

Trüeb RM. Molecular Mechanisms of Androgenetic Alopecia. Experimental Gerontology. 2002;37(8-9):981–90.

Ustuner ET. Cause of Androgenic Alopecia: Crux of the Matter. Plastic and Reconstructive Surgery Global Open. 2013;1(7).

Vierhapper, H; Maier, H; Nowotny, P; et al. Production Rates of Testosterone and of Dihydrotestosterone in Female Pattern Hair Loss. Metabolism. 2003 Jul 1;52(7):927–9.

Vest BE, Krauland K. Malassezia Furfur. [Updated 2023 May 22]. In: StatPearls [Internet]. Treasure Island (FL): StatPearls Publishing; 2023 Jan-. Available from: https://www.ncbi.nlm.nih.gov/books/NBK553091/.

Watson, S. (2010, Jan 7). Hair Problems. WebMD. https://www.webmd.com/skin-problems-and-treatments/hair-loss/hair-problems.

Watson, K (2018, Jun 20). Routine Hair Shedding: Why It Happens and How Much to Expect. Healthline. https://www.healthline.com/health/how-much-hair-loss-is-normal.

Watson, S (2010, Jan 7). Hair Problems. WebMD. https://www.webmd.com/skin-problems-and-treatments/hair-loss/hair-problems.

Webb A, DeCosta B, and Holick M. Sunlight Regulates the Cutaneous Production of Vitamin D3 by Causing its Photodegradation. The Journal of Clinical Endocrinology & Metabolism. 1989;68(5):882–7.

WebMD Connect to Care Staff. (2020, Nov 18). Does Biotin Really Work for Hair Loss Prevention? WebMD. https://www.webmd.com/connect-to-care/hair-loss/does-biotin-really-prevent-hair-loss.

Wikipedia Contributors (2022, Mar 27). Antiandrogen. Wikipedia. https://en.wikipedia.org/wiki/Antiandrogen.

Wikipedia contributors. (2022, Mar 30). Hair Loss. Wikipedia. https://en.wikipedia.org/wiki/Hair_loss.

Yip L, Rufaut N, and Sinclair R. Role of Genetics and Sex Steroid Hormones in Male Androgenetic Alopecia and Female Pattern Hair Loss: An Update of What We Now Know. Australasian Journal of Dermatology. 2011;52(2):81–8.

Young AR, Harrison GI, Chadwick CA, Nikaido O, Ramsden J, and Potten CS. The Similarity of Action Spectra for Thymine Dimers in Human Epidermis and Erythema Suggests that DNA is the Chromophore for Erythema. Journal of Investigative Dermatology. 1998;111(6):982–8.

Chapter 4: Fungus and the Five Whys

Alexander, S. 1968. Loss of Hair and Dandruff. Br. J. Dermatol. 79:549–552.

Bories M, Martini M, Et M, and Cotte J. Effects of Heat Treatment on Hair Structure. International Journal of Cosmetic Science. 1984;6(5):201–11.

Nematian J, Ravaghi M, Gholamrezanezhad A, Nematian E. Increased Hair Shedding May Be Associated with the Presence of Pityrosporum ovale. Am J Clin Dermatol. 2006;7(4):263-6.

Nett CS, Reichler I, Grest P, Hauser B, Reusch CE. Epidermal dysplasia and Malassezia infection in two West Highland White Terrier siblings: an inherited skin disorder or reaction to severe Malassezia infection? Vet Dermatol. 2001 Oct;12(5):285-90.

Machado ML, Ferreiro L, Ferreira RR, Corbellini LG, Deville M, Berthelemy M, Guillot J. Malassezia Dermatitis in Dogs in Brazil: Diagnosis, Evaluation of Clinical Signs and Molecular Identification. Vet Dermatol. 2011; 22(1):46-52. doi: 10.1111/j.1365-3164.2010.00909.x.

Phillips TG, Slomiany WP, and Allison R. Hair Loss: Common Causes and Treatment. American Family Physician. 2017;96(6):371–8.

Tampieri MP. Update on the Diagnosis of Dermatomycosis. Parassitologia. 2004 Jun;46(1-2):183–6.

Tchernev G. Folliculitis Et Perifolliculitis Capitis Abscedens Et Suffodiens Controlled With a Combination Therapy: Systemic Antibiosis (Metronidazole Plus Clindamycin), Dermatosurgical Approach, and High-Dose Isotretinoin. Indian J Dermatol. 2011; 56(3):318-20. doi: 10.4103/0019-5154.82492.

Trüeb RM. Molecular Mechanisms of Androgenetic Alopecia. Experimental Gerontology. 2002;37(8-9):981–90.

Van Neste M. Assessment of Hair Loss: Clinical Relevance of Hair Growth Evaluation Methods. Clinical and Experimental Dermatology. 2002;27(5):358–65.

Chapter 5: How Much Hair Have I Lost?

Ashique K, and Kaliyadan F. Clinical Photography for Trichology Practice: Tips and Tricks. International Journal of Trichology. 2011;3(1):7.

Blume-Peytavi, U; Hillmann, K; Guarrera, M. Hair Growth Assessment Techniques. In Hair Growth and Disorders 2008 (pp. 125–157). Springer, Berlin, Heidelberg.

Dhurat R, and Saraogi P. Hair Evaluation Methods: Merits and Demerits. International Journal of Trichology. 2009;1(2):108.

Draelos ZD. Sunscreens and Hair Photoprotection. Dermatologic Clinics. 2006;24(1):81–4.

Editorial Team. (20 September 2021). Scalp Biopsy: Does it Help Diagnose Hair Loss? Hims. https://www.forhims.com/blog/scalp-biopsy.

Grover C, and Khurana A. Telogen Effluvium. Indian Journal of Dermatology, Venereology and Leprology. 2013;79:591.

Gupta, M; Mysore, V. Classifications of Patterned Hair Loss: A Review. J Cutan Aesthet Surg. 2016 Jan-Mar;9(1):3–12. doi: 10.4103/0974-2077.178536. PMID: 27081243; PMCID: PMC4812885.

Harrison S, and Sinclair R. Telogen Effluvium. Clinical and Experimental Dermatology. 2002;27(5):389–95.

Jackson, AJ; Price, VH. How to Diagnose Hair Loss. Dermatol Clin. 2013 Jan;31(1):21–8. doi: 10.1016/j.det.2012.08.007. Epub 2012 Sep 29. PMID: 23159173.

Lee, SH; & Yang, CS. An Intelligent Hair and Scalp Analysis System Using Camera Sensors and Norwood-Hamilton Model. Int. J. Innov. Comput. Inf. Control. 2018 Apr 1;14(2):503–18.

Miami Hair Institute. (2018, January 10). Hair Evaluation Methods: The Hair Pull Test. https://www.miamihair.com/blog/hair-loss-treatment-2/hair-evaluation-methods-hair-pull-test/.

NYU Langone Health Staff. Diagnosing Hair Loss. NYU Langone Health. https://nyulangone.org/conditions/hair-loss/diagnosis.

TRUTEST Laboratories (n.d.). What Are the Tests to Be Done to Diagnose Hair Loss. https://www.trutestlab.com/blog/what-are-the-tests-to-be-done-to-diagnose-hair-loss.

Van Neste M. Assessment of Hair Loss: Clinical Relevance of Hair Growth Evaluation Methods. Clinical and Experimental Dermatology. 2002;27(5):358–65.

Warner, J (2008, Jun 16). Quick Test May Help Spot Male Hair Loss. WebMD. https://www.cbsnews.com/news/quick-test-may-help-spot-male-hair-loss-16-06-2008/.

Chapter 6: Hiding Hair Loss

Haskin, A; Aguh, C. Ethnic Hairstyling Practices and Hair Prostheses II: Wigs, Weaves, and Other Extensions. In Fundamentals of Ethnic hair 2017 (pp. 53–66). Springer, Cham.

Roberts JL. Androgenetic Alopecia: Treatment Results with Topical Minoxidil. Journal of the American Academy of Dermatology. 1987;16(3):705–10.

Saed, S; Ibrahim, O; Bergfeld, WF. Hair Camouflage: A Comprehensive Review. International Journal of Women's Dermatology. 2016 Dec 1;2(4):122–7.

Sakamoto, K; Lochhead, R; Maibach, H; et al. Cosmetic Science and Technology: Theoretical Principles and Applications. Elsevier; 2017 Apr 6.

Setty, LR. Hair Patterns of The Scalp of White and Negro Males. American Journal of Physical Anthropology. 1970 Jul;33(1):49–55.

Tobin D. Human Hair Pigmentation–Biological Aspects. International Journal of Cosmetic Science. 2008;30(4):233–57.

Chapter 7: Over the Counter Hair Treatments

Anzai A, Pereira AF, Malaquias KR, Guerra LO, and Mercuri M. Efficacy and Safety of a New Formulation Kit (Shampoo+ Lotion) Containing Anti-Inflammatory and Antioxidant Agents to Treat Hair Loss. Dermatologic Therapy. 2020;33(3):e13293.

Banihashemi, M; Nahidi, Y; Meibodi, NT; et al. Serum Vitamin D3 Level in Patients with Female Pattern Hair Loss. International Journal of Trichology. 2016 Jul;8(3):116.

Bater, K & Rieder, E. Over-the-Counter Hair Loss Treatments: Help or Hype? Journal of Drugs in Dermatology: JDD. 2018 Dec 1;17(12):1317–21.

Berthiaume, MD; Merrifield, JH; Riccio, DA. Effects of Silicone Pretreatment on Oxidative Hair Damage. Journal of the Society of Cosmetic Chemists. 1995 Sep 1;46(5):231–46.

Biotin: Fact Sheet for Health Professionals. (2021). https://ods.od.nih.gov/factsheets/Biotin-HealthProfessional/.

Butawan, M; Benjamin, RL; Bloomer, RJ. Methylsulfonylmethane: Applications and Safety of a Novel Dietary Supplement. Nutrients. 2017 Mar;9(3):290.

Cornwell PA. A Review of Shampoo Surfactant Technology: Consumer Benefits, Raw Materials and Recent Developments. International Journal of Cosmetic Science. 2018 Feb;40(1):16–30.

Davidson, K. M. (2020, Apr 20). Can Biotin Help Men Grow Hair? Healthline. https://www.healthline.com/nutrition/biotin-for-men#precautions.

D'Souza, P & Rathi, SK. Shampoo and Conditioners: What a Dermatologist Should Know? Indian Journal of Dermatology. 2015 May;60(3):248.

Elder R. Final Report on the Safety Assessment of Sodium Lauryl Sulfate and Ammonium Lauryl Sulfate. Journal of the American College of Toxicology. 1983;2(7):127–81.

Gade VKV, Mony A, Munisamy M, Chandrashekar L, and Rajappa M. An Investigation of Vitamin D Status in Alopecia Areata. Clinical and Experimental Medicine. 2018;18:577-84.

Gerkowicz A, Chyl-Surdacka K, Krasowska D, and Chodorowska G. The Role of Vitamin D in Non-Scarring Alopecia. International Journal of Molecular Sciences. 2017;18(12):2653.

Goren, A; Sharma, A; Dhurat, R; et al. Low-Dose Daily Aspirin Reduces Topical minoxidil Efficacy in Androgenetic Alopecia Patients. Dermatologic Therapy. 2018 Nov;31(6):e12741.

Gotter, A. (2019, Mar 8). What Is Ketoconazole Shampoo? Healthline. https://www.healthline.com/health/ketoconazole-shampoos#risks.

Grover C, and Khurana A. Telogen Effluvium. Indian Journal of Dermatology, Venereology and Leprology. 2013;79:591.

Guo, EL & Katta, R. Diet and Hair Loss: Effects of Nutrient Deficiency and Supplement Use. Dermatology Practical & Conceptual. 2017 Jan;7(1):1.

Hon, KL; et al. Alopecia Areata. Recent Patents on Inflammation & Allergy Drug Discovery (2011): 5(2): 98–107.

Inui S, and Itami S. Reversal of Androgenetic Alopecia by Topical Ketoconzole: Relevance of Anti-Androgenic Activity. Journal of Dermatological Science. 2007;45(1):66–8.

Kim J, Kim SR, Choi Y-H, Shin Jy, Kim CD, Kang N-G, et al. Quercitrin Stimulates Hair Growth with Enhanced Expression of Growth Factors via Activation of MAPK/CREB Signaling Pathway. Molecules. 2020;25(17):4004.

Labrozzi, A. Nutrients in Hair Supplements: Evaluation of Their Function in Hair Loss Treatment. Hair Ther Transplant. 2020;10(1):1–6.

MacGill, M. (2017, July 28). Male Pattern Baldness: What You Need to Know. Medical News Today. https://www.medicalnewstoday.com/articles/68077.

McElwee KJ, and Shapiro J. Promising Therapies for Treating and/or Preventing Androgenic Alopecia. Skin Therapy Letter. 2012;17(6):1–4.

Messenger, AG; Rundegren, J; Minoxidil: Mechanisms of Action on Hair Growth. Br J Dermatol. 2004 Feb;150(2):186–94. doi: 10.1111/j.1365-2133.2004.05785.x. PMID: 14996087.

Nair, R; & Maseeh, A. Vitamin D: The "Sunshine" Vitamin. Journal of Pharmacology & Pharmacotherapeutics. 2012 Apr;3(2):118.

NULASTIN INC. (2021, June 7). Biotin: Extremely Beneficial or Completely Useless? Here's Your Answer. https://nulastin.com/blogs/news/biotin-extremely-beneficial-or-completely-useless-here-s-your-answer.

Panchaprateep. Suparuj Lueangarun et. col. Efficacy and Safety of Oral Minoxidil 5mg Once Daily in the Treatment of Male Patients with Androgenetic Alopecia: An Open-Label and Global Photographic Assessment. Dermatol Ther (Heidelb) (2020) 10:1345–1357 https://doi.org/10.1007/s13555-020-00448-x Received: August 12, 2020 / Published online: September 24, 2020.

Panico, A; Serio, F; Bagordo, F; et al. Skin Safety and Health Prevention: An Overview of Chemicals in Cosmetic Products. Journal of Preventive Medicine and Hygiene. 2019 Mar;60(1):E50.

Park, SY; Na, SY; Kim, JH; et al. Iron Plays a Certain Role in Patterned Hair Loss. Journal of Korean Medical Science. 2013 Jun 1;28(6):934–8.

Patel DP, Swink SM, and Castelo-Soccio L. A Review of the Use of Biotin for Hair Loss. Skin Appendage Disorders. 2017;3(3):166-9.

Patel, S; Sharma, V; Chauhan, N; et al. (2015). Hair Growth: Focus on Herbal Therapeutic Agent. Current Drug Discovery Technologies. 12. 10.2174/1570163812666150610115055.

Piérard-Franchimont, C; Goffin, V; Henry, F; et al. Nudging Hair Shedding by Antidandruff Shampoos. A Comparison Of 1% Ketoconazole, 1% Piroctone Olamine And 1% Zinc Pyrithione Formulations. International Journal of Cosmetic Science. 2002 Oct;24(5):249–56. doi: 10.1046/j.1467-2494.2002.00145.x. PMID: 18498517. https://pubmed.ncbi.nlm.nih.gov/18498517/.

Praderio, C. (August 24, 2017). Those "Hair and Nail" Vitamins Aren't Doing Anything for Your Hair and Nails. Insider. https://www.insider.com/does-biotin-work-hair-nails-2017-8.

Price VH. Treatment of hair loss. New England Journal of Medicine. 1999;341(13):964–73.

Pumthong G, Asawananonda P, Varothai S, Jariyasethavong V, Triwongwaranat D, Suthipinittharm P, et al. Curcuma Aeruginosa, a Novel Botanically Derived 5α-Reductase Inhibitor in the Treatment of Male-Pattern

Baldness: A Multicenter, Randomized, Double-Blind, Placebo-Controlled Study. Journal of Dermatological Treatment. 2012;23(5):385–92.

Rajput, R. A Scientific Hypothesis on the Role of Nutritional Supplements for Effective Management of Hair Loss and Promoting Hair Regrowth. Journal of Nurtrion Health and Food Science. 2018;6(3):1.

Rasheed H, Mahgoub D, Hegazy R, El-Komy M, Abdel Hay R, Hamid M, et al. Serum Ferritin and Vitamin D in Female Hair Loss: Do They Play a Role? Skin Pharmacology and Physiology. 2013;26(2):101–7.

Saini K, and Mysore V. Role of Vitamin D in Hair Loss: A Short Review. Journal of Cosmetic Dermatology. 2021;20(11):3407–14.

Sanfilippo, A. & English III, Joseph. (2006). An Overview of Medicated Shampoos Used in Dandruff Treatment. P and T. 31. 396–400.

Schweikert HU, and Wilson JD. Regulation of Human Hair Growth by Steroid Hormones. I. Testosterone Metabolism in Isolated Hairs. The Journal of Clinical Endocrinology & Metabolism. 1974;38(5):811–9.

Shanmugam, S; Baskaran, R; Nagayya-Sriraman, S; et al. The Effect of Methylsulfonylmethane on Hair Growth Promotion of Magnesium Ascorbyl Phosphate for the Treatment of Alopecia. Biomolecules & Therapeutics. 2009 Jul 31;17(3):241–8.

Srivilai, J; Phimnuan, P; Jaisabai, J; et al. Curcuma Aeruginosa Roxb. Essential Oil Slows Hair-Growth and Lightens Skin in Axillae; A Randomised, Double Blinded Trial. Phytomedicine. 2017 Feb 15;25:29–38.

Theradome. Frequently Asked Questions. Theradome. Available from: https://theradome.com/frequently-asked-questions.

Trost, LB; Bergfeld, WF; Calogeras, E. The Diagnosis and Treatment of Iron Deficiency and Its Potential Relationship to Hair Loss. Journal of the American Academy of Dermatology. 2006 May 1;54(5):824–44.

Wikramanayake, TC; Villasante, AC; Mauro, LM; et al. Prevention and Treatment of Alopecia Areata with Quercetin in the C3H/Hej Mouse Model. Cell Stress and Chaperones. 2012 Mar;17(2):267–74.

Chapter 8: FDA-Cleared Medications

Adil A, and Godwin M. The Effectiveness of Treatments for Androgenetic Alopecia: A Systematic Review and Meta-Analysis. Journal of the American Academy of Dermatology. 2017;77(1):136-41. e5.

Azadgoli, B; Baker, RY. Laser Applications in Surgery. Annals of Translational Medicine. 2016 Dec;4(23).

Chan L, and Cook DK. Female Pattern Hair Loss. Australian Journal of General Practice. 2018;47(7):459–64.

Faghihi G, Mozafarpoor S, Asilian A, Mokhtari F, Esfahani AA, Bafandeh B, et al. The Effectiveness of Adding Low-Level Light Therapy to Minoxidil 5% Solution in the Treatment of Patients with Androgenetic Alopecia. Indian Journal of Dermatology, Venereology and Leprology. 2018;84:547.

Feldman PR, Gentile P, Piwko C, Motswaledi HM, Gorun S, Pesachov J, et al. Hair Regrowth Treatment Efficacy and Resistance in Androgenetic Alopecia: A Systematic Review and Continuous Bayesian Network Meta-Analysis. Frontiers In Medicine. 2023;9:3800.

German, M & Ortega, A. 6 Most Effective Alternatives to Finasteride Oct 14, 2021.

Hoffmann R. TrichoScan: Combining Epiluminescence Microscopy with Digital Image Analysis for the Measurement of Hair Growth in Vivo. European Journal of Dermatology. 2001;11(4):362–8.

Kaufman KD, Olsen EA, Whiting D, Savin R, DeVillez R, Bergfeld W, et al. Finasteride in the Treatment of Men with Androgenetic Alopecia. Journal of the American Academy of Dermatology. 1998;39(4):578–89.

Libecco JF, and Bergfeld WF. Finasteride in the Treatment of Alopecia. Expert Opinion on Pharmacotherapy. 2004;5(4):933–40.

McClellan KJ, and Markham A. Finasteride: A Review of Its Use in Male Pattern Hair Loss. Drugs. 1999;57:111–26.

Olsen EA, Messenger AG, Shapiro J, Bergfeld WF, Hordinsky MK, Roberts JL, et al. Evaluation and Treatment of Male and Female Pattern Hair Loss. Journal of the American Academy of Dermatology. 2005;52(2):301–11.

Otomo, S. Hair growth effect of Minoxidil. Nihon Yakurigaku Zasshi. Folia Pharmacologica Japonica. 2002 Mar 1;119(3):167–74.

Panchaprateep. Suparuj Lueangarun et. col. Efficacy and Safety of Oral Minoxidil 5mg Once Daily in the Treatment of Male Patients with Androgenetic Alopecia: An Open-Label and Global Photographic Assessment. Dermatol Ther (Heidelb) (2020) 10:1345–1357 https://doi.org/10.1007/s13555-020-00448-x Received: August 12, 2020 / Published online: September 24, 2020.

Rasheed H, Mahgoub D, Hegazy R, El-Komy M, Abdel Hay R, Hamid M, et al. Serum Ferritin and Vitamin D in Female Hair Loss: Do They Play a Role? Skin Pharmacology and Physiology. 2013;26(2):101–7.

Rossi, A; Cantisani, C; Melis, L; et al. Minoxidil Use in Dermatology, Side Effects and Recent Patents. Recent Pat Inflamm Allergy Drug Discov. 2012 May;6(2):130–6. doi: 10.2174/187221312800166859. PMID: 22409453.

Rundegren J. A One-Year Observational Study with Minoxidil 5% Solution in Germany: Results of Independent Efficacy Evaluation by Physicians and Patients 1. Journal of the American Academy of Dermatology. 2004;50(3):P91.

Rushton D, Norris M, Dover R, and Busuttil N. Causes of Hair Loss and the Developments in Hair Rejuvenation. International Journal of Cosmetic Science. 2002;24(1):17–23.

Suchonwanit P, Rojhirunsakool S, and Khunkhet S. A Randomized, Investigator-Blinded, Controlled, Split-Scalp Study of the Efficacy and Safety of a 1550-Nm Fractional Erbium-Glass Laser, Used in Combination with Topical 5% Minoxidil Versus 5% Minoxidil Alone, for the Treatment of Androgenetic Alopecia. Lasers in Medical Science. 2019;34:1857–64.

Suchonwanit P, Thammarucha S, and Leerunyakul K. Minoxidil and Its Use in Hair Disorders: A Review [Corrigendum]. Drug Design, Development and Therapy. 2020;14:575–6.

Tanaka Y, Aso T, Ono J, Hosoi R, and Kaneko T. Androgenetic Alopecia Treatment in Asian Men. The Journal of Clinical and Aesthetic Dermatology. 2018;11(7):32.

Theradome. Frequently Asked Questions. Theradome. Available from: https://theradome.com/frequently-asked-questions.

Vanderveen, EE; Ellis, CN; Kang, S; et al. Topical Minoxidil for Hair Regrowth. Journal of the American Academy of Dermatology. 1984 Sep 1;11(3):416–21.

Van Neste, D; Fuh, V; Sanchez-Pedreno, P; et al. Finasteride Increases Anagen Hair in Men with Androgenetic Alopecia. British Journal of Dermatology. 2000 Oct;143(4):804–10. doi: 10.1046/j.1365-2133.2000.03780.x. PMID: 11069460.

Zito PM, Bistas KG, Syed K. Finasteride. [Updated 2022 Aug 25]. In: StatPearls [Internet]. Treasure Island (FL): StatPearls Publishing; 2023 Jan-. Available from: https://www.ncbi.nlm.nih.gov/books/NBK513329/.

Chapter 9: Off-Label Treatments

Almohanna, HM; Ahmed, AA; Tsatalis, JP; et al. The Role of Vitamins and Minerals in Hair Loss: A Review. Dermatology and Therapy. 2019 Mar;9(1):51–70.

Ayatollahi A, Hosseini H, Gholami J, Mirminachi B, Firooz F, and Firooz A. Platelet Rich Plasma for Treatment of Non-Scarring Hair Loss: Systematic Review of Literature. Journal of Dermatological Treatment. 2017;28(7):574–81.

Chaffer CL, Brueckmann I, Scheel C, Kaestli AJ, Wiggins PA, Rodrigues LO, et al. Normal and Neoplastic Nonstem Cells Can Spontaneously Convert to a Stem-Like State. Proceedings of the National Academy of Sciences. 2011;108(19):7950–5.

Elghblawi, E. Platelet-Rich Plasma, the Ultimate Secret for Youthful Skin Elixir and Hair Growth Triggering. Journal of Cosmetic Dermatology. 2018 Jun;17(3):423–30.

Gentile P, Dionisi L, Pizzicannella J, de Angelis B, de Fazio D, and Garcovich S. A Randomized Blinded Retrospective Study: The Combined Use of Micro-Needling Technique, Low-Level Laser Therapy and Autologous Non-Activated Platelet-Rich Plasma Improves Hair Re-Growth in Patients with Androgenic Alopecia. Expert Opinion on Biological Therapy. 2020;20(9):1099–109.

Gentile P, Garcovich S, Bielli A, Scioli MG, Orlandi A, and Cervelli V. The Effect of Platelet-Rich Plasma in Hair Regrowth: A Randomized Placebo-Controlled Trial. Stem Cells Translational Medicine. 2015;4(11):1317–23.

John Hopkins Medicine. Platelet-Rich Plasma (PRP) Injections). Retrieved from https://www.hopkinsmedicine.org.

Justicz, N; Chen, JX; Lee, LN. Platelet-Rich Plasma for Hair Restoration. Hair Transplant Surgery and Platelet Rich Plasma. 2020:113–21.

Katzer T, Leite Junior A, Beck R, and da Silva C. Physiopathology and Current Treatments of Androgenetic Alopecia: Going Beyond Androgens and Anti-Androgens. Dermatologic Therapy. 2019;32(5):e13059.

Kubicka, B. (2015, Jul 7). The Mesotherapy Story. Medical Use. Clinicbe. Available from: https://www.clinicbe.com/the-mesotherapy-story/.

Li, ZJ; Choi, HI; Choi, DK; et al. Autologous Platelet-Rich Plasma: A Potential Therapeutic Tool for Promoting Hair Growth. Dermatologic Surgery. 2012 Jul;38(7pt1):1040–6.

Mysore V. (2010). Mesotherapy in Management of Hairloss – Is it of Any Use? International Journal of Trichology, 2(1), 45–46. https://doi.org/10.4103/0974-7753.66914.

Sakamoto, K; Lochhead, R; Maibach, H; et al. Cosmetic Science and Technology: Theoretical Principles and Applications. Elsevier; 2017 Apr 6.

Stanczak, M. Is Platelet Rich Plasma Injection an Effective Treatment for Hair Loss in Androgenetic Alopecia and Alopecia Areata? (2017). PCOM Physician Assistant Studies Student Scholarship. 415. https://digitalcommons.pcom.edu/pa_systematic_reviews/415.

TrichoCentre Staff. (2021, Sep 1). Platelet-Rich Plasma (PRP) and Laser Phototherapy (LPT) - Blog. TrichoCentre. https://www.trichocentre.com/an-integrative-therapy-for-the-successful-treatment-of-hair-loss/.

Watson, S. (2018, Aug 22). What Is Mesotherapy? Healthline. https://www.healthline.com/health/mesotherapy#hair-loss.

Chapter 10: Debunked Treatment Choices

Patel, S; Sharma, V; Chauhan, N; et al. (2015). Hair Growth: Focus on Herbal Therapeutic Agent. Current Drug Discovery Technologies. 12. 10.2174/1570163812666150610115055.

Population Inversion. Physics and Radio Electronics. Available from: https://www.physics-and-radio-electronics.com/physics/laser/laser-populationinversion.html.

Sebetić, K; Sjerobabski Masnec, I; Cavka, V; et al. UV Damage of The Hair. Collegium Antropologicum. 2008 Oct;32 Suppl 2:163–5. PMID: 19138021.

Chapter 11: And the Undisputed Champion Is . . .

Sinclair R, Patel M, Dawson Jr T, Yazdabadi A, Yip L, Perez A, et al. Hair Loss in Women: Medical and Cosmetic Approaches to Increase Scalp Hair Fullness. British Journal of Dermatology. 2011;165(s3):12–8.

Chapter 12: Laser Phototherapy and Laser Phototherapy Devices

Afifi L, Maranda EL, Zarei M, Delcanto GM, Falto-Aizpurua L, Kluijfhout WP, et al. Low-Level Laser Therapy as a Treatment for Androgenetic Alopecia. Lasers in Surgery and Medicine. 2017;49(1):27–39.

Akhondzadeh S. The Importance of Clinical Trials in Drug Development. Avicenna J Med Biotechnol. 2016 Oct-Dec;8(4):151. PMID: 27920881; PMCID: PMC5124250.

Albini A. Some Remarks on the First Law of Photochemistry. Photochemical & Photobiological Sciences. 2016;15:319–24.

AlGhamdi MAI. Comparative Effectiveness Research in Photodynamic Therapy for Oral Lichen Planus. University of California, Los Angeles; 2016.

Algorri JF, Ochoa M, Roldán-Varona P, Rodríguez-Cobo L, and López-Higuera JM. Light Technology for Efficient and Effective Photodynamic Therapy: A Critical Review. Cancers. 2021;13(14):3484.

Ash C, Dubec M, Donne K, and Bashford T. Effect of Wavelength and Beam Width on Penetration in Light-Tissue Interaction Using Computational Methods. Lasers in Medical Science. 2017;32:1909–18.

Avci P, Gupta GK, Clark J, Wikonkal N, and Hamblin MR. Low-Level Laser (Light) Therapy (LLLT) for Treatment of Hair Loss. Lasers in Surgery and Medicine. 2014;46(2):144–51.

Avram MR, and Rogers NE. The Use of Low-Level Light for Hair Growth: Part I. Journal of Cosmetic and Laser Therapy. 2009;11(2):110–7.

Choi MS, and Park BC. The Efficacy and Safety of the Combination of Photobiomodulation Therapy and Pulsed Electromagnetic Field Therapy on Androgenetic Alopecia. Journal of Cosmetic Dermatology. 2023;22(3):831–6.

Chung, PS; Kim, JW; Lee, JO; et al. The Effect of Low-Power Laser on the Murine Hair Growth. Archives of Plastic Surgery. 2005;32(2):149–54.

Chung PS, Kim YC, Chung MS, Jung SO, and Ree C. The effect of low-power laser on the murine hair growth. Journal of the Korean Society of Plastic and Reconstructive Surgeons. 2004;31:1–8.

De Jode M, Mcgilligan J, Dilkes M, Cameron I, Hart P, and Grahn M. A Comparison of Novel Light Sources for Photodynamic Therapy. Lasers in Medical Science. 1997;12:260–8.

Delaney SW, and Zhang P. Systematic Review of Low-Level Laser Therapy for Adult Androgenic Alopecia. Journal of Cosmetic and Laser Therapy. 2018;20(4):229–36.

Enwemeka CS. Standard Parameters in Laser Phototherapy. Photomedicine and Laser Surgery. 2008;26(5):411–2.

Federal Court Rules That 510(k) Clearance Relates to Safety and Effectiveness | Drug & Device Law. Available from: https://www.druganddevicelawblog.com/2018/06/california-district-court-rules-that-510k-clearance-relates-to-safety-and-effectiveness.html.

Fixler D, Duadi H, Ankri R, and Zalevsky Z. Determination of Coherence Length in Biological Tissues. Lasers in Surgery and Medicine. 2011;43(4):339–43.

Fushimi T, Inui S, Ogasawara M, Nakajima T, Hosokawa K, and Itami S. Narrow-Band Red LED Light Promotes Mouse Hair Growth through Paracrine Growth Factors from Dermal Papilla. Journal of Dermatological Science. 2011;64(3):246–8.

Guo Y, Qu Q, Chen J, Miao Y, and Hu Z. Proposed Mechanisms of Low-Level Light Therapy in the Treatment of Androgenetic Alopecia. Lasers in Medical Science. 2021;36:703–13.

Gupta AK, and Foley KA. A Critical Assessment of the Evidence for Low-Level Laser Therapy in the Treatment of Hair Loss. Dermatologic Surgery. 2017;43(2):188–97.

Greguss, P. Biostimulation of Tissue by Laser Radiation. Proc. SPIE 1353, First International Conference on Lasers and Medicine (1990): 79.

Han, L; Liu, B; Chen, X; et al. Activation of Wnt/β-catenin Signaling Is Involved in Hair Growth-Promoting Effect of 655-Nm Red Light and LED in in Vitro Culture Model. Lasers in Medical Science. 2018 Apr;33(3):637–45.

Jimenez JJ, Wikramanayake TC, Bergfeld W, Hordinsky M, Hickman JG, Hamblin MR, et al. Efficacy and Safety of a Low-Level Laser Device in the Treatment of Male and Female Pattern Hair Loss: A Multicenter, Randomized, Sham Device-Controlled, Double-Blind Study. American Journal of Clinical Dermatology. 2014;15:115–27.

Kim, TH; Kim, NJ; Youn, JI. Evaluation of Wavelength-Dependent Hair Growth Effects on Low-Level Laser Therapy: An Experimental Animal Study. Lasers in Medical Science. 2015 Aug;30(6):1703–9.

Kim H, Choi JW, Kim JY, Shin JW, Lee Sj, and Huh CH. Low-Level Light Therapy for Androgenetic Alopecia: A 24-Week, Randomized, Double-Blind, Sham Device–Controlled Multicenter Trial. Dermatologic Surgery. 2013;39(8):1177–83.

Laakso EL, Cramond T, Richardson C, and Galligan JP. Plasma ACTH and β-endorphin Levels in Response to Low Level Laser Therapy (LLLT) for Myofascial Trigger Points. Laser Therapy. 1994;6(3):133–41.

Leal ECP, Lopes-Martins RÁB, Frigo L, De Marchi T, Rossi RP, De Godoi V, et al. Effects of Low-Level Laser Therapy (LLLT) in the Development of Exercise-Induced Skeletal Muscle Fatigue and Changes in Biochemical Markers Related to Postexercise Recovery. Journal of Orthopaedic & Sports Physical Therapy. 2010;40(8):524–32.

Leal Junior ECP, Lopes-Martins RÁB, Baroni BM, De Marchi T, Taufer D, Manfro DS, et al. Effect of 830 nm Low-Level Laser Therapy Applied Before High-Intensity Exercises on Skeletal Muscle Recovery in Athletes. Lasers in Medical Science. 2009;24:857–63.

Leavitt M, Charles G, Heyman E, and Michaels D. HairMax LaserComb® Laser Phototherapy Device in the Treatment of Male Androgenetic Alopecia: A Randomized, Double-Blind, Sham Device-Controlled, Multicentre Trial. Clinical Drug Investigation. 2009;29:283–92.

Martínez-Pizarro S. Low-Level Laser Therapy for Androgenetic Alopecia. Actas Dermo-Sifiliograficas. 2020;112(2):99–102.

Munck A, Gavazzoni MF, and Trüeb RM. Use of Low-Level Laser Therapy as Monotherapy or Concomitant Therapy for Male and Female Androgenetic Alopecia. International Journal of Trichology. 2014;6(2):45.

Nichols, E. Understanding FDA Cleared vs Approved vs Granted for Medical Devices. Greenlight Guru. Available from: https://www.greenlight.guru/blog/fda-clearance-approval-granted.

Photochemistry. Chaudhary Charan Singh University. Available from: https://ccsuniversity.ac.in/bridge-library/pdf/Bsc-IV-sem-physical-chem-Unit-IV.pdf.

Photochemistry. Michigan State University. Available from: https://www2.chemistry.msu.edu/faculty/reusch/virttxtjml/photchem.htm.

Qadri T, Bohdanecka P, Tunér J, Miranda L, Altamash M, and Gustafsson A. The Importance of Coherence Length in Laser Phototherapy of Gingival Inflammation—A Pilot Study. Lasers in Medical Science. 2007;22:245–51.

Qiu J, Yi Y, Jiang L, Miao Y, Jia J, Zou J, et al. Efficacy Assessment for Low-Level Laser Therapy in the Treatment of Androgenetic Alopecia: A Real-World Study on 1383 Patients. Lasers in Medical Science. 2022;37(6):2589–94.

Rushton D, Gilkes J, and Van Neste D. No Improvement in Male-Pattern Hair Loss Using Laser Hair-Comb Therapy: A 6-Month, Half-Head, Assessor-Blinded Investigation in Two Men. Clinical And Experimental Dermatology. 2012;37(3):313–5.

Satino JL, and Markou M. Hair Regrowth and Increased Hair Tensile Strength Using the Hairmax Lasercomb For Low-Level Laser Therapy. International Journal of Cosmetic Surgery and Aesthetic Dermatology. 2003;5(2):113–7.

Scarpim AC, Baptista A, Magalhães DSF, Nunez SC, Navarro RS, and Frade-Barros AF. Photobiomodulation Effectiveness in Treating Andro-genetic Alopecia. Photobiomodulation, Photomedicine, and Laser Surgery. 2022;40(6):387–94.

Sinclair R, Patel M, Dawson Jr T, Yazdabadi A, Yip L, Perez A, et al. Hair Loss in Women: Medical and Cosmetic Approaches to Increase Scalp Hair Fullness. British Journal of Dermatology. 2011;165(s3):12–8.

Vijayananthan A, and Nawawi O. The Importance of Good Clinical Prac-tice Guidelines and Its Role in Clinical Trials. Biomedical Imaging and Intervention Journal. 2008;4(1).

WHITE P. The Treatment of Androgenetic Alopecia with LLLT Devices.

Wikramanayake TC, Rodriguez R, Choudhary S, Mauro LM, Nouri K, Schachner LA, et al. Effects of the Lexington LaserComb on Hair Regrowth in the C3H/Hej Mouse Model of Alopecia Areata. Lasers in Medical Science. 2012;27:431–6.

Wikramanayake TC, Villasante AC, Mauro LM, Nouri K, Schachner LA, Perez CI, et al. Low-level Laser Treatment Accelerated Hair Regrowth in a Rat Model of Chemotherapy-Induced Alopecia (CIA). Lasers in Medical Science. 2013;28:701–6.

Chapter 13: Show Me the Science: An Evidence-Based Guide to LPT

AL-MUTAIRI N. 308-nm Excimer Laser for the Treatment Of Alopecia Areata. Dermatologic Surgery. 2007;33(12):1483–7.

Conlan MJ, Rapley JW, and Cobb CM. Biostimulation of Wound Healing by Low-Energy Laser Irradiation a Review. Journal of Clinical Periodon-tology. 1996;23(5):492–6.

Feuerstein, O. Light Therapy: Complementary Antibacterial Treatment of Oral Biofilm. Advances in Dental Research. 2012 Sep;24(2):103–7.

Ghanaat M. Types of Hair Loss and Treatment Options, Including the Novel Low-Level Light Therapy and Its Proposed Mechanism. Southern Medical Journal. 2010;103(9):917–21.

Ginani F, Soares DM, Barreto MPEV, and Barboza CAG. Effect of Low-Level Laser Therapy on Mesenchymal Stem Cell Proliferation: A Systematic Review. Lasers in Medical Science. 2015;30:2189–94.

Greguss P. Interaction of Optical Radiation with Living Matter. Optics & Laser Technology. 1985;17(3):151–8.

Guarrera, M; Cardo, P; Arrigo, P; et al. Reliability of Hamilton-Norwood Classification. International Journal of Trichology. 2009 Jul;1(2):120.

Gundogan C, Greve B, and Raulin C. Treatment of Alopecia Areata with the 308-nm Xenon Chloride Excimer Laser: Case Report of Two Successful Treatments with the Excimer Laser. Lasers in Surgery and Medicine. 2004;34(2):86–90.

Gupta A, and Carviel J. Meta-Analysis of Photobiomodulation for the Treatment of Androgenetic Alopecia. Journal of Dermatological Treatment. 2021;32(6):643-7.

Hamblin, MR. Photobiomodulation or Low-Level Laser Therapy. Journal of Biophotonics. 2016 Dec;9(11–12):1122.

Jacques SL. How Tissue Optics Affect Dosimetry of Photodynamic Therapy. Journal of Biomedical Optics. 2010;15(5):051608-6.

Joulai Veijouye S, Yari A, Heidari F, Sajedi N, Ghoroghi Moghani F, Nobakht M. Bulge Region as a Putative Hair Follicle Stem Cells Niche: A Brief Review. Iran J Public Health. 2017 Sep;46(9):1167-1175. PMID: 29026781; PMCID: PMC5632317.

Junior, AB. Laser Phototherapy in Dentistry. Photomedicine and Laser Surgery. 2009 Aug 1;27(4):533–4.

Kalia S, and Lui H. Utilizing Electromagnetic Radiation for Hair Growth: A Critical Review of Phototrichogenesis. Dermatologic Clinics. 2013;31(1):193–200.

Karu TI. Cellular and Molecular Mechanisms of Photobiomodulation (Low-Power Laser Therapy). IEEE Journal of Selected Topics in Quantum Electronics. 2013;20(2):143–8.

Kawalek AZ, Spencer JM, and Phelps RG. Combined Excimer Laser and Topical Tacrolimus for the Treatment of Vitiligo: A Pilot Study. Dermatologic Surgery. 2004;30(2):130–5.

Lanzafame RJ, Blanche RR, Bodian AB, Chiacchierini RP, Fernandez-Obregon A, and Kazmirek ER. The Growth of Human Scalp Hair Mediated by Visible Red Light Laser and LED Sources in Males. Lasers in Surgery and Medicine. 2013;45(8):487–95.

Lanzafame RJ, Blanche RR, Chiacchierini RP, Kazmirek ER, and Sklar JA. The Growth of Human Scalp Hair in Females Using Visible Red Light Laser and LED Sources. Lasers in Surgery and Medicine. 2014;46(8):601–7.

Lee JH, Eun SH, Kim SH, Ju HJ, Kim GM, and Bae JM. Excimer Laser/Light Treatment of Alopecia Areata: A Systematic Review and Meta-Analyses. Photodermatology, Photoimmunology & Photomedicine. 2020;36(6):460–9.

Liu K-H, Liu D, Chen Y-T, and Chin S-Y. Comparative Effectiveness of Low-Level Laser Therapy for Adult Androgenic Alopecia: A System Review and Meta-Analysis of Randomized Controlled Trials. Lasers in Medical Science. 2019;34:1063–9.

Measuring Laser Beam Divergence. Web Archive. Available from: https://web.archive.org/web/20151120123452/http://www.uslasercorp.com/envoy/diverge.html.

Munck, A; Gavazzoni, MF; Trüeb, RM. Use of Low-Level Laser Therapy as Monotherapy or Concomitant Therapy for Male and Female Androgenetic Alopecia. International Journal of Trichology. 2014 Apr;6(2):45.

Plikus MV, and Chuong C-M. Complex Hair Cycle Domain Patterns and Regenerative Hair Waves in Living Rodents. Journal of Investigative Dermatology. 2008;128(5):1071–80.

Roberts DB, Kruse RJ, and Stoll SF. The Effectiveness of Therapeutic Class IV (10 W) Laser Treatment for Epicondylitis. Lasers in Surgery and Medicine. 2013;45(5):311–7.

Rompolas, P; & Greco, V. Stem Cell Dynamics in the Hair Follicle Niche. Seminars in Cell & Developmental Biology, 25–26, 34–42. https://doi.org/10.1016/j.semcdb.2013.12.005.

Suchkov S, and Herrera AS. The Role of Human Photosynthesis in Predictive, Preventive and Personalized Medicine. EPMA Journal. 2014;5(Suppl 1):A146.

Takac S, and Stojanović S. Characteristics of Laser Light. Medicinski Pregled. 1999;52(1–2):29–34.

Vedantu. (2022, Apr 27). Transparent, Translucent, and Opaque Objects. https://www.vedantu.com/physics/transparent-translucent-and-opaque-objects.

WHITE P. The Treatment of Androgenetic Alopecia with LLLT Devices.

Xu C, Zhang J, Mihai DM, and Washington I. Light-Harvesting Chlorophyll Pigments Enable Mammalian Mitochondria to Capture Photonic Energy and Produce ATP. Journal of Cell Science. 2014;127(2):388–99.

Young AR. Chromophores in Human Skin. Physics in Medicine & Biology. 1997;42(5):789.

Zarei M, Wikramanayake TC, Falto-Aizpurua L, Schachner LA, and Jimenez JJ. Low Level Laser Therapy and Hair Regrowth: An Evidence-Based Review. Lasers in Medical Science. 2016;31(2):363–71.

Chapter 14: Dispelling Myths About Laser Phototherapy

Gupta A, and Carviel J. Meta-Analysis of Photobiomodulation for the Treatment of Androgenetic Alopecia. Journal of Dermatological Treatment. 2021;32(6):643–7.

Grymowicz M, Rudnicka E, Podfigurna A, Napierala P, Smolarczyk R, Smolarczyk K, et al. Hormonal Effects on Hair Follicles. International Journal of Molecular Sciences. 2020;21(15):5342.

Jenkins PA, and Carroll JD. How to Report Low-Level Laser Therapy (LLLT)/Photomedicine Dose and Beam Parameters in Clinical and Laboratory Studies. Photomedicine and Laser Surgery. 2011;29(12):785–7.

Knappe, V; Frank, F; Rohde, E. Principles of Lasers and Biophotonic Effects. Photomedicine and Laser Surgery. 2004 Oct 1;22(5):411–7.

Laser Therapy Compared to LED Therapy. Available from: https://www.proughchiro.com/storage/app/media/compared_led_therapy.pdf.

Minvaleev RS, Bogdanov RR, Bahner DP, and Levitov AB. Headstand (Sirshasana) Does Not Increase the Blood Flow to the Brain. The Journal of Alternative and Complementary Medicine. 2019;25(8):827–32.

Moreno-Arias G, Castelo-Branco C, and Ferrando J. Paradoxical Effect after IPL Photoepilation. Dermatologic Surgery. 2002;28(11):1013–6.

Nistico, SP; Del Duca, E; Farnetani, F; et al. Removal of Unwanted Hair: Efficacy, Tolerability, and Safety of Long-Pulsed 755-Nm Alexandrite Laser Equipped with a Sapphire Handpiece. Lasers in Medical Science. 2018 Sep;33(7):1479–83.

Rochkind S, Nissan M, and Lubart A. A Single Transcutaneous Light Irradiation to Injured Peripheral Nerve: Comparative Study with Five Different Wavelengths. Lasers in Medical Science. 1989;4:259–63.

Ryer, A. Light U, Light V. Light Measurement Handbook. Available from: https://cgvr.informatik.uni-bremen.de/teaching/cg_literatur/ILT-Light-Measurement-Handbook.pdf.

Texas Heart Institute Staff. (2021, December 3). Vasculature of the Head. Texas Heart Institute. https://www.texasheart.org/heart-health/heart-information-center/topics/vasculature-of-the-head/.

Tobin DJ. The Cell Biology of Human Hair Follicle Pigmentation. Pigment Cell & Melanoma Research. 2011;24(1):75–88.

UMass Chan Medical School. (2015, July 21). Brain Circulation. Available from: https://www.umassmed.edu/strokestop/modules/module-3-the-blood-supply-of-the-brain/brain-circulation/.

Vest BE, Krauland K. Malassezia Furfur. [Updated 2023 May 22]. In: StatPearls [Internet]. Treasure Island (FL): StatPearls Publishing; 2023 Jan-. Available from: https://www.ncbi.nlm.nih.gov/books/NBK553091/.

Yamazaki M, Miura Y, Tsuboi R, and Ogawa H. Linear Polarized Infrared Irradiation Using Super Lizer™ Is an Effective Treatment for Multiple-Type Alopecia Areata. International journal of dermatology. 2003;42(9):738–40.

Chapter 15: Is LPT Right for Me?

Agaiby A, Ghali L, and Dyson M. Laser Modulation Of T-Lymphocyte Proliferation in Vitro. Laser Therapy. 1998;10(4):153–8.

Edelson R, Berger C, Gasparro F, Jegasothy B, Heald P, Wintroub B, et al. Treatment of Cutaneous T-Cell Lymphoma by Extracorporeal Photochemotherapy. New England Journal of Medicine. 1987;316(6):297–303.

Qadri T, Bohdanecka P, Tunér J, Miranda L, Altamash M, and Gustafsson A. The Importance of Coherence Length in Laser Phototherapy of Gingival Inflammation—A Pilot Study. Lasers in Medical Science. 2007;22:245–51.

Chapter 16: Meet the Team: Hair Loss Professionals and their Specialties

Dias MFRG. Hair Cosmetics: An Overview. International Journal of Trichology. 2015;7(1):2.

Elewski BE. Journal of Investigative Dermatology Symposium Proceedings. Elsevier; 2005:190–3.

Gianfaldoni, S; Tchernev, G; Wollina, U; et al. An Overview of Laser in Dermatology: The Past, the Present and … the Future (?). Open Access Macedonian Journal of Medical Sciences. 2017 Jul 23;5(4):526–530. doi: 10.3889/oamjms.2017.130. PMID: 28785350; PMCID: PMC5535675.

Hair Conditions. The Institute of Trichologists. Available from: https://trichologists.org.uk/conditions/hair-conditions/.

Meyer-Gonzalez, T; Bacqueville, D; Grimalt, R; et al. Current Controversies in Trichology: A European Expert Consensus Statement. Journal of the European Academy of Dermatology and Venereology. 2021 Nov;35:3–11.

Revital Tricology. (2020, Dec 2). 60 Seconds Hair Loss Test. Available From: https://www.revitaltrichology.com/60-seconds-hair-loss-test.php.

Scalp Conditions. The Institute of Trichologists. Available from: https://trichologists.org.uk/conditions/scalp-conditions/.

Schweikert HU, and Wilson JD. Regulation of Human Hair Growth by Steroid Hormones. I. Testosterone Metabolism in Isolated Hairs. The Journal of Clinical Endocrinology & Metabolism. 1974;38(5):811–9.

Trüeb, RM; Vañó-Galván, S; Kopera, D; et al. Trichologist, Dermato-trichologist, or Trichiatrist? A Global Perspective on a Strictly Medical Discipline. Skin Appendage Disorders. 2018;4(4):202–7.

What is Trichology? The Institute of Trichologists. Available from: https://trichologists.org.uk/conditions/.

Chapter 17: Frequently Asked

Chamberlain AJ & Dawber RP. Methods of Evaluating Hair Growth. Australasian Journal of Dermatology. 2003 Feb;44(1):10–8.

Cohen B. The Cross-Section Trichometer: A New Device for Measuring Hair Quantity, Hair Loss, and Hair Growth. Dermatologic Surgery. 2008;34(7):900–11.

Hoffmann R. TrichoScan: Combining Epiluminescence Microscopy with Digital Image Analysis for the Measurement of Hair Growth in Vivo. European Journal of Dermatology. 2001;11(4):362–8.

Kalfalah F, Seggewiß S, Walter R, Tigges J, Moreno-Villanueva M, Bürkle A, et al. Structural Chromosome Abnormalities, Increased DNA Strand Breaks and DNA Strand Break Repair Deficiency in Dermal Fibroblasts from Old Female Human Donors. Aging (Albany NY). 2015;7(2):110.

Lodewijckx J, Robijns J, Claes M, Pierson M, Lenaerts M, and Mebis J. The Use of Photobiomodulation Therapy for the Management of Chemotherapy-Induced Alopecia: A Randomized, Controlled Trial (HAIR-LASER trial). Supportive Care in Cancer. 2023;31(5):1–11.

Whitting DA, Blume-Peytavi U, Hillmann K, and Guarrera M. Hair Growth Assessment Techniques. Hair Growth and Disorders. 2008:125–57.

Chapter 18: The Future of Laser Phototherapy

Chow RT, Johnson MI, Lopes-Martins RA, and Bjordal JM. Efficacy of Low-Level Laser Therapy in the Management of Neck Pain: A Systematic Review and Meta-Analysis of Randomized Placebo or Active-Treatment Controlled Trials. The Lancet. 2009;374(9705):1897–908.

Data Reportal. Digital Around the World. Available from: https://datareportal.com/global-digital-overview#:~:text.

Dodd EM, Winter MA, Hordinsky MK, Sadick NS, and Farah RS. Photobiomodulation Therapy for Androgenetic Alopecia: A Clinician's Guide to Home-Use Devices Cleared by the Federal Drug Administration. Journal of Cosmetic and Laser Therapy. 2018;20(3):159–67.

Elman, M; Lebzelter, J. Light Therapy In the Treatment of Acne Vulgaris. Dermatologic Surgery. 2004 Feb;30(2):139–46.

Glickman, G; Byrne, B; Pineda, C; et al. Light Therapy for Seasonal Affective Disorder with Blue Narrow-Band Light-Emitting Diodes (Leds). Biological Psychiatry. 2006 Mar 15;59(6):502–7

Gupta AK, and Bamimore MA. Factors Influencing the Effect of Photobiomodulation in the Treatment of Androgenetic Alopecia: A Systematic Review and Analyses of Summary-Level Data. Dermatologic Therapy. 2020;33(6):e14191.

Hamblin, MR. Photobiomodulation or Low-Level Laser Therapy. Journal of Biophotonics. 2016 Dec;9(11–12):1122.

Hsieh, RL; Lee, WC. Short-Term Therapeutic Effects of 890-Nanometer Light Therapy for Chronic Low Back Pain: A Double-Blind Randomized Placebo-Controlled Study. Lasers in Medical Science. 2014 Mar;29(2):671–9.

Kemper, KJ. Let There Be Light. Research on Phototherapy, Light Therapy, and Photobiomodulation for Healing-Alternative Therapy Becomes Mainstream. Complementary Therapies in Medicine. 2018 Dec;41:A1–6.

Lam; et al. Laser Stimulation of Collagen Synthesis in Human Skin Fibroblast Cultures. Lasers in the Life Sciences (1986): 1: 61–77

Mignon C, Botchkareva NV, Uzunbajakava NE, and Tobin DJ. Photobiomodulation Devices for Hair Regrowth and Wound Healing: A Therapy Full of Promise But a Literature Full of Confusion. Experimental Dermatology. 2016;25(10):745–9.

Morimoto, Y; et al. Low Level Laser Therapy for Sports Injuries. Laser Therapy (2013): 22(1): 17–20.

Okuni; et al. Low-Level Laser Therapy (LLLT) for Chronic Joint Pain of the Elbow, Wrist and Fingers. Laser Therapy (2012): 21(1): 33–37.

Olivieri, L; et al. Efficacy of Low-Level Laser Therapy on Hair Regrowth in Dogs with Noninflammatory Alopecia: A Pilot Study. Veterinary Dermatology (2015): 26(1): 35–39, e11.

Rosner M, Solomon A, Assia E, Belkin M, Caplan M, Cohen S, et al. Dose and Temporal Parameters in Delaying Injured Optic Nerve Degeneration by Low-Energy Laser Irradiation. Lasers in Surgery and Medicine. 1993;13(6):611–7.

Stelian, J; Gil, I; Habot, B; et al. Improvement of Pain and Disability in Elderly Patients with Degenerative Osteoarthritis of the Knee Treated with Narrow-Band Light Therapy. Journal of the American Geriatrics Society. 1992 Jan;40(1):23–6.

Waiz M, Saleh AZ, Hayani R, and Jubory SO. Use of the Pulsed Infrared Diode Laser (904 Nm) in the Treatment of Alopecia Areata. Journal of Cosmetic and Laser Therapy. 2006;8(1):27–30.

GLOSSARY

5-alpha reductase: An enzyme produced in follicles with the genetic "code" for hair loss. It converts testosterone to dihydrotestosterone (DHT), which is responsible for the shrinkage of hair follicles and shortening of hair.

Acid: Chemically, an acid is any substance that gives off hydrogen ions in water. Acids usually form salts by combining with certain metals and alkalis. Acids have a sour taste and turn certain dyes red. Common examples include Hydrochloric acid, Sulphuric acid, etc.

Acne: An inflammation of the skin that occurs when the hair follicles become plugged with oil, sebum, and dead skin cells. It often presents in the form of pimples and is associated with hormonal (testosterone) levels and the sebaceous glands.

Adenosine triphosphate (ATP): Organic molecule found in the cells of all living organisms responsible for storing and transferring energy in the cell. It is the major source of energy for cellular reactions and is referred to as the energy currency of the cell.

Adrenal glands: Small, triangular-shaped glands located on top of both kidneys. They produce hormones that help regulate the body's metabolism, immune system, blood pressure, response to stress, and other essential functions.

Alopecia areata (AA): An autoimmune disorder that usually results in unpredictable hair loss in patches. It occurs due to an abnormality in the immune system that damages hair follicles leading to hair loss.

Alopecia universalis: An advanced form of alopecia areata that is characterized by the complete loss of hair on the scalp and body.

Alzheimer's disease: A common type of dementia that affects memory, thinking, and behavior, eventually destroying the ability of a person to carry out the simplest tasks.

Anagen phase: Also known as the "growth phase" or "active phase" of the hair growth cycle. During this phase the cells in the root of the hair are rapidly dividing so more new hair is formed. The length of this phase varies from individual to individual, lasting somewhere between three to five years.

Androgen hormones: Group of sex hormones responsible for the growth and development of the male reproductive system and masculine characteristics. Testosterone is the most common androgen hormone.

Androgenetic alopecia: Also known as male pattern hair loss (MPHL) or female pattern hair loss (FPHL). It is primarily a genetic disorder characterized by progressive hair loss from the scalp due to abnormal levels of androgen and thyroid hormones.

Anemia: A blood disorder in which the body lacks enough healthy red blood cells to carry adequate oxygen to the body's tissues.

Anesthetics: Medicines that produce general or local loss of sensation in the body and are usually used to prevent pain during surgery or medical procedures.

Angiogenesis: Process of formation and growth of new blood vessels from the existing vessels. In hair transplants (HT), this process is very important so that the donor hairs can attached to the scalp. Proper angiogenesis is vital for a successful HT procedure.

Anthralin: Medicine isolated from the Araroba tree. It is used to treat skin/scalp conditions like psoriasis and alopecia areata.

Anti-androgen drugs: Drugs that work by minimizing the effects of androgen hormones, such as testosterone. These drugs are used for many purposes like slowing prostate cancer, managing ovarian tumors, diabetes, heart diseases, etc.

Anti-apoptotic: Any drug, chemical, or physical agent that prevents apoptosis. Apoptosis is a programmed process in which a series of molecular steps in a cell leads to its death.

Antibody: Special proteins produced by the body's immune system to protect itself from foreign substances.

Antifungal: Drug or chemical that kills or stops the growth of fungi that cause infections.

Anti-inflammatory agents: Substances that reduce inflammation (redness, swelling, and pain) in the body.

Anti-nuclear antibody (ANA): Antibodies that destroy the cells by targeting the proteins within the nucleus of a cell. The presence of a large number of these antibodies indicates autoimmune diseases.

Antioxidants: Substances that protect cells from the damage caused by free radicals (unstable molecules made by the process of oxidation during normal metabolism). Common examples are vitamin C, vitamin E, Selenium, etc.

Apoptosis: A programmed process in which a series of molecular steps in a cell leads to its death.

Arrector pili muscles: Small muscles that are attached to hair follicles in mammals. Contraction of these muscles causes the hairs to stand and causes goosebumps.

Aspirin: Also known as acetylsalicylic acid. It is a medicine commonly used to reduce fever and relieve pain. One of the oldest pain reliever medicines (over 3,500 years) and originally sourced from the bark from the willow tree now chemically synthesized.

Assyrians: People who have lived in the Middle East (Assyria) since ancient times. Today, they can be found all over the world.

Astaxanthin: A red pigment that belongs to a group of chemicals called carotenoids. It occurs in certain algae and also protects human cells from damage. They are used for many purposes like the treatment of Alzheimer's disease, aging skin, muscle soreness from exercise, and reducing brain damage from stroke.

Asthma: A long-term disease of the lungs that causes airways to get inflamed and narrow making it difficult to breathe. It results in wheezing, breathlessness, chest tightness, and coughing.

Atom: Smallest particle of an element that can exist independently. An atom consists of a central nucleus that is surrounded by electrons.

ATP (adenosine triphosphate): Organic molecule found in the cells of all living organisms responsible for storing and transferring energy in the cell. It is the major source of energy for cellular reactions and is referred to as the energy currency of the cell.

Autism: A developmental disability caused by differences in the brain and characterized by challenges with social skills and repetitive behaviors. People with autism have problems with social communication and restricted behaviors or interests.

Autoimmune disease: A disease in which the body's immune system attacks its own healthy cells by mistake. Common examples include lupus, rheumatoid arthritis, Crohn's disease, Graves' disease, ulcerative colitis, etc.

Babylonians: Inhabitants of Babylonia: an ancient cultural region and state based in the city of Babylon in central-southern Mesopotamia.

Bacteria: A group of single-celled, microscopic organisms that exist in their millions in almost every environment on Earth, most of which cause diseases in humans and animals.

Beam divergence: Angular measure of increase in the diameter of the beam with distance from the optical aperture from which the beam emerges. It relates to the width of a beam. A narrower beam generally means a lower divergence.

Beta-carotene: Colorful pigments present in plants, fruits, and vegetables that give them their characteristic and bright colors. Beta-carotenes are precursors of vitamin A and are metabolized by the body to obtain vitamin A.

Biomedical engineer: Biomedical engineers focus on advances in technology and medicine to develop new devices and equipment for improving human health.

Biopsy: Removal of a piece of tissue or a sample of cells from the body for examination.

Biostimulation: The process of stimulating cells or micro-organisms to enhance their growth by modification and addition of materials to their environment. This technique is used in hair loss treatments to increase hair growth by stimulating the mitochondria in the hair cells with light energy.

Biotin: Also known as vitamin B7. It is found in foods like eggs, milk, and bananas. It plays important functions in the body such as the conversion of food into energy, strengthening of hair and nails, etc. Although an extremely rare condition, biotin deficiency can cause thinning of the hair and a rash on the face.

Bipolar disorder: A mental disorder that causes intense shifts in mood, energy levels, and behavior. It is caused by chemical imbalances in the brain.

Blemishes: Marks, spots, discolorations, or flaws on the skin that are usually benign, harmless, and not life-threatening.

Bloodwork: Also known as a blood test is a regular checkup and testing of blood that helps in the diagnosis of certain diseases and conditions.

Broadband polarized light therapy: It involves the use of visible light for the healing of wounds and other clinical applications.

Bulge: The region of the hair follicle that contains all the stem cells for that hair follicle. The function of these bulge stem cells is to form new hair follicles. The bulge region is located between the opening of the sebaceous gland and the attachment site of the arrector pili muscle.

Camouflage: A way of hiding something by painting it in such a way that when placed against a background, it makes the thing difficult or impossible to see.

Cancer: A disease of uncontrolled cell division in a part of the body resulting in the development of abnormal cells or tumors. It can also spread to other parts of the body.

Cardiologist: A specialized doctor of heart who diagnoses and treats various heart conditions.

Cardiovascular disease: A group of disorders or conditions that affect the heart and blood vessels. They include heart attack, stroke, arrhythmia, etc.

Carotenoids: Carotenoids are pigments found in plants, algae, and bacteria that give bright yellow, red, and orange colors. They are also present in the eyes.

Castration: The process of removal of reproductive organs (testes and ovaries) in males and females to stop the production of sex hormones.

Catagen phase: One of the three phases of the hair growth cycle. It is a transitional phase between the anagen (growing) and the telogen (resting). In this phase, although the hair is not growing, it's still visible coming out of the follicle.

Cauterization: The technique of burning a part of a body or wound to stop it from bleeding or getting infected, or to remove harmful cells.

Cellulose: A polysaccharide consisting of a chain of several hundred to many thousands of glucose units. It is an important component of the cell wall in plants.

Central centrifugal cicatricial alopecia: Central centrifugal cicatricial alopecia (CCCA) is a form of scarring alopecia on the scalp that clinically presents as patches of permanent hair loss.

Centrifuge: A device that spins at a very high speed and separates substances according to their density. It is used in various laboratories to separate fluids, gases, or liquids.

Chemo-induced alopecia: Hair loss that occurs due to chemotherapy treatments. It is one of the most dramatic and distressing side effects of chemotherapy.

Chemotherapy: Method of treatment of cancer that uses powerful medicines to kill fast-growing cancerous cells in the body.

Chlorophyll: A green pigment present in the leaves of plants that captures sunlight and converts it into chemical energy which is stored as food.

Chromophores: Unique light-absorbing pigments (like chlorophyll) present in mammals. They absorb sunlight and convert it into energy. The most common example is melanin which gives color to eyes, hair, and skin.

Circadian rhythm: A twenty-four-hour cycle that is controlled by the body's internal clock. It is a natural, internal process that regulates the sleep-wake cycle and repeats roughly every twenty-four hours.

Coal tar: A dark viscous liquid that is formed by strong heating of coal in the absence of air. It contains many useful organic compounds.

Coherent light: Light waves having the same color and frequency. Coherent light is used in fiber optics, medical diagnostics, and lasers.

Collagen: The most abundant protein in the body. It provides support and strength to the skin, muscles, and bones.

Colorectal cancer: Also known as colon cancer or rectal cancer. It is a disease in which cells in the colon or rectum grow rapidly without any control and form abnormal cells.

Corticosteroids: Also known as steroids. They are used to reduce inflammation and suppress the immune system. They are also found to be effective in the treatment of alopecia areata.

Cortisol: A hormone produced by adrenal glands that are located on top of the kidneys. It increases the level of sugar (glucose) in the blood.

Cranium: The part of the skull that encloses the brain. It is made up of eight bones called cranial bones and protects the brain from any damage.

C-reactive protein (CRP): A protein formed by the liver. Its level increases due to inflammation in the body. CRP test is used to indicate inflammation caused by infection, injury, or chronic diseases like rheumatoid arthritis or lupus.

Cuticle: The outermost part of the hair strand. It is composed of overlapping dead cells and protects hair from damage.

Cyclosporine: A drug used to suppress the immune system to prevent the rejection of organs after transplantation. It is also effective in the treatment of alopecia universalis.

Cysts: Abnormal, fluid-filled sacs formed on the skin or in any part of the body. Generally, they are harmless but sometimes, they can cause cancer.

Dandruff: A condition in which dry skin cells on the scalp are shed and are clumped together to form white flakes. It is harmless and sometimes causes itchiness. It can be treated with medicated shampoo.

Dapsone: A drug used to treat leprosy. It works by decreasing swelling (inflammation) and stopping the growth of bacteria. It is also used in the treatment of dissecting cellulitis of the scalp.

Dermatology: The branch of medicine that is concerned with various skin conditions. It involves the diagnosis and management of any health condition that may affect the skin, hair, and nails.

Dermatotrichology: A discipline in which board-certified dermatologists also deal with the scientific study and treatment of the hair, scalp, and their associated diseases.

Diabetes: A chronic disease in which the body can't produce enough insulin or the body cannot make good use of the insulin it produces. Due to a lack of insulin, the blood sugar level rises which leads to many other disorders and complications. Skin disorders and hair loss can be a symptom of diabetes.

Diabetic ulcers: Wounds or sores usually found on the bottom of feet that occur in people with diabetes. The healing process is slow and they can lead to lower limb amputation.

Dibutylester: A diester (a compound derived from two acids) obtained by the condensation of the carboxy groups of phthalic acid. It is generally used as insect repellent and as a solvent for perfume oil and resins. It is also effective in the treatment of alopecia universalis.

Dihydrotestosterone (DHT): When the enzyme 5 alpha-reductase combines with the male hormone testosterone, the result is dihydrotestosterone. It is involved in the development of male characteristics and the sexual differentiation of organs. DHT is the specific hormone that starts the hair loss process in those follicles which have the genetic message for hair loss.

Diphenylcyclopropenone: Also known as diphencyprone. It is a drug used for treating alopecia areata and alopecia universalis.

Dissecting Cellulitis of the scalp (DCS): Also known as Hoffman disease. It is an inflammatory disorder of the scalp that is often associated with patchy hair loss.

Dimethyl sulfoxide (DMSO): A chemical solvent that is used to reduce inflammation and pain It is also used in chemotherapy treatment.

Dormant phase: Time during the life cycle of an organism or cell in which there is no active growth. It is a state of reduced metabolic activity adopted under difficult environmental conditions.

Eczema: A skin disorder also known as atopic dermatitis that can manifest as anything from simple itching and inflammation to an eruption with a crusty, scaly residue. Eczema is more of a symptom than a disease and can be caused by irritants like soap, dampness, pollens, molds, etc.

Edge emitting laser diodes (EEL diodes): They are the most commonly used laser diodes in which the laser beam is issued from the side surface of the LD chip in them. They are used for consumer applications such as CD-ROMs, DVDs, Laser pointers, and barcode scanners.

Electrical charge: The property of matter that causes it to experience a force when placed in an electromagnetic field. It can be positive or negative. It is the number of electrons that pass from one body to another in different modes.

Electromagnetic (EM) energy: Also known as radiant energy or electromagnetic radiation. It is the energy carried by electromagnetic waves during their propagation from one place to another.

Electromagnetic field: It is the region where the electromagnetic force produced by accelerated charges is present. It is actually a combination of invisible electric and magnetic fields of force.

Electron microscope: The type of microscope that uses a beam of electrons to produce highly magnified images of very small objects. It has a very high resolution than an ordinary optical microscope.

Electronics: A branch of physics that deals with the emission, behavior, and effects of electrons using various electronic devices. It usually deals with electrical circuits.

Emulsifier: Food additives used to mix two substances that are typically immiscible (like oil and water) and separate them when they are combined.

Endocrine system: The system of the glands and tissues that produce hormones in the human body. It controls and regulates metabolism, energy level, reproduction, growth, and development of the body.

Endoscopy: A non-surgical process used to examine the internal organs of the body. It consists of a long, thin tube with a small camera inside (endoscope) which is passed into the body through the mouth.

Energy: Ability or capacity of something to work. It is a basic physical quantitative property related to activity and is measured in joules.

Enzyme: Specialized proteins that speed up the rate of chemical reactions inside the body. They are not destroyed during the reaction and can be used over and over.

Epidermal growth factor (EGF): A protein that stimulates cell growth and differentiation in various epidermal and epithelial tissues. It is used in medicine to speed up wound recovery. However, it causes suppression of normal hair growth.

Erectile dysfunction: Also known as impotence. It is defined as difficulty in getting and keeping an erection that's firm enough for intercourse.

Erythema: Redness of the skin caused by injury or another inflammation-causing condition. It is considered to be an allergic reaction to medicine or an infection.

Estradiol (E2): Primary form of estrogen (female sex hormone) in the human body. It is involved in the development of the female reproductive system and the regulation of the menstrual cycle.

Estrogen: Female sex hormone produced by ovaries. It plays an important role in the regulation of the menstrual cycle by developing the walls of the uterus. It also regulates the growth and development of the body especially female reproductive parts.

Food and Drug Administration (FDA): A US federal agency responsible for ensuring safety standards in the food, drug, and cosmetics industries.

Female pattern hair loss (FPHL): Pattern of hair loss in women with androgenetic alopecia and is characterized by progressive hair thinning and shedding. It occurs due to hormones, aging, and genetics and can be treated by the drug Minoxidil, Finasteride, and laser phototherapy.

Ferritin: A protein inside cells that stores iron. The amount of iron can be found by ferritin level test. The lower amount of ferritin indicates a lower level of iron in the blood which can result in anemia.

Fibroblast: A type of cell that is involved in the formation of connective tissues. They are large, flat, elongated cells that play an important role in the healing of wounds.

Finasteride: Also known as Propecia. It is a drug that is used to prevent hair loss but it can cause erectile dysfunction, depression, anxiety, and other neurological issues.

Fitzpatrick IV system: A classification system based on a person's skin color. There are six different skin types on the basis of responses to sun exposure in terms of the degree of burning and tanning according to this system.

Fluence: The amount of optical energy that is applied or delivered per square centimeter surface area of tissue. It is measured in watts per square centimeter.

Folate (vitamin B9): Naturally occurring form of vitamin B9. It is necessary for the healthy growth of cells.

Follicular unit extraction (FUE): A hair restoration technique in which individual hair follicles are removed from the back of the head and are grafted onto the thinning parts of the scalp. This is a no scarring method but scalp must be shaven prior to procedure.

Follicular unit transplantation (FUT): A hair restoration technique in which strips of the scalp containing hair follicles are removed from the back of the head and are grafted onto the absent or thinning parts of the scalp. This technique does leave a scar from the removed strip section.

Folliculitis: Inflammation of hair follicles caused by an infection with bacteria. It can occur anywhere on hair-covered skin.

Free radicals: Unstable molecules made by the process of oxidation during normal metabolism.

Frequency: The number of light waves passing a fixed point in a specific time interval or the number of cycles per second. It is one of the parameters in the selection of lasers for therapeutic purposes. It is measured in hertz (Hz).

Frontal fibrosing alopecia: Frontal fibrosing alopecia (FFA) is a form of lichen planopilaris (LP)—a scalp condition that causes inflammation in the scalp and hair follicles leading to permanent hair loss.

Gastrointestinal tract (GI tract): Also called the alimentary canal or digestive system. It is a long tube that consists of organs and glands involved in the digestion of food including the stomach, small intestine, etc. GI starts in the mouth and ends at the rectum.

Genes: Parts of DNA that consist of specific codes for the synthesis of proteins in the body. They are called the basic unit of inheritance. They are passed from parents to offspring and contain the information needed to specify physical and biological traits.

Genetic traits: Specific characteristics of an individual that are passed by parents to their children such as eye color, skin color, blood type, etc.

Genetics: Branch of biology that deals with the study of genes and their transmission from parents to their children.

Glands: Specialized organs or groups of cells that produce and release substances that carry out specific functions in the body. There are two types of glands: endocrine glands, and exocrine glands.

Hair follicles: Tube-like structures in the outer layer of the skin that surround the root and strand of a hair. They anchor each hair into the skin and contribute to the growth of the hair strand.

Hair weaving: A non-surgical process that involves attaching hair extensions to the existing hair to provide the appearance of a full crown and voluminous hair.

Hemoglobin: A specialized protein present in red blood cells that carries oxygen from the lungs to all parts of the body.

Hormones: Specialized chemical messengers that are produced and released by various glands of the endocrine system. Hormones control the various body functions and are carried by the bloodstream to their target sites.

Hyaluronic acid: Also called hyaluronan. It is a substance found in the fluids in the eyes and joints. It acts as a cushion and lubricant in the joints and is also helpful in preventing hair loss.

Hyperandrogenism: Overproduction of male sex hormones (androgens) like testosterone in females. It can lead to excessive hair growth on the face and other parts of the body.

Hyperkeratotic buildup: Excessive buildup of keratin protein that leads to the thickening of the outer layer of the skin. It occurs due to inflammation, irritation of the skin, and genetic mutations.

Hypothalamus: Part of the brain that keeps the body's internal conditions at a constant level by regulating various processes such as heart rate and body temperature. It also produces some hormones.

International Association of Trichologists (IAT): An international corporation of trichologists that promotes the study of and research in all aspects of the treatment and care of the human hair and scalp in health and disease.

Immune system: The body's natural defense system that protects the body against many infections and diseases. It is a complex network of organs, cells, and proteins. White blood cells are a major component of the immune system.

Immunosuppressants: Drugs that are used to control or keep a check on the body's immune system. These drugs suppress and reduce the strength of the immune system. Commonly, they are used to prevent the rejection of the transplanted organ by the immune system.

Incandescent: Something emitting light and glowing extremely bright like an LED or bulb, uses a metal filament to produce light.

Incision: A wound that is made by a surgeon during surgery to perform an operation.

Inflammatory bowel disease: A disease that causes inflammation in the gastrointestinal tract (digestive system). It can also cause pain, cramps, diarrhea, weight loss, and extreme tiredness.

Infrared light: A portion of the electromagnetic spectrum that has lower energy than the red end of visible light. It is invisible to human eyes and has many applications like in night vision devices.

Ischemic heart disease: Also known as coronary heart disease. It results in the weakening of heart muscles due to reduced blood flow caused by narrowed heart arteries.

IV Infusions: Stands for intravenous infusion. It is a method of drug infusion to the body by directly putting liquid into the bloodstream.

Keratinocytes: Primary type of cell found in the epidermis (the outermost layer of the skin). In humans, they constitute 90% of the epidermal skin cells. They act as a barrier and play an essential role in protection by preventing foreign substances from entering the body.

Ketoconazole: A drug used to treat infections caused by fungi on the skin. It can also be used to control hair loss and regrow the hair on the scalp by fighting dandruff and the fungi that cause dandruff.

Kingdom Animalia: Group of organisms that are eukaryotic (having a nucleus in cells), multicellular, and heterotrophic (obtaining their food by eating other organisms). It is the largest Kingdom and includes all animals, birds, and insects.

Kingdom Plantae: Group of organisms that are eukaryotic (having a nucleus in cells), multicellular, and autotrophic (making their own food by photosynthesis). It is the second-largest kingdom and includes all plants.

Krebs cycle: Also known as the citric acid cycle. It is a cyclic process occurring in living cells by which glucose molecule is broken down and their energy is stored in the form of ATP.

LASER: Stands for Light Amplification by Stimulated Emission of Radiation. A laser is a coherent and focused beam of photons produced from a laser diode. It is used in eye surgery, cutting, engraving, drilling, hair loss treatment, etc.

Laser diode: A semiconductor device that converts electrical energy into light energy to produce high-intensity coherent light i.e., a laser. It is used in fiber optic communications, barcode readers, laser printing, and laser scanning.

Laser phototherapy (LPT): Non-invasive treatment that uses lasers as the coherent light source to stimulate the growth of cells and hair follicles, reduce pain and inflammation, and improve tissue healing. It helps to combat hair loss and improve the appearance of hair.

LED: Stands for Light Emitting Diode. It is a semiconductor device, which emits light when an electric current passes through it. It is used in digital devices, traffic signals, camera flashes, toys, etc.

Lichen planopilaris: An autoimmune disorder that causes inflammation in the scalp and hair follicles leading to permanent hair loss.

Lichen planus: A condition that is associated with hepatitis C and can cause swelling and irritation in the skin, hair, nails, and inside the mouth.

Loose anagen syndrome: An inherited hair disorder in which the hair strands are not firmly attached to the scalp and can be painlessly pulled from the scalp.

Low-level light therapy (LLLT): Low-level light therapy is a form of light therapy that utilizes non-coherent or coherent focused light from non-ionizing forms of light sources including lasers, LEDs, and broadband light, in the visible and near-infrared spectrum to stimulate a process, especially during medical treatment.

Lupus: Autoimmune disease that can cause joint pain, skin rashes tiredness, and organ damage. It also causes hair loss.

Luteal phase: Phase that occurs in the second half of the menstrual cycle after ovulation. It prepares the uterus for a possible pregnancy by thickening its walls.

Lycopene: A antioxidant carotenoid that is related to beta carotene and gives the red color to some vegetables and fruits like tomatoes carrots and watermelons.

Lymph: Fluid that flows in the vessels of the lymphatic system.

Lymphatic system: A complex network of tissues, organs, and vessels that contain fluid called lymph. Its function is to maintain fluid levels in tissues by returning all fluid that leaks out of the blood vessels back to blood circulation. It also has an important role in the body's defense system.

Lymphocytes: The type of white blood cells that form the body's immune system and help the body fight infection and disease. There are two types of lymphocytes: b lymphocytes and t lymphocytes.

Macular degeneration: An eye disease that can blur your central vision and it happens when aging causes damage to the macula—the part of the eye that controls sharp, straight-ahead vision.

Malassezia furfur (MF): Species of yeast that makes up over 80% of the fungi that live on human skin and causes many common skin diseases, such as psoriasis and dermatitis. One such condition is seborrheic dermatitis, which causes dandruff.

Marginal alopecia: Also called traction alopecia. It is an acquired hair loss caused by prolonged tension and repeatedly pulling on the hair. It results from regularly wearing tight weaves, and braids, and using hair extensions, chemical relaxers, and rollers.

Melanin: Pigment in the body that gives color to hair, eyes, and skin. The more melanin produced by the body, the darker the skin gets.

Melanoma: The most dangerous type of skin cancer that develops from pigment-producing cells called melanocytes. It grows quickly and can spread to any other organ.

Menopause: Complete stoppage of the menstrual cycle in females. It begins between the ages of forty-five to fifty-five years.

Mesotherapy: A non-invasive, non-surgical technique that uses injections of vitamins, enzymes, hormones, and plant extracts to treat pain, injuries, infections, and vascular diseases. It is also effective in the treatment of various skin conditions and hair loss.

Metabolic syndrome: A collection of conditions that increase the risk of heart disease, diabetes, stroke, and other serious problems. These conditions include increased blood pressure, high blood sugar, excess body fat, etc.

Metabolism: The sum of all processes occurring inside the body. It involves the changes of food and drink into energy. It has two types: catabolism, and anabolism.

Methylprednisolone: An anti-inflammatory drug that is used to treat conditions such as blood disorders, arthritis, severe allergic reactions, certain cancers, and eye conditions.

Methylsulfonylmethane (MSM): A chemical that occurs naturally in humans and some green plants and animals. It is used for conditions like pain, swelling, and aging. It is also beneficial for hair growth.

Microscope: A device used to examine extremely small objects. It produces magnified images of objects that are too small to be seen by the naked eye such as cells of our body.

Microwaves: A type of electromagnetic radiation having a high frequency and wavelength ranging from about one meter to one millimeter. They are used in communication, radar, and cooking (microwave ovens).

Millennia: A period of one thousand years.

Minoxidil (Rogaine): A drug used to stimulate hair growth in men and women. It is also used for the treatment of high blood pressure and pattern hair loss.

Mitochondria: Also known as the powerhouse of cells. They are double membrane-bound organelles present inside the cells. They release energy from food materials by a process called respiration and store it in the form of ATP.

Monochromatic: Light consisting of a single wavelength and only one color.

Messenger RNA (mRNA): Single-stranded molecule formed from DNA by a process called transcription. It carries the information necessary for the production of proteins from DNA to ribosomes.

Nanometer: A unit of length in the metric system, equal to one-billionth of a meter.

NASA: Stands for National Aeronautics and Space Administration. It is an agency that is responsible for various space studies and space programs in the USA.

Neonatal jaundice: The type of jaundice that occurs in newborn babies. It is a condition in which a child's skin appears yellow due to elevated levels of bilirubin within the first few days of life. It is common and usually harmless.

Nervous system: A complex system consisting of the brain, spinal cord, and a complex network of nerves. Its main function is to transmit signals between the brain and the rest of the body and to provide coordination to our bodies.

Neurosurgery: Medical specialty concerned with the diagnosis and surgical treatment of people with various nerve injuries, especially brain disorders.

Nitric oxide (NO): A colorless poisonous gas formed by oxidation of nitrogen or ammonia that is present in the atmosphere and also in mammals. It acts as a vasodilator and as a mediator of cell-to-cell communication.

Non–scarring alopecia: A type of hair loss that occurs without any scarring being present. The hair is usually lost in round or oval patches initially. This lost hair usually grows back without any other problems or any further hair loss.

Norwood–Hamilton Scale: Classification system used to measure the stages and extent of male pattern hair loss. It was devised by James Hamilton in the 1950s.

Nutrient: Chemical substance necessary for an organism to survive, grow and reproduce. The main nutrients required by humans are proteins, fats, carbohydrates, vitamins, and minerals.

Obesity: Accumulation of abnormal or excessive fat in the body. It is a leading cause of a large number of diseases like hypertension, diabetes, and coronary artery disease.

Ophthalmology: Branch of medicine that deals with the diagnosis and treatment of eye disorders.

Optical Power Output: This is defined as the power of the light coming out of the end of a laser diode. It is usually specified in watts or joules per second. The higher the optical power output the more dosage or fluence that laser diode can deliver.

Optics: Branch of physics that deals with the study of production, behavior propagation, and the properties of light, along with its interactions with matter and the construction of instruments that use or detect it.

Orthostatic hypotension: Sudden decrease in blood pressure while standing and sitting down. It causes dizziness or lightheadedness and fainting. It is most commonly caused by loss of fluid within the blood vessels.

Osteoporosis: Disorder in which bones become weak and porous. Bones become so weak and brittle that a fall or even mild stresses such as bending or coughing can break them. It occurs in men and women in old age.

Ovulation: Phase in the menstrual cycle in which a mature egg is released from the ovary. Normally, it occurs on the fourteenth day of each cycle.

Oxidation: Loss of electrons during a chemical reaction by a molecule. It is also the removal of oxygen and the gain of hydrogen by atoms or molecules.

Oxidative stress: Disturbance in the balance between the free radicals and antioxidants in the body which can cause damage to cells.

Ozone layer: Part of Earth's atmosphere that contains a high concentration of ozone molecules. It absorbs most of the sun's ultraviolet radiation and protects us from various skin diseases.

Pacemaker: Device that helps to control and maintain the heartbeat. It is surgically implanted in the chest region of the body. It sends electrical pulses to keep the heart beating at a normal rate and rhythm.

Papilla: Small projection of tissue at the base of a hair or tooth or feather. It is made up of cells that play a key role in regulating hair growth.

Parabens: Chemicals often used as preservatives in cosmetics, foods pharmaceuticals, and beverages. They can cause irritation and allergy to the skin.

Parkinson's disease: A brain disorder that causes shaking, loss of muscle control, and difficulty with balance and coordination. It is caused by the degeneration of nerve cells in the brain.

Pathology: Branch of biology that deals with the study of causes and effects of disease or injury. It involves the diagnosis of disease through the examination of surgically removed organs.

Pericardial Effusion: A disease associated with the presence of an abnormal amount of fluid (pericardial fluid) between the layers surrounding the heart.

Pernicious anemia: Disease that occurs due to a deficiency of vitamin B12 in the body. It results in a decrease in the number of red blood cells when the intestines can't properly absorb vitamin B12.

Pharmacology: Branch of medicine that deals with the sources, chemical composition, and action of drugs on the systems and processes of living animals.

Photobiostimulation: Process of stimulating biological tissue and inducing biological reactions by use of low-powered light.

Photochemical reaction: The chemical reaction that is initiated by the absorption of energy in the form of light such as ultraviolet, visible, or infrared radiation.

Photonic pathway: Pathway followed by plants to convert light energy into glucose.

Photons: Tiny packets of energy that comprise waves of electromagnetic radiations of light. Light travels in the form of these small wave packets and they are the basic unit of all light.

Photosynthesis: The process by which plants use carbon dioxide and water to produce their food (glucose) in the presence of sunlight and release oxygen as a by-product.

Phthalates: A group of chemicals that are added to make plastics more durable and used as ingredients for shampoo and conditioners.

Physiology: Branch of biology that deals with the study of functions and mechanisms of different organs of the body.

Pigments: Substances that are intensely colored and, when added, give colors to other materials. They are completely or partially insoluble in water.

Piroctone olamine: Drug that is used to kill fungus. It increases the thickness of hair and reduces hair loss.

Pituitary gland: A major gland located at the base of the brain. It produces hormones that control other glands of the endocrine system. It also regulates growth, metabolism, and reproduction.

Placenta: The organ that provides a connection between the fetus and the wall of the uterus of the mother during pregnancy. It provides oxygen and nutrients to the fetus.

Polycystic ovary syndrome (PCOS): A condition in which ovaries produce male hormones higher than their normal amounts. It causes irregularity in the menstrual cycle, excess hair growth, and infertility.

Polyps: Small, mushroom-like tissue growths that are caused by abnormal production of cells.

Postpartum alopecia: A type of hair loss that occurs after childbirth. It usually starts about three months after giving birth and can last up to six months.

Power: The rate at which energy is transferred or converted. It is measured in watts.

Power density: It is the measure of the intensity of power output per target area.

Prednisone: Medicine used to suppress the immune system and decrease inflammation. It is used to treat rashes, inflammatory bowel disease, asthma, and dissecting cellulitis of the scalp (DCS).

Progesterone: A hormone that plays an important role in the menstrual cycle. It is released by the corpus luteum in the ovary. It is also necessary for the maintenance of pregnancy.

Prolactin: Hormone made by the pituitary gland. It is involved in the development of breasts and the production of milk in women.

Propecia (Finasteride): A drug that is used to prevent hair loss but can cause erectile dysfunction, depression, anxiety, and other neurological issues.

Propylene glycol: Viscous, colorless liquid that is used to mix water and oils. It absorbs extra water and maintains moisture in certain medicines.

Prostate gland: Gland located just below the urinary bladder and produces fluid that nourishes sperm and makes up a part of semen.

Prototype: A preliminary version, model, or release of a device made to test a concept and from which other forms are developed.

Pseudopelade: A rare form of permanent hair loss from the scalp, the cause of which is unknown.

Psoriasis: Skin disease that causes a rash with itchy, scaly patches, most commonly on the knees, elbows, trunk, and scalp.

Puberty: The transitional period of development between childhood and adulthood. It is the time in someone's life when he or she becomes sexually mature. It happens between ages eight to thirty years in females and between nine and fourteen years in males.

Pulmonary hypertension: A condition in which there is high blood pressure in pulmonary arteries, which carry blood from the heart to the lungs. It can damage the right-hand side of the heart.

Pulsing: Rapidly turning ON and OFF of a device or light source.

Quercetin: An anti-inflammatory substance found in leaves, flowers, and fruits. It is used for protection against heart disease and cancer. It is also effective against alopecia areata.

Radiation/rays: Energy or waves that are emitted from a source and travel at the speed of light. There are four types: alpha, beta, neutrons, and electromagnetic waves. They are very useful in X-ray machines and the treatment of cancer.

Rayon: A fiber derived from wood pulp. Its composition is the same as cellulose which is present in cell walls of plants. It is used to make various articles of clothing and hair fibers which are applied on the scalp.

Receptors: Various cells and organs in the body that detect specific stimuli like heat, light, etc., and send the signals to the brain to produce a response to those stimuli.

Red blood cells: Also known as erythrocytes. They are the type of blood cells that carry oxygen from the lungs to all parts of the body. They are formed by red bone marrow and have a life span of about four months.

Refraction: Bending or change in direction of waves as they enter from one medium into another. It is caused by the change in the speed of the wave due to a change in the intensity of the medium.

Retina: Part of the eye which captures light and sends signals to the brain to form images. It is the light-sensitive layer of tissue containing millions of cells at the back of the eyeball near the optic nerve.

Retinoids: Chemical compounds that are derivatives of vitamin A. They are very beneficial for the skin and are used in cosmetics to help reduce wrinkles and signs of aging. They are also used to treat various diseases like dissecting cellulitis of the scalp (DCS).

Rheumatoid arthritis: An autoimmune disease that causes pain, swelling, and stiffness in joints.

Ringworm: A skin infection caused by fungi living on the dead tissues of skin, hair, and nails. It causes a red and itchy circular rash. It is also one of the causes of hair loss in humans.

RNA: Stands for ribonucleic acid. It is a single-stranded molecule that is formed by DNA in the cell through a process called transcription. It has three types and is involved in the formation of proteins.

Rosacea: A skin condition that causes redness on the skin and a rash. It usually occurs on the nose and cheeks.

Salicylic acid: A compound found in most plants. It removes thick, scaly skin and damaged cells of the scalp. It belongs to a class of medications called keratolytic agents.

Saline solution: A mixture of salt and water used in cleaning wounds, treatment of dehydration, storage of contact lenses, and hair transplant surgery.

Savin–Ludwig Scale: Classification system used to measure the stages and extent of female pattern hair loss. It was devised by Dr. Ronald Savin in 1996.

Scalp: The layer of skin and tissue that covers the bones of the cranium. It is the thickest skin of the body. It is rich in blood vessels and has an abundance of hair follicles.

Scaly skin: Skin with dry, rough, cracked, and flaky patches. It occurs when the skin loses moisture and hydration. It is common in people living in cold climates or low-humidity areas.

Scanning transmission electron microscope: The type of electron microscope used to view the structure of tissue and molecules. The electrons are passed through the specimen and generate the image.

Seasonal Affective Disorder (SAD): The type of depression related to changes in seasons and usually occurs in winter. Less exposure to sunlight is one of the main causes of SAD.

Sebaceous glands: Glands present in the skin (also in hair follicles) and secrete sebum which lubricates and waterproofs the skin.

Seborrheic dermatitis: A skin condition that affects the scalp. The fungus Malassezia furfur (MF) is its main cause. It causes an itchy rash, flaky scales, and dandruff on the scalp.

Sebum: An oily, waxy substance produced by the body's sebaceous glands in the skin. It coats, moisturizes, and protects the skin from friction and dehydration.

Sham device: A medical device substitute with the only purpose of acting as a placebo in controlled clinical trials or product testing.

Silicones: Silicones are artificial compounds that act as sealant, adhesive, or coating to protect electronics. They are also used in hair conditioners to give a silky-smooth appearance by covering hair shafts and locking in moisture.

Small intestine: Narrow, coiled tube present between the stomach and large intestine. It is involved in the digestion and absorption of food. Its length is about seven meters.

Smallpox: An infectious disease caused by the variola virus. It causes rashes on the skin which leave scars. It was the leading cause of death in the past.

Sodium lauryl sulfate (SLS): A surfactant used in cosmetics, personal care products, and as a cleaning agent in household cleaning products. It can irritate the eyes, skin, and lungs.

Sparse hair: Hair has less density and thickness than normal hair and is caused by a decrease in active hair follicles.

Speckling: Formation of light patterns when a highly coherent light beam such as a laser is diffusely reflected at a surface with a rough structure, such as a piece of paper, white paint, a display screen, or a metallic surface. Only laser sources can generate speckling effect.

Spectrum: A band of colors obtained by splitting white light into its constituent colors when it passes through a prism.

Spironolactone: A drug used to treat high blood pressure, heart failure, and kidney diseases. It is also effective in the treatment of androgenetic alopecia.

Squaric acid: Medication used in the treatment of alopecia areata. It is also used to treat common warts.

Starvation: Condition of having no food for a long period. It is an extreme hunger resulting due to a lack of essential nutrients leading to death.

Stem cells: Undifferentiated cells in the body that can be specialized into various types of cells. They repair, restore, and replace damaged cells in different parts of the body.

Steroids: Steroids are chemicals or hormones, that are naturally formed in the body. They are used as medicines to reduce inflammation in the body.

Sub-cellular level: Smaller than a normal cell such as cell organelles like mitochondria, chloroplast, nucleus, etc.

Surfactants: Substances that are used to reduce the surface tension of liquids. They are used in detergents and shampoos. They increase the wetting property of shampoo but can cause skin dryness and irritation.

Tanning: A process in which skin color is darkened by exposure to ultraviolet (UV) radiation from the sun. It increases the melanin pigment in the skin.

Telogen phase: One of the three phases of the hair growth cycle. In this phase, the follicles are resting, and hair does not grow but stays attached to the follicle. Approximately 10–15% of all hair is in this phase at any one time and this phase lasts around three months.

Telogen effluvium: Telogen effluvium is a temporary hair loss due to excessive shedding of resting hair observed after having a high fever or recovering from an illness. Telogen effluvium sheds about 300–400 hairs per day which is three to four times more than normal hair loss and normally lasts for around two months following acute illness or stress.

Terminal hair: The thick, coarse hair that is seen on a normal, adult head, beard, underarms, makes up eyelashes, and eyebrows. It is thick, coarse, pigmented hair unlike vellus hair, which is short, thin, light-colored hair found on the heads of newborn babies and the scalp of bald men.

Testosterone: Male sex hormone produced inside the testicles. It regulates sexual development, muscle mass, and red blood cell production. A normal level of testosterone is sufficient to cause hair loss in men with genetic tendencies. Women also produce a small amount of testosterone.

Therapeutic window: The range of dosage that provides a safe and effective response without significant adverse effects.

Thyroxine (T4): Also called thyroid hormone. It plays an important role in body metabolism and functions of different organs such heart, digestive tract, muscles, brain, and the maintenance of bones.

Topicals: Drugs or products that are applied directly to the surface of the body (skin or scalp), such as shampoos or conditioners. They only affect the part of the skin to which they are applied.

Traction alopecia: Traction alopecia is an acquired hair loss caused by prolonged tension and repeatedly pulling on the hair. It results from regularly wearing tight weaves, and braids, and using hair extensions, chemical relaxers, and rollers.

Translucent: Any substance that allows some light to pass through but objects on the other side can't be seen clearly. Often described as semi-transparent.

Trauma: A physical injury caused by an accident or attack. Also referred to as a very depressing or disturbing experience that may cause psychological damage.

Traumatic brain injury (TBI): Sudden Injury to the brain caused by a blow or bump on the head and leads to disruption in the normal function of the brain.

Trichogram: Semi-invasive technique for the evaluation of patients with hair loss that involves the microscopic examination of hair shafts.

Trichologist: A professional who specializes in hair and scalp care and helps people with the treatment of the associated problems.

Trichotillomania: Also known as "hair-pulling disorder." It is a psychological disorder in which the patient pulls out the hair on their head or in other places, such as their eyebrows or eyelashes.

Triiodothyronine (T3): Hormone produced by the Thyroid gland and plays an important role in the body's metabolism, heart, and digestive functions, muscle control, brain development and function, and the maintenance of bones.

Trimester: Period of three months, especially as a division of the duration of pregnancy.

Tumors: An abnormal mass of tissue that forms when abnormal cells group together. A tumor can be cancerous (malignant) or noncancerous (benign).

Ultraviolet (UV) light: A portion of the electromagnetic spectrum that has a shorter wavelength and higher energy than visible light. It is invisible to the human eye and overexposure to these UV radiations can lead to serious health issues, including cancer.

Vellus hairs: Also known as "peach fuzz." These are short, thin, light-colored hairs that grow on most of the body. They are also found on the heads of newborn babies and the scalp of bald men.

Vertigo: Often described as dizziness. It is a feeling of spinning, even when a person is not moving.

Watt: The SI unit of power, equivalent to one joule per second.

Wavelength: The distance between two successive points on a wave that is characterized by the same phase of the oscillation. The absorption properties of a laser depend on its wavelength. The unit of measurement of the wavelength is the nanometer (nm).

Alternative Terms for Laser Phototherapy (LPT)

Below are some various names for the phenomena of applying energy to tissue.

Bio stimulating Laser
Bioluminescence
Bioregulating Laser
Biostimulation (BIOS)
Cold laser therapy
Laser Phototherapy (LPT)
Low-Level Light Therapy (LLLT)
Low-Level Laser Therapy
Low Power Laser Therapy
Low-Level Laser
Low Power Laser
Low-energy Laser
Low Intensity Light Therapy (LILT)
Low-intensity-level Laser
Low-reactive-level Laser
Medical Laser

Mid-Laser
Phototherapy
Photobiostimulation
Photobiomodulation Laser
Photobiology
Photobiomodulation
Photochemotherapy
Photonic stimulation
Photomedicine
Photophysics
Photochemistry
Photosynthesis
Photonics
Red light therapy
Soft Laser
Therapeutic Laser

About the Author

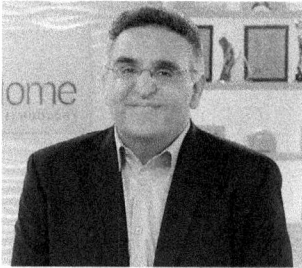

Sayyid Tamim Hamid is the inventor of the world's first FDA-cleared, wearable, phototherapy device to prevent hair loss, and thicken and regrow hair. After receiving undergraduate and graduate degrees in electrical engineering, computer engineering and biomedical engineering, Tamim designed and implemented innovative tools at NASA to improve astronaut safety and efficiency in space shuttle operations. While there, he implemented various lasers and photonics systems which gave him the intricate knowledge necessary to implement cool lasers into Theradome.

His professional history includes growing the revenue of multimillion dollar international corporations and serving as senior executive in companies that were sold to GE Medical and Johnson & Johnson.

Tamim used his laser knowledge, fine-tuned at NASA, and combined it with his driving passion for helping others to pursue a lifelong mission in the field of hair loss and restoration. He is now one of the world's leading experts.

Currently, Tamim works diligently to make the Theradome laser hair restoration device a household name by educating medical professionals and the public about the safety and benefits of this technology.

Tamim lives with his wife of thirty-three years outside San Francisco, CA. in his rare free time, Hamid enjoys tending to his olive orchard and pressing artisanal dipping olive oil.

Take The TheraQuiz For Free!

Congratulations, you've read the book and now it's time to find out if LPT is right for you.

TheraQuiz, your first step to stop hair loss and grow back your hair.

TheraQuiz is a simple, yet thorough quiz developed by a certified Trichologist, or hair and scalp expert, to determine the health of your hair and scalp. It's a great place to start your hair growth journey. By taking this quiz, you will be armed with the knowledge you need to take the next steps to take control of your hair loss issues.

It's easy to get started. Simply scan the TheraQuiz QR code below. Here's how:

1. Open the Camera app from your smart phone home screen, control center, or lock screen.
2. Select the rear facing camera. Hold your device so that the TheraQuiz QR code below appears in the viewfinder in the Camera app. Your device will automatically recognize the TheraQuiz QR code and will show a notification.
3. Tap the notification to open the link associated with the TheraQuiz QR code. You will be taken directly to the TheraQuiz webpage.
4. You can also visit the TheraQuiz directly: **www.theraquiz.com**.

www.ingramcontent.com/pod-product-compliance
Lightning Source LLC
Chambersburg PA
CBHW070049030426
42335CB00016B/1839